NURSING ETHICS, 1880s TO THE PRESENT

This important text draws on decades of research, arguing that modern nursing germinated and grew an ethics from its own native soil, which is rich, fulsome, and philosophically informed, grounded in the tradition and practice of nursing.

It is an ethics with a positive agenda for the good nurse, a good society, a healthy people, and human flourishing. This native nursing ethics was forgotten, creating space for a foreign bioethics' colonization of nursing in the second half of the twentieth century. Drawing from a wide range of sources from the USA, the UK, Canada, and Ireland, the book addresses the early and enduring ethical concerns, values, and ideals of nursing as a profession that engages in direct clinical practice and in developing policy. Fowler calls for reclaiming and renewing nursing's ethical tradition.

This systematic and comprehensive book is an essential contribution for students and scholars of nursing ethics.

Marsha Fowler is Emerita Professor of Ethics. She holds the honorific "Code Scholar and Historian" for her foundational and ongoing work on the Code of Ethics for Nurses (American Nurses Association). She was also a consultant for the most recent International Council of Nursing Code of Ethics for Nursing (2021).

"A thorough and fascinating account of the evolution of nursing ethics. Fowler interweaves real-life stories about the people who shaped the early foundation of the discipline, with her sharp-witted analysis of how their wisdom can inform today's nursing practice. This book provides an inspiring story of how nursing ethics emerged, distinct from bioethics, and why this matters in our quest to provide humane, compassionate care for those we serve."

Peggy L. Chinn, RN, PhD, DSc (Hon), FAAN
Professor Emerita, University of Connecticut
Editor Emerita, Advances in Nursing Science
Nursology.net

"In this innovative and engaging text, Marsha integrates disparate histories, previously disconnected, illuminating the rich and complex backdrop to the development of nursing ethics. These histories foreground nursing ethics as a social ethics and nurse leaders as trailblazers committed to remedying social injustice, the histories of exemplary women and of the value(s) of nursing. A recommended read for all interested in past, present, and future of care and nursing ethics."

Professor Ann Gallagher PhD MA BA (Hons)
PGCEA RMN SRN FRCN FAAN
Head of Department of Health Sciences
Brunel University London
Editor-in-Chief, Nursing Ethics

"This impressive historical account of the birth of nursing ethics skillfully highlights and contrasts the education and evolution of nursing ethics before the emergence of bioethics. The voices and engaging vignettes are particularly compelling, making this book a valuable resource for anyone seeking a deeper understanding of role of ethics in nursing."

Liz Stokes, PhD, JD, RN
Director, Nursing Programs & Center for Ethics and Human Rights
American Nurses Association

"Marsha Fowler's treatise on the history of nursing ethics makes for a marvellous read. She guides her reader through an intricate and complex history of how nurses and those who write for and about them have wrestled with the ideas of fairness, equity, truth and virtue, critically reflecting on the history and evolution of thought from a perspective that is only accessible to a seasoned scholar with a wicked wit."

Sally Thorne, RN, PhD, FAAN, FCAHS, FCAN, CM
Professor, School of Nursing, University of British Columbia, Canada
Editor, Nursing Inquiry

NURSING ETHICS, 1880s TO THE PRESENT

An Archaeology of Lost Wisdom and Identity

Marsha Fowler

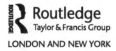
Routledge
Taylor & Francis Group

LONDON AND NEW YORK

Designed cover image: © Marsha Fowler

First published 2024
by Routledge
4 Park Square, Milton Park, Abingdon, Oxon OX14 4RN

and by Routledge
605 Third Avenue, New York, NY 10158

Routledge is an imprint of the Taylor & Francis Group, an informa business

British Library Cataloguing-in-Publication Data
A catalogue record for this book is available from the British Library

Library of Congress Cataloging-in-Publication Data
Names: Fowler, Marsha Diane Mary, author.
Title: Nursing ethics, 1880s to the present: an archaeology of lost wisdom and identity / Marsha Fowler.
Description: Abingdon, Oxon; New York, NY: Routledge, 2024. |
Includes bibliographical references and index.
Identifiers: LCCN 2023042263 | ISBN 9781032200729 (hardback) |
ISBN 9781003262107 (ebook)
Subjects: LCSH: Nursing ethics—History.
Classification: LCC RT85 .F69 2024 | DDC 174.2/9073—dc23/eng/20231102
LC record available at https://lccn.loc.gov/2023042263

ISBN: 978-1-032-20072-9 (hbk)
ISBN: 978-1-032-20071-2 (pbk)
ISBN: 978-1-003-26210-7 (ebk)

DOI: 10.4324/9781003262107

Typeset in Times New Roman
by codeMantra

Fæder ūre þū þe eart on heofonum
sī þīn nama ġehālgod

CONTENTS

TABLES

ACKNOWLEDGMENTS

Acknowledgments are difficult for fear of omitting someone to whom one is indebted, though it is impossible to measure the depth and breadth of indebtedness any researcher and scholar has. I supposed I should start by mentioning Zenodotus (Ζηνόδοτος) of Ephesus, the first known librarian from whom all librarians descend. Certainly librarians have been a constant transfusion for me throughout my career. My only and admittedly insufficient way to repay this debt of gratitude is to offer a book of my own making, and their nurture, for their shelves. I am especially indebted to Alice at LA County School of Nursing Library, Ann at City of Hope Library, Denise at my university library, Helen at the University of Surrey Archives, and Dawn at the Royal College of Nursing Library Archives.

I am grateful for the colleagues and friends in ethics who have journeyed with me, several of whom have written a narrative for this book's final chapter, several of whom are now of blessed memory, several of whom have reached a period of frailty. I am grateful for their friendship and colleagueship, and episodic rollicking good times.

I am grateful to Professors Sally Thorne, Peggy Chinn, and Martha Turner for their review of this work, and for their encouragement, support, challenge, reflection, and continuing good humor all along the way.

I am grateful to my longtime friends for unflagging encouragement, to Jo, Karen, Katie, Patricia, Pearl, Thea, Verena, and my personal meteorologist Justin. And my beloved cousin Karen. And Anne. And my Wednesday coffee klatch.

I am grateful to those who kept me stocked with groceries and greens and human contact during the Covid-19 lockdown—Katie, Pearl, and Jo—and who enabled me to keep writing with much less worry.

I am grateful to my publisher, and editor Amy for her forbearance, in the midst of myriad besetting woes for the publishing industry that so earnestly supports the advance and preservation of knowledge. I am grateful to Bethany and Pam for help with manuscript cleanup—a yeoman's task.

I am grateful for the providence that has given me a life of the mind, a garden, a bicycle, a bread oven, and a quirky, more or less sane galère with whom I share twisted strands of DNA.

Marsha Fowler
Feast of the Transfiguration, August, 2023

INTRODUCTION

I have spent most of my life in the Republic of California. In the mid-1800s, the Bear Flag Republic was an unrecognized Alta California breakaway state from Mexico. It ruled a segment of Northern California, above San Francisco, for all of 25 days, after which the United States claimed the territory. A grizzly bear and the words "California Republic" still adorn the state flag. In 1890, the California State Floral Society chose the California poppy, or golden poppy (*Eschscholzia californica*), as the California state flower. In the spring and summer its silky, brilliant, golden-orange flowers and frilly, pale blue-green foliage grace the rolling hills of the state in massive meadows of floral gold carpet. The California poppy is a tough, fast-growing, self-seeding, drought-tolerant, resilient native flower with a long taproot that thrives in poor, sandy soils. Its petals close at night and in cold windy weather, staying closed in cloudy weather, but opening again to a morning's warmth. The fruit of the poppy is a slender capsule 1.2 to 3.5 inches long, which, when the seed is ripe, suddenly dehisces (you can hear them pop) and explosively ejects the tiny seeds, effectively self-scattering them up to six feet away. There are circuitous laws that prevent trampling poppy fields and if you pluck a poppy flower, you will be disappointed – its petals will fall off. Poppies feed the

DOI: 10.4324/9781003262107-1

ecosystem's critters—birds, small herbivores, butterflies, moths, bees, and other pollinators. *E. californica*'s beauty, hardiness, toughness, drought-tolerance, and sustenance of the ecosystem that envelops it derive from being a native plant in its native soil.

NURSING ETHICS IS THE NATIVE WILDFLOWER OF THE SOIL OF NURSING

It has a breathtaking beauty, a deep taproot, nourishingly interacts with the environment around it, and it thrives in its own soil. That's what this book is about: digging into the soil of nursing, finding its seeds, and enjoying the elegant, bold, golden flowers of its native ethics.

Preface before the Introduction

I have spent the past 50 years researching the history and development of nursing ethics, which has resulted in a massive collection of source material written by women for women, and by nurses for nurses. Well, actually, there are a few priests, pastors, and physicians who sneak into the mix, and one psychologist. This source material covers the period from the 1880s to 1965 as one body of literature, then from 1965 onward as a second wave of material. The first purpose of this book is to make this largely lost or forgotten mass of ethics material accessible to researchers for their own scholarly purposes.

Three Phases of This Undertaking

There have been three phases of research that have been tied to my own bumbling evolution.

The First Phase

This phase occurred while working on my dissertation in the early 1980s. My dissertation looked at the development of successive iterations of the American Nurses Association's *Code of Ethics for Nurses*, including the precursor codes and the Florence Nightingale Pledge. In the process, I stumbled across a huge body of nursing ethics literature, in textbooks, articles, International Council of Nurses (ICN) addresses, commencement speeches, curricular requirements, and much more, of which I had been unaware. While Isabel Hampton Robb's book *Nursing Ethics for Hospital and Private Use* (1900) was known in our nursing ethics circles, little of the other approximately 100 books and editions was. The first phase of this research was to identify, find, and collect this body of literature in the 1980s, specifically prior to the existence of the internet. Because these were early works, especially those from the 1870s to 1930s, stray references to them were informal; that is, without the full bibliographic citations that are conventional today. Finding these works meant moving from one book to the next looking for mentions, writing letters or telephoning librarians across the US to obtain a book via postal service, rummaging through jumble sales and estate sales, all in the hopes that someone's beloved nurse Aunt Tilley had socked away her nursing textbooks in her attic. These works have been brought together as the *Nursing Ethics Heritage Collection* in an archival library in the UK. The collection is open to researchers and scholars and is of special interest to those in nursing ethics and history, but also to those in literary criticism, women's, feminist, and intersectional studies, politics, and women's history.

The Second Phase

This phase involved a survey of the nursing ethics literature for its content, themes, continuous threads, and vocabulary over its evolving social setting. This phase is largely *descriptive* in nature though with some beginning analysis. In and of itself, this has been a massive task to which most of my research and scholarship has been devoted. By creating a working typology of domains of interest, I hope that it will allow future scholars to home-in on more discrete and tractable glugs from this overflowing flagon. I hope that what I have done in the first phase (identification and collection) and second phase (comprehensive description) will position others to work on the source material.

The Third Phase

This phase will extend beyond my lifetime. It is the *analysis* of our nursing ethics heritage. Analysis is beyond the compass of my own career, for there is more source material here than any one career can apprehend. This, then, gives rise to the overriding purpose of the book: to make the source material available and accessible to other researchers and scholars, to move the cause of nursing ethics forward.

The Actual Introduction

Clarifying the Terminology of This Book—Nursing Ethics, Not Bioethics

This literature is about what I designate *nursing ethics*. The earliest modern nursing ethical discourse must be distinguished from the ethical discourse that arose in the mid-1960s and 1970s called in succession *medical ethics*, *biomedical ethics*, and *bioethics*. *Biomedical ethics* was imported into nursing from the 1970s forward. In the *bioethics* period, the mid-1980s onward, the field became increasingly interdisciplinary, not always including nursing. In the bioethics period, nurses began to incorporate bioethics into nursing, largely via nursing's own growing body of literature. Bioethics in nursing came to grapple with the inadequacies and ill-fittingness of bioethics in addressing nursing concerns, and gave rise to several approaches to ethics that encompass feminist concerns and an ethics of caring literature, but they did not reclaim nursing ethics in the process. In this text, *nursing ethics* refers to the nursing ethics heritage literature of the past and its reclamation for the present and future.

Periodization of Terminology

Within the bioethics literature, the terminology relating to ethics in nursing and medicine varies by period and by author. For clarity, I assign a specific meaning to each term. While medical ethics reaches back to Hippocrates, for clarity, we will deal with terminology pertaining to the modern professions of medicine and nursing. The terms as used in this work are:

TABLE I.1 Terms used

Term	Dates	By and For
Nursing Ethics	Mid-1800s to mid-1960s And renewing	Promulgated by nurses and their guild for nurses, and specific to nursing practice in all its relationships. Nursing's professional ethics. Includes codes of ethics. Taught by nursing faculty. Its potential is for reclamation and renewal for contemporary and future use.
Ethics in Nursing	Mid-1800s to mid-1960s	Promulgated by non-nurses for nurses, mostly by clergy, a few philosophers, physicians and a psychologist/ philosopher. With the exception of the psychologist, these works engage with nursing only nominally.
Medical Ethics	1800s to present	Promulgated by physicians and their guild for physicians, and specific to medical practice. Medicine's professional ethics taught by physicians. Includes codes of ethics. Has ancient origins.
Biomedical Ethics	Mid-1960s to 1980s	Period of emergence, transition, and coalescence. Promulgated by theologians, philosophers, and physicians, and related to medical practice and research.
Bioethics	Late 1980s forward	Promulgated by philosophers, theologians, physicians, attorneys, sociologists, and anthropologists, et al.: expanded to be interdisciplinary, yet often excluding nurses. Incorporates medical practice, research, and health policy concerns. Taught by philosophers and physicians.
Bioethics in Nursing, or Nursing Bioethics	Mid-1970s to present	Initially entailed the application of *medical ethics* to nursing, then evolved as *biomedical ethics* and became *bioethics*. Now draws upon the largely medico-centric bioethics literature, modifying and applying it to nursing and generating a *nursing bioethics* literature. Taught by nursing faculty to nursing students, and at conferences and workshops. Has its own body of literature.

Three Purposes of the Book

The first purpose of this book, then, is to gift this resource of nursing ethics literature to the reader and scholars of nursing bioethics for their own research and scholarship. As much as is possible, within the strictures of the publisher's word-count limitation, I have included early nursing ethics source documents in full.

The second purpose of this book is to present a descriptive analysis of the content of the first hundred years of nursing ethics, prior to the rise of bioethics. This analysis will draw primarily from the US and UK textbooks, spokes-journals, and collateral materials such as ICN speeches. Distinctions will be made between the nurse and non-nurse-authored nursing ethics textbooks. Many far-flung resources remain to be accessed that I simply could not get to (e.g., the Royal College of Nursing (RCN) archives in Edinburgh), but suggestions for source material that remains to be collected or examined, and their locations, will be given.

The third purpose of this book is to describe the loss of the ethical wisdom of the first hundred years of nursing ethics, and the colonization of nursing ethics by bioethics as it arose in the mid-1960s. Bioethics is not a solo voice; there is a choir of voices, and yet none of those capture the ground-note of the nursing ethics that had been lost. I hope that that ground-note can be sounded sufficiently herein, in order to reclaim and renew nursing ethics in a way that engages with other approaches to ethics in nursing today. If successful, it will have the power to address nursing-specific concerns that are not the focus of other disciplines (or bioethics), and to highlight the values, ideals, aspirations, nursing identity, and *the good* in and of nursing.

A Caveat on the Period Literature in This Book

The early works in nursing ethics are not easy literature for modern readers. Early nursing was developed as a profession for women, and its literature was written by women for women and by nurses for nurses. As such, the literature uses the exclusive language of female pronouns. In addition, much of this literature is written in the style of late Victorian women's literature that, to today's reader, can feel antiquated, classist, genteel, rambling, a bit stream-of-consciousness, and frustrating in its indirectness, prolixity, and circumlocution. It has a certain charm and turn of phrase, but is admittedly an acquired taste. It also means that the nature of the rhetoric—its indirectness, circumlocutions, prolixity, loquacious and meandering style—requires significantly longer quotes to capture its point; succinct, it is not.

It is also necessary to mention that English is a living language, where words may have a sense-evolution, so that care must be taken to understand various words in the sense that the author intended, not necessarily in their contemporary usage. For example, the word *naughty* first meant a person with *naught* or nothing, not one who was ill-behaved, or as having any allusion to sex. Where source material is quoted in this book, it will be left as written—pronouns, misspellings, variant spellings, erratic punctuation, and all. Where a pivotal word has undergone significant sense evolution, an accompanying "translation" will be provided.

Uncovering this literature also involved developing a lexicon of terms that were used in their period for which another term would be used today. This is important as a portion of this literature has been digitized and some of it is searchable, but it will not be able to be searched using contemporary terms. For example, a *toddler* was a *runabout child*, *aging* was termed *senile decay*, *nurse exploitation* was termed *nurse sweating*, and someone who had *naught* was termed a *pauper*, *mendicant*, or *almsman*. It should also be noted that considerable ink has been cast upon parchment that distinguishes between *ethical* and *moral*. Herein, I will use standard conventions and not labor over whether *moral philosophy* as a field should really be called *ethical philosophy*, or whether one's *moral compass* is really an *ethical compass*. There are bigger fish to fry.

Fiddly Stuff

Direct quotations will be left as they were originally written; pronouns will not be changed, spelling and punctuation will not be altered or corrected even where spelling changes within a single quote. The intent here is that the reader read what the author wrote, not what an editor changed.

Declaration of Conflict of Interest: I Am a Nurse—Authorial Perspectives, Biases, Standing, and Limitations

The situatedness of the author gives rise to the work's limitations that will need to be overcome by others. To start, there are always some hazards associated with recollecting events in which one has participated, both because of the vagaries of memory over time, but also because life and education trains one to see through specific lenses, in my case those of nursing and social ethics. It is important to note, too, that I am not a formally trained historian so, *ab initio*, I beg the forbearance of my nurse-historian colleagues for any historiographic errors arising from my ignorance.

I have been an active participant and observer in many of the historical changes and circles that this work addresses, including the dramatic changes that have taken place in women's history, nursing history, technological and scientific development, clinical changes, and of course the rise of bioethics as a discipline and discourse. As a hospital-based, diploma-school graduate, I was a registered nurse (RN) before *Roe v. Wade*, and before the internet was invented. I participated in the movement of nursing into colleges and universities in the 1960s. I participated in the marches and protests of second-wave feminism for women's rights, reproductive rights (birth control and abortion), and environmental concerns. Envision love beads, bell-bottoms, crocheted vests, macrame, guitars, and protest folk songs. I also participated in civil rights protests, in the development of intensive care units, in the specializations in both nursing and medicine, and in the rise of bioethics and its colonization of nursing, and more. A number of my observations derive from first-hand experience and thus a portion of this work is inextricably autobiographical. Furthermore, while I am a consumer of nursing philosophy, I am neither a nursing philosopher, nor a nursing theorist. My doctorate is not in nursing, it is in ethics, specifically in social ethics and *bioethics*—as *nursing ethics* no longer existed in nursing's consciousness during my doctoral studies in the early 1980s.

In addition, I am an old, white, short, American, second-wave feminist, Christian woman. "Old" means that I have lived through extraordinary changes within nursing. I initially graduated from a diploma school attached to a hospital medical center in a large urban area in California. It represented the best of advancing nursing education, as well as the throwback strictures on single women living together in a hospital-school dormitory. I lived through the 1965 American Nurses Association (ANA) position paper that called for the movement of nursing education out of diploma programs and into colleges and universities at a time when there were no continuation mechanisms for diploma nurses to become baccalaureate prepared. These are two different nursing worlds and two different educational worlds. I have participated in the emergence of bioethics for approximately 50 years. As a consequence, "old" also means that I have lived long enough that my views have evolved and developed, and have become both more nuanced and stubborn. My later writings differ from my earliest ones. We should all live so long that our earlier writings become an embarrassment to us. It also means that I have come to a place in life that I prefer to be myself, idiosyncrasies and all. Given that there is a degree of autobiography herein, in embarking upon this project, I decided to write in my own voice and not that of desiccated academic rhetoric: the reader will hear my voice in the way that I have written this book. To quote England's soccer goalkeeper Mary Earps, "Be unapologetically yourself." This is not unprecedented, for this is the voice used by our early nursing ethicists in their ethics textbooks.

"White" means that I cannot speak for nurses or persons of color even though I know that there is much work to be done in ethics in nursing as it relates to persons of color who would have chosen nursing, who choose nursing, and to graduate nurses of color. In particular, research on race, class, and gender in nursing is in far too short a supply. It also means that I must acknowledge that I have my own social, generational, and racial-ethnic blind spots that I war against. I do fail but am thankful for those who help to remove the scales from my eyes.

"Short" is both a reality and a metaphor. Several years after completing my PhD in social ethics, and having some recognition in the field by then, I was at a meeting peopled by white male ethicists. We stood in a circle as we chatted. The men were all a foot or more taller than me. As we chatted, or more accurately, as they chatted over my head, never making eye contact with me, but connecting with one another, passing by what I said and subsequently saying it themselves as if their own thought, I was the little woman who was not recognized as present. Nursing has often been the short, voiceless, little woman in the bioethics circle.

"American" probably means some of usual buccaneering behavior for which Americans are infamous and rightly reviled, but also that the book reflects English-language (and American-language) literature and history of the Anglo-American nursing body. There are significant differences between and among nursing communities in the English-speaking countries, and the sources herein are drawn chiefly from the US, UK (some), Canada (in token), and Ireland (a smidge) but are principally American (for which I apologize). In addition, ethics in nursing in Europe is different and dismayingly cannot be addressed within the scope of this book, nor can ethics in nursing in the global nursing community. I recognize this deficit but must leave it for others to take up the task.

"Second-wave feminist" means an author who marched and protested for women's reproductive freedom, for pay equity, and for women's rights in general—and a nurse who cared for patients who had, in desperation, attempted "coat-hanger" self-abortion—in part, the genesis of my interest in ethics in the mid-1960s. A 1960s second-wave feminism coupled with nursing experience generates a range of specific sensibilities and allegiances—and now worries for the future.

"Christian," with a Jewish heritage as well, means a particular set of sensibilities and allegiances and, in my case, in the direction of social criticism, social justice, social advocacy, and the common good—as a clergywoman and pastor. My own Reformed Tradition, arising in the Protestant Reformation in the 1500s, has an enduring concern for the shape of society as it affects human flourishing, well-being, and safety, but I acknowledge has had its own historical foibles and inertias.

"Woman" means that as I view the span of modern nursing, from the mid-1800s to the present, I see the costs to early nursing leaders in forming the profession against social and legal odds. I have also seen the social resistance, as well as some professional ambivalence, toward the entry of men into the profession, and the increasing numbers of men doing so.

As I dive into the nursing ethics literature, I have a pride-of-profession even while I acknowledge that while the ethical values and ideals of nursing are stunning, in reality individual nurses, and nursing as a profession, do not always live up to those values and ideals. I acknowledge the flawed nature of humanity, and the grievous errors individual nurses and organized nursing have made over the decades, yet I remain proud of the values, ideals, and aspirations of the profession and its members for healing; and for compassionate, caring service to individuals and society, whatever our patients' personal attributes or situation in life, and however imperfectly those moral ideals may have been realized.

And Finally, the Roadmap for the Book Chapters

The chapters are interrelated but not co-dependent, and each one can stand alone. On the assumption that readers may read individual chapters out of sequence, there is a small amount of redundancy, and a few of the key quotations may reappear in another chapter, though sometimes for a different purpose. These are the 11 chapters. Here, in brief, is where we are going so that we do not get lost along the way, organized in clusters for reading, followed by a more expanded roadmap:

Reading Clusters:

- **Chapters 1–3:** early ethics education requirements for nursing students and the extensive nursing ethics literature in books, chapters, articles, and more.
- **Chapter 4:** the beginnings of nursing and nursing ethics as social ethics, and the interrelations between social issues that affected women and women's education and shaped nursing ethics from the start. Coordinates with Chapter 10.
- **Chapters 5–6:** the rise of the field of bioethics, from a nursing perspective, first within its social context (Chapter 5) and then within its health-care context (Chapter 6) and its movement into nursing.
- **Chapters 7–9:** an overview of the development of nursing ethics in the UK (and a bit in Canada; Chapter 7) and the US (Chapter 8). Patricia Benner picks up many of the threads of previous chapters and examines virtue and care ethics and the ethics internal to nursing practice (Chapter 9).
- **Chapter 10:** examines the discipline of *social ethics* in greater depth. Coordinates with Chapter 4 which is its *in vivo* exemplar.
- **Chapter 11:** Concludes the book with personal narratives from ethics friends and colleagues who have accompanied me along the way.
- **Afterword:** The Nurses Are Up to Something

Here Is the Expanded Roadmap

Chapter 1: Education in Nursing Ethics: Sturdy Standards: We begin with nursing education in ethics at the start of modern nursing. In 1915, the NLNE (National League for Nursing Education—later NLN) established curricular requirements for the education of nursing students. These requirements are rigorous, philosophically informed, and demanding. The chapter looks at each of the textbooks recommended for faculty teaching ethics and the additional recommended readings. The chapter looks at the philosophical influences upon the ethics requirements, in the context of the Progressive Era and the philosophy of Pragmatism. The work of James, Pierce, and Dewey on education also shapes how nurses and ethics should be taught. The chapter also contains the current American Association of Colleges of Nursing (AACN) ethics requirements for comparison.

Chapter 2: An Archaeology of the Nursing Ethics Literature: Digging Up Textbooks: There was an extensive publishing industry surrounding the formation of nursing education in its early years. An astonishing number of nursing ethics textbooks and editions were available to nursing students in the 1900s. The chapter divides the textbooks by nurse vs. non-nurse authors, mostly priests, then looks at the categories more critically. The nurse-authored books are evaluated individually. The reader is directed to the best among the sources, and I indicate which sources are less adequate and the basis for that estimation. Some of these works are commended for use today.

Chapter 3: The Nursing Ethics Literature: More to Read: There is a massive body of ethics literature beyond the textbooks. This chapter examines "first chapters," that is, the first chapter of medical-surgical textbooks from the late 1800s, as the first chapter was always about moral character and duty. It also examines the first extant dissertation on nursing ethics—Vaughan's incidence of moral concerns in nursing practice, 1935. The chapter also looks at other ethics literature that is not textbooks, not journal articles—such as NLN Minutes, ICN speeches, graduation speeches, etc.

Chapter 4: Nursing Ethics as Social Ethics: Moral Courage on the March: It is not possible to disentangle the rise of nursing and nursing education from issues of the social location of women and their legal liabilities that hampered the foundation of a profession for women. Thus, a book on nursing ethics must begin with social ethics. This chapter focuses on how, from the start, women's suffrage, the social location of women, issues of the Progressive Era, and the bicycle-shaped early nursing ethics as a *social ethics* engaged with social and health policy and social activism. Nursing's own class structure also affected its ethics and voice. Nursing social ethics was concerned for ways in which social conditions and injustices generated ill health and a range of additional injustices and oppressions. The chapter uses venereal disease as an exemplar issue for nursing's social ethics.

Chapter 5: An Unauthorized Biography of Bioethics: Its Social Context: As nursing moves into colleges and universities, it "loses" its native ethics at the same time that bioethics emerges as a field. Since bioethics diverts nursing ethics, it is important to look at its rise before returning to a survey of nursing ethics. This chapter examines the broader social forces and events surrounding the emergence of bioethics and how it shaped the questions bioethics was interested in (and not interested in). The chapter picks up on social context that other histories neglect, and how they influence the emerging bioethics—e.g., the consumer movement, second-wave feminism, the Beecher and Pappworth reports, the coalescence of medical sovereignty, whistleblowers and the widespread betrayal of social trust, sociological critiques of medicine of the period, the "technological imperative" discourse of the period, and the "we kill babies" discourse of the period. This chapter is socially focused and defers both bioethical concern for clinical or practice issues and the movement of bioethics into nursing to the next chapter.

Chapter 6: Nursing's Nescient Embrace of a Nascent Bioethics: This chapter is parallel to Chapter 5 but fixes on the specifically medical context of the rise of bioethics, e.g., the Seattle Hemodialysis case, the Karen Quinlan and Tony Bland cases, the Baby Doe cases, the thalidomide tragedy, the DES scandal, and the male body as normative in medicine. This chapter includes the religiogenesis of bioethics, then its subsequent secularization, and the exclusion of religion in the same ways that nursing has been excluded. Attention is given to building the bioethical-medical-industrial complex and the role of the Kennedy family in the generation of foundational bioethical structures. The Kennedy Fellowships in Medical Ethics for Nurses facilitated the movement of bioethics into nursing.

Chapter 7: Nursing Ethics in the United Kingdom, 1888 to 1960s (with a Nod to Canada): This chapter looks at the early nursing ethics literature in the UK (journal articles, books) and its emphasis on "character" and "virtues" sometimes called "personality" and other terms, as well as social issues. Specific ethical themes throughout the early UK literature are identified and explored. The chapter concludes with a brief examination of the general (non-topical) ethics literature.

Chapter 8: Nursing Ethics before Bioethics: Prologue to the Future: This chapter moves into the content and structure of nursing ethics in the US, its relational nature, its preventive ethics through relationship preservation, and the norms that shape practice. It looks at the practice-generated norms that arise from within the "classes" of nursing relationships, the concept of military etiquette, specific duties within each of the specified relationships, and the *Code of Ethics for Nurses* as an anomalous remnant of nursing ethics.

Chapter 9: Studying Expert Ethical Comportment and Preserving the Ethics of Care and Responsibility Embedded in Expert Nursing Practice: This chapter is generously contributed by Professor Patricia Benner. Her chapter is a rich, dense, chocolaty brownie—compared with my popcorn—cooked with the lid off. Her chapter is about nursing practice at the intimate, ethics-enacting, level of the nurse–patient relationship. Drawing from MacIntyre, Taylor, Dunne, Dreyfus, and her own research on nursing practice, her chapter explores nursing practice itself as a source of ethics. Contrasting her findings with the received bioethics, she examines how taken-for-granted self-understandings disrupt *virtue and care ethics*, *care traditions*, and the *caring practices* of expert nurses. As a renewal of virtue ethics for nursing practice today, her chapter fills the gap between saying that nursing ethics is virtue-based, and demonstrating how, in nursing practice itself, that is the case.

Chapter 10: A Closet Full of Ethics for Seasonal Wear: This chapter addresses the development of the field of social ethics from the later 1800s into the twentieth century and forward. It looks at the nominal assertion of a social ethics in bioethics that focuses on distributive justice, against the three periods of social ethics in the US. In particular, social ethical voices that have gone unheard, or have been silenced, or pushed to the margins, are brought forward for their potential contributions to nursing ethics today. The chapter also introduces the important debate in the philosophy of law, the Hart–Devlin debate, on the legislation of morality. It is a debate that raises important questions for nursing, questions of social policy and informed voting.

Chapter 11: Voices and Vignettes: This chapter consists of personal narratives of friends and colleagues who have been and are engaged in bioethics in nursing.

They include Anne Davis, Christine Grady, Emiko Konishi, Pamela Grace, Miriam Hirschfield, Peggy Chinn, Verena Tschudin, Elizabeth Peter, Patricia Benner, Janet Storch, Laurie Badzek, and Andrew Jameton. These narratives speak to why or how these persons devoted themselves to ethics in nursing. It is hoped that their stories will inspire others to do so as well.

Afterword: The Nurses Are Up to Something: This takes note of four women who, together, disrupted, upended, subverted, and reclaimed philosophy at Oxford University. The "women were up to something," just as nurses could be up to something. This Afterword is intended to provoke thinking about the way forward in nursing ethics, toward building a future for nursing ethics that meets contemporary needs in addressing the ethical concerns of nurses and the nursing profession.

Conclusion

In the process of writing this book, it became apparent that the sheer volume of research material I had accumulated would far exceed the publisher's allotted book length. I was not far into the writing when I realized that decisions had to be made as to what to cut or exclude. A chapter on codes of ethics for nurses, another on religion and religious ethics in nursing, another on ethics and internationalism, on global nursing, another on evil in nursing, another on diverse ethical theories employed in nursing, and others were worthy of inclusion but had to be deferred. Certainly nursing needs a book on the history and development of nursing ethics from every continent, every nation, every culture and tradition. I hope that, one day, such a project will be undertaken by others in their respective countries, for the enrichment—and unity—of the nursing world, and for the continued development of ethics education in nursing. For now, however, it is my hope that *nursing ethics* will make its way back into the hearts and minds and identity of nurses, for the profound, trenchant, perspicacious, and capacious wisdom that it offers.

1

EDUCATION IN NURSING ETHICS

Sturdy Standards

Nursing History as Entangled History

Many of the histories of nursing that were written in the 1900s and into the twenty-first century were largely insular, national histories. Where they covered world nursing, they did so nation-by-nation, taking nation-states as their meaningful boundaries. Nursing history is, however, *entangled history*. As a methodology, *entangled history* examines the complex ways in which aspirations, ideas, cultural matter, and people cross national borders. Entangled history is by nature transcultural; it examines cultural interconnectedness, interdependencies, interferences, facilitations, mutualities, power dynamics, entanglements, exchanges, and more. It recognizes the multidirectional nature of transfers and their mutations and accommodations. As an example of an entangled history, Ann Taylor Allen writes about the development of the kindergarten. Importantly, Allen indicates, the interchange of ideas and cooperation can end abruptly when politics intervenes:

> The kindergarten—a new kind of early childhood education... was at first rejected in Germany... but found a much warmer reception when German political exiles brought it to the United States. Although invented by a man, the kindergarten was developed by women, who established one of the earliest and most successful transnational networks. After the kindergarten was reestablished in Germany, an American-German dialogue influenced both the institution itself and the careers of its promoters in both countries. This is an "entangled" history that traces the complex ways in which ideas and people cross national boundaries. The kindergarten offered women opportunities for professional employment, social-reform activism, and intellectual recognition. The story covers three generations of women and ends in 1917 with the rupture of the German-American network during the First World War.[1]

DOI: 10.4324/9781003262107-2

It would seem odd to raise the issue of early childhood education, other than as an example of entangled history. Yet nursing and childhood education are more closely related than is apparent on the surface: as the two earliest "women's professions," they are considered together in early works on the analysis of professions.[2] Establishing kindergarten as a new form of early childhood education and establishing nursing and its education have much in common, but with significant differences. Both, novelly, afforded women paid work outside the home, but nurses worked with (and touched) strangers who were adults, including adult males, as well as children. Before it moved outside the domestic setting, both early childhood education and care of the ill largely took place within the home and fell to the lot of women. While the kindergarten was a new form of education external to the home, nursing had long existed in structured public settings such as hospitals, convent hospices, and workhouses. In addition, both nursing and kindergarten teaching gathered educated women to a paid occupation, and social reform. As World War I brought an abrupt end to the German–American kindergarten network, so too, as Aeleah Soine writes, the same war wrought a precipitous decline of the US–UK–German "collaborative and interrelated nature of nursing reform."[3]

As the putative founder of modern nursing *education*, Florence Nightingale's reach was long, though not all encompassing. The Nightingale School for Nurses, established at St Thomas' Hospital in London in 1860, did stimulate the growth of nursing schools well beyond the waters that surround the UK. The first modern Canadian schools of nursing, on a modified Nightingale model,[4] were established at General and Marine Hospital in St. Catharines, Ontario, in 1874; the Toronto General Hospital (1881) and Montreal General Hospital (1890). In 1868, Nightingale sent Lucy Osburn to Australia to establish a nursing school at the Sydney Hospital site. The US also adopted a modified Nightingale model. The first three "training schools" of nursing (all established in 1873, all attached to a general hospital) were the New York Training School at Bellevue Hospital, the Connecticut Training School for Nurses at the State Hospital (later New Haven Hospital), and the Boston Training School at Massachusetts General Hospital. Nightingale also sent some of her graduates to the US, and US nurse leaders traveled to the UK to confer with nurse educators and leaders there. Wellington Hospital was the first to open a Nightingale model training school for nurses in New Zealand, 1883. However, Jamaica followed another path, similar to the German deaconess tradition, which differed significantly from the Nightingale model. Archbishop (Church of England) Enos Nuttall founded an order of deaconesses in Jamaica in 1890. The Deaconesses established the first training school for nurses, associated with Kingston Public Hospital.[5,6,7] In some instances, where the Deaconess tradition was in place, schools of nursing that subsequently developed in universities adopted a Nightingale model which was preferred by physicians for their own self-interest.

Historiographies for Nursing

More recent or emergent perspectives in historiography, such as *entangled history*, can offer nursing-focused insights into its history and development.[8] Feminist perspectives have of course fruitfully made their way into nursing with concepts and categories that have helped nursing articulate its past and present situation. Postcolonial,[9,10,11,12,13] intersectional, and critical race and other critical theories are contributing to nursing's social self-understanding, and have helped to elucidate its history and blind spots. Additional historiographic perspectives such as cultural transfer history,[14] borderland history,[15] *histoire croisée*,[16,17] and transnational history,[18,19] global history,[20] entangled history[21,22] and the "spatial turn" in history,[23,24,25] among others, will prove fruitful in years to come as nursing expands its self-analysis in relation to global nursing, nurse migration, cultural and technological transfer, and more. Many of these methodologies arose within a specific discipline, then developed across disciplines. For example, postcolonial theory begins in literary criticism with Edward Said's *Orientalism*,[26] and subsequently explodes into other disciplines in the social sciences, humanities, theology, the arts, and more. These more recent perspectives in historiography have moved history from the humanities to the social sciences, and have made disciplinary boundaries as permeable as national boundaries in scholarly research. What this means is that any consideration of nursing history must look well beyond nursing and may derive its insights from an unusual domain of scholarship, such as linguistics, diplomatic relations, music, and architecture. It is beyond the scope of this chapter and book (and author) to delve into an analysis of historiographic methods. They are, however, a means of enriching our understanding of the ethics of the profession and enable us to look more closely at the entangled histories that knit an early modern nursing, its education, its practice, and its ethics.

Nursing Curriculum as Entangled History

To remain, here, with the perspective of nursing history is an entangled history, the story of the development of nursing, nursing education, and organizations serves to display that entanglement. The export of Nightingale and Deaconess nursing education models and movements, and the formation of the International Council of Nurses, are major elements of nursing's entangled history, as are the establishment of widely shared nursing journals, international congresses, and the transnational work of early nursing leaders. As nursing came to grips with attempting to standardize nursing education curricula in the late 1800s, there was considerable interchange between and amongst nursing leaders, through the vehicles of international congresses, publications, personal letters, visits, and more. Isabel Robb (née Hampton), at the International Congress of Charities, Correction and Philanthropy (Section III, 1893), presented a paper calling for educational standards for nursing education. Deploring the current lack or diversity of educational standards, or the medical profiteering in creating private schools to serve as cheap labor, Robb writes:

> A "trained nurse" may mean anything, everything, or next to nothing, and with this state of affairs the results are far from what they should be, and public criticism is frequently justly severe upon our shortcomings...[27]

The Congress was "international," though that largely meant Europe and North America. The major contingents from all sections (including medical and nursing) were from the UK and the US with speakers from Scotland (identified separately), France, Germany, Switzerland, the Netherlands, Canada, Japan, and Chile. Papers were delivered in English, French, and German. The nursing section itself was largely weighted toward the UK and US participation, with papers on nursing education, practice, midwifery, legislation, standards, social ethics, health policy, and more, followed by a discussion of every paper with respondents as well as questions from participants. Some years hence, the ICN would provide a similar forum for international exchange and collaboration.

Untangling the influences upon curriculum would seem a Gordian knot. However, in their work on transnational entanglements in social reform, Leonards and Randeraad developed a novel approach.

Who were the people at the cutting edge of social reform in Europe between 1840 and 1880, and how were they connected? This article proposes a method to locate a transnational community of experts involved in social reform and focuses on the ways in which these experts shared and spread their knowledge across borders. After a discussion of the concepts of social reform, transnationalization, and transfer, we will show how we built a database of visitors to social reform congresses in the period of 1840–1880, and explain how we extracted the core group of experts from this database. This "congress elite"... we discuss their travels, congress visits, publications, correspondence, and membership of learned and professional organizations. We argue that individual members of our elite, leaning on the prestige of their international contacts, shaped reform debates in their home countries. We conclude by calling for further research into the influence that the transnational elite were able to exert on concrete social reforms in different national frameworks in order to assess to what extent they can be regarded as an "epistemic community in the making."[28]

In a similar manner, we might ask: "Who were the nurse leaders at the cutting edge of nursing educational and social reform, between 1865 and 1910, and how were they connected?" How were their ideas exchanged and who informed and influenced whom, and how did that shape nursing curriculum, education, ethics and social engagement? The list of nursing's elite, in both middle and upper classes, is long, but the Leonards and Randeraad method would seem a good starting place, especially since many of the necessary historical documents for nursing organizations are now available digitally. The same method might be used and questions asked for the narrower domain of nursing ethics education.

The battle for nursing authority over nursing education, for the standardization of entrance requirements and program length, and for the standardization of curriculum was a shared, international struggle, shepherded in part by the ICN, which is well described in most nursing history books and need not be repeated here. What is less well known are the ethics curricular requirements that were established early on for nursing education.

The transnational entanglement of nursing ethics is most evident in nursing's social ethics, with its focus on moral character (virtue), and in the development of a whole-person approach to ethics. There was a less specific or direct effect upon ethics education requirements per se, other than the shared emphases on society, community, character (virtue), a whole-person ethics, and duties to self. Our entangled ethics history is most evident in nursing engagement in social reform. Now, however, our focus is on curricular requirements, which is foundational to our subsequent consideration of the nature and scope of nursing ethics.

Nursing Ethics Curriculum

In the United States, in 1915, the National League for Nursing Education (NLNE; later National League for Nursing, NLN) established curricular requirements that included specific requirements for ethics curriculum. These requirements were mandated for nursing education in American schools. While there was a specific section of the curriculum devoted entirely to ethics (an "ethics course"), ethics was also mandated to be taught throughout the curriculum. The heaviest emphasis, outside the ethics course itself, is found in the "Social and Professional Subjects" section, and the section titled "History (including Ethical and Social Principles)." These ethics requirements for 1915–1919 are transcribed here.[29] Note that the term *principles*, or phrase *principles of ethics*, should be understood in a generic sense, not as it is understood in contemporary bioethics.

The Standardized and Mandated NLNE Ethics Requirements for Nursing Education, 1915–1919

These are the remarkable requirements in their unedited original (including incomplete sentences, etc.), transcribed below. I have inserted the uncited sources for the requirements within the document itself in bold.

Principles of Ethics **[course]**
  Time: 10 hours. Classes and conferences conducted by the superintendent of nurses or a special lecturer. Given in the second year.

Objects of the Course

1. To follow up the work of the first year in the historical and social aspects of nursing by a fuller discussion of the principles of behavior, their origin, meaning and practical bearings on the common experiences and problems of life.

---

2. To try to lead the pupil to formulate more clearly and definitely her philosophy of life, to stimulate her in the formation of the right kind of personal habits, to help her in building up a strong and an attractive personality, and to give her a vision of what a full, happy, useful, and well-ordered life may be.

3. The effort is made here to build up broad general principles which equally apply well to all phases of life and all types of people, rather than to emphasize a special code which is restricted to one group and one type of occupation.

Outline of Classes

I.   Introduction—Customary Morality **[drawn from Dewey & Tufts, Chapters 3, 4]**
     Meaning and derivation of ethics, morals, customs. Distinguish from etiquette, manners, religion. Kind of problems considered in a study of ethics (give concrete examples). Basis of all behavior found in the original nature of man with its equipment of instincts and tendencies. These neither good nor bad in themselves, but become good or bad according to their effect on other human beings. Repetition and resulting satisfaction the conditions of development. Four levels of stages of conduct: (1) Instincts, controlled and influenced only by physical pains and pleasures; (2) modified by rewards and punishments; (3) controlled by the thought of praise or blame; (4) Conduct regulated by a personal ideal which enables one to do right even when it entails personal suffering and the condemnation of society. First stage non-moral, represented by infants and mental defectives. Most people in second and third stages—where custom and tradition are principal guides to conduct (group or customary morality). Customs and laws gradually built up by the social group for its on welfare and protection, and habits enforced through ritual and ceremony, force of public opinion or physical force. Weakness and limitations in this kind of morality.

II. Personal or Reflective Morality **[drawn from Dewey & Tufts, Chapters 5, 9]**
     Personal as opposed to group or customary morality involves free choice and independent moral judgment, instead of unreasoning acceptance of custom or slavish imitation of others. Social habits and customs still determine conduct to a large extent but the individual is responsible and accountable for his own actions. His conduct becomes purposeful, voluntary, and spontaneous, as opposed to impulsive or forced conduct. Laws, which he first obeyed mechanically, he learns to obey rationally.

In this stage of conduct, morals are differentiated from manners, conscience substituted for custom, and principles for rules of conduct. Personal or reflective morality has three aspects: (1) right feeling or a delicate sensitiveness to ethical ideals and an ardent desire to realize them; (2) right thinking or sound moral judgement; (3) right doing or the vigorous carrying out of one's purposes and ideals. This is conscientiousness or obedience to the inward law "where the person himself sets up the ideal standard, judges his conduct by it, holds himself responsible to himself and seeks to do justice." **[Dewey & Tufts, 182]** Conscience is not infallible—needs constant enlightenment and training, must be kept sensitive and responsive, and must be obeyed as the highest moral law which the individual knows.

III.   Ethical Ideals and Standards **[drawn from Dewey & Tufts, Chapters 6–8]**

Ethical ideals are the product of all the preceding ages and of all one's experiences in life. The body of accepted moral and ethical principles have very slowly accumulated and are constantly undergoing changes and modifications. Each age works out a different conception of moral worth or goodness. Great moral leaders are those who break through traditions and customs, and establish new ideals of conduct. They are the prophets, saints, martyrs, and reformers. Moral ideals are embodied in art, literature, religion, law, etc. Earliest ethical principles of high value found in Hebrew and Greek literatures. The Roman law and the Christian Church, the main sources of later ethical standards and the great conservative forces in preserving old standards. Examples of early ethical teachings are seen in the ten commandments, the golden rule, proverbs, fables, etc., ethical influence of great characters in history, biography, fiction, and contemporary life.

IV.   Moral Judgment **[drawn from Dewey & Tufts, Chapters 9, 11, 16, 19]**

The second essential to reflective morality is sound moral judgment or wisdom, "the parent or nurse of all the virtues."[30] Element of choice and moral valuation implies capacity for reflection, discrimination and sound thinking as well as an adequate body of knowledge to guide one's decision. Imagination needed to forecast possible results of any given choice and to see the wider and more remote as well as the immediate results. Sympathetic insight into others' lives and a wide acquaintance with human nature necessary to insure just judgments. Wisdom needed in deciding means to be used as well as ends to be realized. Wisdom means insight, sagacity, sanity, and common sense, not to be confused with mere knowledge. Moral judgment not essentially different from judgments required in business or professional matters. Ability to judge wisely in some degree inherited, but may be developed by exercise and self-criticism. Impulsive, capricious, or "snap" judgments likely to be superficial and unreliable. Prejudice and strong emotion warp judgment. Dogmatism and intolerance usually based on narrow range of facts, and shallow thinking. Until facts can be obtained, judgment should be suspended.

V. Conduct and Character **[drawn from Dewey and Tufts, Chapters 13, 14]**

The third essential—will power or moral energy to control vagrant or selfish impulses and carry out one's purpose and ideals. High ideals and thoughtful decisions are ineffective unless put into practice. Those who profess fine ideas and emotions without doing anything to carry them out are called sentimentalists or hypocrites. Motive power comes from the emotions and sentiments which are the springs of action as well as the key to character. What a person is, is shown by what he desires most, what annoys, pains, or grieves him, in what he finds satisfaction. Disposition and temperament are largely inherited, but character is made. It is the result of all one's choices and actions, of all one's physical, mental, or moral habits. Important to make allies instead of enemies of one's habits. Rules for habit-formation (see James). Action must be vigorous and forceful as well as rightly directed—must be applied consistently in all the affairs of everyday life.

VI. The Place of "the Self" in the Moral Life **[drawn from Dewey & Tufts, Chapters 18, 19]**

Virtues are habits of will or modes of conduct which tend to promote the welfare of the individual and collective life. Vices are abnormal developments of the will that tend to enslave and destroy life. The normal impulse of individuals is to satisfy the desires and claims of self. The higher welfare of the self includes the welfare of the larger group. Involves struggle between egoism and altruism, between narrow selfishness and benevolence. Self-control the mainspring of character—mastery of the lower by the higher impulses. Suppression and eradication of natural impulses and emotions and extreme self-renunciation as advocated by ascetics tend to cripple and narrow life. Self-expression and self-development to be emphasized, as well as self-denial and self-sacrifice. Courage or persistent natural vigor needed to resist lower desires and give moral power to meet pain, danger, and public disapproval, when necessary. Strong character implies virility, vigor, and strong moral fibre, not negative, spineless "goodyness." Modesty (freedom from false pride and excessive desires), chastity, self-possession, perseverance, fortitude, patience, constancy—all aspects of self-control and courage. A high conception of individual honor, self-respect, and wholesome ambition, essential to complete development of the self. Vanity, servility, aggressiveness, etc. are perversions of the impulse to further self's welfare and development.

VII. The Social Virtues. **[drawn from Dewey & Tufts, Chapters 8, 18, 19, 24]**

The parental or "motherly" instinct—the main root of the social virtues. Tenderness, compassion, sympathy, pity, benevolence, and helpfulness, generally expressed in various forms of charity and philanthropy, such as caring for children, the sick, helpless, and dependent. Unless safeguarded by knowledge and good judgment, benevolence may be injurious to oneself and others. Good will, or love of one's neighbor, is incompatible with envy, malice, and all the subtle as well as active forms of cruelty and selfishness. Patriotism or love of one's country—another form of benevolence. Justice a fundamental social virtue, representing the ideas of equity, rectitude, fairness, impartiality, honesty as opposed to exploitation, oppression or injustice of all kinds. Veracity implies frankness, fidelity, and sincerity in all human relationships as opposed to lying, flattery, slander, and misrepresentation. Social virtues of cooperation, good-will, fair play, give and take, enter into every phase of human life and work.

VIII. Ethical Principles as Applied to Community Life **[drawn from Dewey & Tufts, Chapters 20, 21]**

The growth of democracy in modern life. Result of growing belief in the worth and possibilities of the individual and his right to self-expression and development. Danger of over emphasis on individual rights and neglect of obligations. New emphasis on social ends or group welfare, not incompatible with individual development. Social efficiency—the modern ideal—highest self-realization and self-expression through service for the common good. Wide variation in types of service and ability needed for community service. Public-spiritedness and patriotism expressed in the faithful doing of inconspicuous and common tasks as well as heroic deeds. Importance of training and efficiency as well as good-will. Recent changes in the status of women and new possibilities of public service opened up. Local questions of family and community welfare discussed from the ethical point of view with practical suggestions for useful service.

IX. Principles of Ethics Applied to One's Work or Profession **[Shift from Dewey & Tufts to nursing ethics textbooks by nurses Robb, Parsons, et al.]**

The relation of various forms of occupation to community welfare. Ideals and traditions of service developed by such professions as the church, the army, medicine, etc. The spirit of the craftsman or artist in relation to his art. Putting one's soul into one's work. The value of work as a means of happiness, personal satisfaction, and development. Growth in independence, integrity, industry, and self-respect through work. The "business-like" qualities and virtues—system, thoroughness, promptness, alertness, economy, reliability, and persistence. Qualities demanded in working with others—loyalty and intelligent cooperation with those in charge, trustworthiness, ability to do good team-work, spirit of courtesy and helpfulness, a sense of humor, discretion. Qualities necessary in leading and guiding others—good judgment, justice, dignity, generosity, initiative, enthusiasm, self-reliance, and the ability to take responsibility. Dangers of narrowness and stagnation in relation to one's occupation; of materialism, cynicism, and mechanical routine. Effects of over-fatigue, and over-work as well as idleness in breaking down moral resistance, decreasing moral sensitiveness, and sapping energy and spirit.

X.   Principles of Ethics as Applied to One's Personal Life **[reflecting nursing: Nightingale, Robb, Parsons, et al.]**

The importance of having definite purposes to work towards, laws to obey, ideals to follow. Self-direction and self-mastery achieved through concentration and practice. The place of religion in the building of character, and the development of one's spiritual life. Essentials of an attractive, wholesome, and strong personality. Its influence on others. Possibilities of strengthening weak moral fiber and cultivating hidden resources of personality and ability in others. The ability to meet moral crises in one's own life and the lives of others. Provision for growth. What we mean by self-government. Application of foregoing principles to special problems, especially those involved in recreation, amusements, and social life, dress and the expenditure of money, relations between men and women, friendships, etc.

Methods of Teaching **[drawn in part from William James]**

1. The practice of ethics is a matter of attitude, spirit, and will more than knowledge. Teaching will never be effective in changing behavior unless it is backed up by the example and personality of the teacher and by the atmosphere and influences which surround the pupil every day. Every subject taught in the training school should be a medium for teaching ethics, and every problem which the pupil meets in her daily work should be an opportunity for practice in ethics. The social life of the pupil nurse is a particularly strong influence in shaping her ideals and developing her

powers. Emphasis should be laid on the foundation of habits of positive service and helpfulness rather than merely the correction of faults and the observation of rules and regulations; on the strengthening of character through complete development rather than the repression and elimination of them or undesirable traits. If the principles of student government are in force in the Nurse's Home, it will give a much better opportunity for exercising the qualities of self-direction and self-control in regard to the pupil's personal life.

2. In teaching ethics, concrete examples should be given to illustrate every point, or to lead up to the discussion. These examples will be found in history and standard literature, poetry, current fiction, newspaper items or personal experiences. It is better not to draw too many examples from hospital life but to give as broad a point of view as possible. Pupils should be asked to bring in examples and to contribute to the discussions in every possible way. The course should be tied up with the earlier course in the historical and social aspects of nursing and to psychology if this is given. It might follow the course in psychology or be combined with it if there is not time for both.

3. If possible, personal conferences might supplement such a course. The teacher could thus get into closer touch with the pupils and could help them better in working out their individual problems.

Text and Reference Books **[readings for those nursing faculty teaching ethics]**

Robb: Ethics of Nursing. **[*Nursing Ethics*, misnamed]**
Parsons: Nursing Problems and Obligations.
Nightingale: Notes on Nursing.
Nightingale: Talks to Pupil Nurses.
Osler: Æquanimitas.
Dewey and Tufts: Ethics.
Mackenzie: Manual of Ethics.
McDougall: Social Psychology.
James: Talks to Teachers.
McCunn: Making of Character.
Emerson: Essays.
Cabot, (E. L.): Every-Day Ethics.
Cabot, (Richard): What Men Live By.

See also under Historical, Ethical and Social Aspects of Nursing, Psychology and Problems of Professional Life.[31]

Sources That Informed the NLNE Requirements

The standards for nursing education contain hints of external, specifically philo-sophical, influences. In their speeches and writings, nursing leaders cite a range of authors, and a range of genres, even poetry. These leaders wax eloquent in their discussion of the content of nursing education, and in many places there are trace elements of external contributions to their thinking that are not cited, though oc-casionally they are. Nurse-historians have written that early nursing leaders were influenced by the Progressive Era movement and the philosophy of Pragmatism that were prevalent (dominant) in the US in that era.[32,33] While some of the early books on nursing education have the scent of pragmatism, Annie W. Goodrich's book *The Social and Ethical Significance of Nursing* is clearly steeped in the work of the Pragmatists, especially the works of John Dewey and William James, both of whom she quotes and cites from several of their books and articles.[34]

Much of what is written on early nursing's engagement with pragmatism has not taken a deep dive into specific works that were influential and the particular ways in which Pragmatism influenced nursing thought or theory. In relation to the program of establishing nursing education and curriculum, with Annie Goodrich's book, for example, we see that she drew concepts and quotes from Dewey's *Reconstruction in Philosophy*,[35] *Experience and Nature*,[36] *The Quest for Certainty*,[37] and his articles in *The New Republic*, "American Education and Culture,"[38] and "Individuality, Equality, and Superiority."[39] She also quotes his definition of *art* (without a citation).[40] Identifying the specific influences of Pragmatism on the de-velopment of nursing's philosophy, theory, educational structures, and curriculum is an under-researched domain.

Even less research has been done on external sources that have informed nurs-ing ethics. Similar to the nursing education books and speeches, the early nursing ethics textbooks only hint at sources that informed their writers. While there are some attributions in-text, many of the earlier works lack bibliographic citations or narrative attributions, which is consistent with the era. As with Goodrich, even direct quotes may not have a citation or attribution. As a whole, the ethics writ-ings have more than a pinch of philosophy, sociology, education, and psychology kneaded into the flour of nursing. The ethics writings, too, reflect the tradition of the American Pragmatists, and John Dewey in particular, Jane Addams as well, and William James to a lesser degree. However, unattributed, definitive evidence of that association appears throughout the NLNE ethics requirements.

The Influence of Pragmatism

Pragmatism arises as an American philosophical tradition in the 1870s, concurrent with the rise of modern nursing education. Histories have customarily named its forefathers as Charles Sanders Peirce (1839–1914), William James (1842–1910), and John Dewey (1859–1952) while neglecting the fact that there were foremoth-ers who influenced these men (e.g., Alice Chipman Dewey (1858–1927), John

Dewey's wife) or who promulgated the pragmatist philosophical theory in their own right (e.g., Jane Addams of Hull House, 1860–1935). Dewey became its most prominent representative and a renowned public intellectual in the US. Pragmatism was the homegrown, dominant, philosophical tradition in the US until the rise of analytic philosophy, which (arguably) eclipsed Pragmatism. In recent years, there has been a renewed interest in and adoption of Pragmatism, particularly among feminists, Black ethicists, and Black radical feminists.

Pragmatism, as a philosophy, has had ebbs and flows both in the US, Canada, and the UK. Initially it was less well received in the UK, though it did make inroads and in recent decades has seen renewal.[41,42,43,44]

Social Context

The task here is to explain why Pragmatism became important in nursing education and ethics, rather than to explicate or argue Pragmatism per se.[45] Setting aside consideration of the Crimean War (1853–1856) and American Civil War (1861–1865), there are many historical forces, in the second half of the 1800s into the 1900s, that converge and incubate major social movements. This was the period of the philosophy of Pragmatism, the establishment of modern nursing education and practice, the Progressive Era (1890s–1920s), the women's rights movement, the first-wave feminist movement; the Niagara Movement and the founding of the National Association for the Advancement of Colored People (NAACP); the Social Gospel movement of the US, Canada, UK, and a number or European countries, which advanced a social ethics for social justice; the earlier Industrial Revolution that led to urbanization and conurbation acceleration in the late 1800s and early1900s; the Labor movement; the efficiency movement; the settlement movement; a rise in immigration (resulting in exclusion laws) in the late 1900s and again around World War II; the development of medicine including germ theory, the discovery of antibiotics (Salvarsan), and the development of vaccines; the development of pharmacology, psychoanalysis, and more; the development of Darwin's theory of evolution; and Marxist and socialist critiques of capitalism; and the development of the pneumatic tire and steel tubing for bicycles which, oddly, played an important role in the women's rights movement as well as district nursing. The movements of this period are too numerous to list. While elements of this (such as the founding of the NAACP) are distinctly American, a number of these movements also manifest in the UK and Canada in their own distinctive forms, such as the Canadian Laurier Era. However, some of these movements—women's rights and suffrage in particular—not only occur across nations, but involve close, transnational, collaboration among women and nurses.

Why Pragmatism?

These movements converge, in part, because of an overlapping set of concerns. There were shared concerns for economic reform, in reaction to political corruption from the concentration of power in big business, monopolies, and wealth among a social elite. Labor rights, including unionization for worker protection and security, and child labor were an attendant concern. Urban squalor, and its unsanitary conditions, and poverty, including poverty among regional, racial, and immigrant populations, and social welfare structures were yet an additional set of concerns. Nursing faced these issues both in terms of social policy concerns, and more directly in nursing practice which largely took place in homes. Rank and file nurses traversed urban neighborhoods and rural villages; they acquired a direct, intimate knowledge of the health effects of poverty. Nursing had a natural concern, then, for these issues. However, as nurses and nursing leaders were women, the disenfranchisement of women had a direct effect upon the formation of nursing as a profession, the establishment and standardization of its education, and the regulation of entry into practice. Thus, the issues of suffrage had a direct effect upon women and nurses-as-women. Labor law also affected nurses so that many of the concerns faced by the recipients of nursing also affected nurses themselves. Pragmatism dives and bobs in this social milieu.

The philosophy of Pragmatism was the most influential philosophy in the late nineteenth- and early twentieth-century US. As a philosophy it is action oriented, emphasizing experience over *a priori* reasoning (including *a priori* abstract rules and principles). William James writes that Pragmatism

> turns away from abstraction and insufficiency, from verbal solutions, from bad *a priori* reasons, from fixed principles, closed systems, and pretended absolutes and origins.... [and] turns towards concreteness and adequacy, towards facts, towards action.... It means the open air and possibilities of nature, as against... dogma, artificiality, and the pretence of finality in truth.[46]

Pragmatism provided a foundational philosophy for social reform, and philosophers of pragmatism took up an enormous range of social causes. Pragmatism, thus, entered into law, education, political and social theory, economics, psychology, art, religion—and nursing. The social concerns of pragmatism overlapped with the personal commitments of nursing's leaders, and with the social forces that affected nursing as an emerging profession, and nurses as they engaged in nursing labors and patient care. Pragmatism and nursing had (and have) a natural affinity. Beyond that affinity, however, many of the leaders in the Progressive movements and Pragmatist Philosophy were friends and colleagues—John Dewey, Lavinia Dock, Lillian Wald, Jane Addams, Adelaide Nutting, and others.

The NLNE Ethics Curricular Requirements

The earliest nursing textbooks, that is, medical-surgical type nursing textbooks, generally contained a first chapter that related specifically to the moral duties and character of the nurse. These works significantly predate the 1908 ethics text by Dewey and Tufts, as does Isabel Robb's 1900 book *Nursing Ethics*. Nursing's ethical corpus, while initially uninfluenced by Dewey and Tufts, did address issues, concerns, and values that had great synchrony with those of Dewey and Tufts' work that followed. By 1915, the ethics curricular requirements had become heavily reliant upon Dewey and Tufts' book *Ethics*[47] as its philosophical-ethical joists.

As noted in the transcribed requirements above, individual sections of the ethics course, specifically sections one through eight, rely heavily on specific chapters in Dewey and Tufts, though with modification. The teaching approaches are influenced by the educational theories of William James and John Dewey.[48] Sections nine and ten are not related to Dewey and Tufts' work at all but are, instead, informed by both pre-existing and contemporaneous, independent, nursing ethics literature.

Summative Comments

Overall, these NLNE ethics requirements are exceptionally strong, coherent, well informed in ethics, comprehensive, and commendable requirements for ethics education, both then and even now (with modernizing modification). A few general comments are in order:

- The incomplete thoughts and sentences are difficult to follow but are "bookmarks" to the Dewey and Tufts book.
- There are elements that are captive of their day, though perhaps not obvious to a modern reader, such as the reflection of the long-standing debate over nature versus nurture, influenced by James' notion of *instincts*[49] (Section IV, "Ability to judge wisely in some degree inherited..."), and the efficiency movement of the late 1800s (e.g., Section VIII, "Importance of training and efficiency as well as good-will ...").
- The vocabulary, too, is dated: for example, the contemporary word *empathy* was not in common use then, so that *sympathy* stands in its place.
- Its emphasis on practice is a part of the experience and action orientation of the philosophy of Pragmatism, as well as its harmony with pivotal elements of the lifeworld of the nurse.
- Though drawn from Dewey and Tufts, Section VI is entirely consistent with the nursing ethics literature that predates it.
- Though this is written during the first wave of feminism, Section VII is prescient in its anticipation of second-wave feminism.
- Sections IX and X are not a part of Dewey and Tufts' work: they are entirely drawn from the nursing ethics literature and the nursing ethics tradition (see, for example, both Robb's and Parson's books in the requirements list).

Rejection of Medical Ethics

At the time that the NLNE formulated their requirements, there was an ample body of literature on medical ethics that could have been relied upon to frame or structure their nursing ethics content. They intentionally and consciously chose not to use any medical-ethical material per se, so that what is here in these requirements draws upon the formal philosophical discipline of ethics itself, with reference to nursing practice alone. It is not in any way derived from or similar to the then current medical ethics. (They made the same choice with the eventual ANA Code of Ethics for Nurses, though for reasons of aspiration-to-professional-status, some medical ethics did intrude.)

The Textbooks

The textbook list is evenly divided between British and American writers. All of the books are authored by well-recognized, acknowledged scholars in their respective fields. Its list includes physician William Osler's *Æquanimitas: With Addresses to Medical Students, Nurses and Practitioners of Medicine*,[50] but does not draw from it in the requirements. The book does contain two talks given to nurses, and an interesting chapter on medical chauvinism that decries nationalism, provincialism, parochialism, and a host of other ills such as pecuniary interest in medicine. Richard Chabot's book *What Men Live By: Work, Play, Love, Worship*[51] supplements the requirements but is not directly drawn upon. Both Osler and Chabot were noted physicians given to broader reflection on the nature of medicine and medical practice. While Dewey and Tufts' book is used to structure the NLNE ethics requirements, John Mackenzie's book *A Manual of Ethics*[52] provides supplemental material that is woven into the Dewey and Tufts material. Mackenzie was a renowned British philosopher; his book is a comprehensive, systematic, deeply substantive, academic book on ethics, with a precision of content. It provided a solid resource for the curricular requirements. Though these ethics requirements are for American schools, the book list is another example of transnational interaction in its use of scholars from both the US and UK.

Ethical Orientation

As their third object of the course makes clear, they intended a "whole life" approach to ethics, not simply a professional ethics that would drive an untenable wedge between the personal and the professional. This framing of ethics saw the personal and professional as one, but also demonstrated a concern for the well-being of the nurse so that she might have (in object number two) "a vision of what a full, happy, useful, and well-ordered life may be."[53] It is an important consistency that if nursing's focus of concern is the whole person of the patient, nursing ethics should be concerned for the whole person of the nurse.

In Section I of the requirements is a nascent theory of moral development that prefigures Kohlberg's sequential stages of moral development.[54] Kohlberg's work was popular in bioethics in nursing in the 1990s. Section I stages of conduct/development are:

Four levels of stages of conduct: (1) Instincts, controlled and influenced only by physical pains and pleasures; (2) modified by rewards and punishments; (3)

controlled by the thought of praise or blame; (4) Conduct regulated by a personal ideal which enables one to do right even when it entails personal suffering and the condemnation of society.

It is noteworthy, however, that the fourth stage is regulated by an *ideal*, not an *a priori*, abstract principle of *justice* navigated through moral reasoning, as is found in Kohlberg. Kohlberg's work was, famously, critiqued by Carol Gilligan[55] as gender-biased such that women, with an orientation toward *care* over *justice*, would assess at a lower level of his stages. Kohlberg disagreed, claiming that many studies found no difference in gender scores, and that where differences were demonstrated, they were a consequence of education, work experiences, and social roles that were taken on, but not gender.[56] The problem with his response is that education, social roles, work experiences, life opportunities, and more are profoundly affected, socially and legally, by gender. By rooting the fourth stage in a *personal ideal*, not principles, (more specifically not a principle of justice), Dewey and Tufts did not fall into the gender trap and could even allow for a personal ideal rooted in one's professional identity.

Section II, on personal and reflective morality, addresses a number of important issues such as the social conditioning of moral behavior and ideals. Accountability and responsibility are included and are found (in varying degrees and ways) in the current ANA *Code of Ethics for Nurses with Interpretive Statements*,[57] the Canadian Nurses Association (CNA) Code of Ethics,[58] the Royal College of Nursing (RCN) *Code of Conduct*,[59] and the Nursing and Midwifery Council (NMC) *The Code*.[60] This section also covers autonomy versus heteronomy, the role of conscience, and moral fiber in the "vigorous pursuing of one's purposes and ideals"—which is essential to addressing today's situations of potential moral distress in practice. In addition, the three aspects of personal or reflective morality in this section have significant correlation with Benner's three apprenticeships for nursing education. Benner writes of three apprenticeships essential to all practice professions:

> All practice professions must address the following three professional apprenticeships:
>
> (a) The cognitive apprenticeship: intellectual training that provides: (i) the academic and theoretical knowledge base required for practice in the discipline; (ii) the capacity to think in ways important to the profession.
> (b) The practice apprenticeship: clinical reasoning and clinical practice skilled know-how that teaches students how to think and solve problems in actual clinical situations. Learning how to reason across time through changes in the patient and/or changes in the clinician's understanding of the patient's condition and concerns.
> (c) Formation and ethical comportment apprenticeship: an apprenticeship to the ethical standards, social roles, and responsibilities of the profession,

through which the novice is introduced to the meaning of an integrated practice of all dimensions of the profession, grounded in the profession's fundamental purposes.[61]

More will be said of the three apprenticeships anon. (See Chapter 9.)

Section III deals with topics that barely receive passing attention in today's bioethical discourse—moral exemplars, ideals, and the arts and humanities that are the repositories that express and teach the values of civilizations and societies, and the models who embody them. The loss of the humanities in nursing, and their reflection upon human experience, is a tragic loss of expressions of the profession's values as well as the heroism, courage, despair, and suffering nurses encounter every day. Consider, for example, Amy Haddad's book of poetry *An Otherwise Healthy Woman*,[62] an intimate portrait of the yearning for compassion, of meeting suffering, of joy—hardly the substance of medical-surgical nursing textbooks.

Section IV explores sound moral judgment as *wisdom*. More specifically it explores the relationship between wisdom and virtue. "Wisdom means insight, sagacity, sanity, and common sense, not to be confused with mere knowledge." Here, reliance upon abstract, noncontextual, *a priori* principles (e.g., "principles of biomedical ethics") is specifically eschewed in favor of *phronesis*, practical reasoning, a form of reasoning that must be developed through experience. This chapter stands as a counterpoint to contemporary bioethics, particularly principlism. Section V largely expands Section IV with a discussion of how ideals, values, virtues, and thoughtful decisions are habituated. Section VI extends the discussion of virtue to character development and the balance of individuality with the common good, and what it takes to strengthen moral fiber. The chapters build and move sequentially in a coordinated and contiguous manner in dealing with the whole person as a moral agent.

Section VII addresses "the social virtues" that move toward social justice: "justice a fundamental social virtue, representing the ideas of equity, rectitude, fairness, impartiality, honesty as opposed to exploitation, oppression or injustice of all kinds." Here we have an anticipation of today's discussion of structures of oppression, racism, and discrimination and the social ills that give rise to health disparities. Section VIII extends this discussion into community life. It looks at the balancing act of democracy—individual rights balanced with group ends, social welfare, and service. Specific attention is given to the status of women and social changes that opened up opportunities for women in society.

When we arrive at Sections IX and X, we move away from Dewey and Tufts and into the nursing ethics literature that had developed and was growing with vigor. These two chapters are different as they specifically rely upon the nursing ethics literature, written by experienced nurses, for nurses, thus focusing—targeting even—nurses, nursing, and nursing practice. This will become apparent in a subsequent discussion of the nursing ethics textbooks.

These ethics curricular requirements were supplemented by other ethics content requirements that further expand these in relation to particular areas of nursing ethical concern. These requirements are such that they work to form the nurse in her identity as a nurse, where the values, aspirations, ideals and commitments of nursing are interiorized and welded to the nurse's DNA. This course is not simply "book-learning." The teaching methods stipulate modeling of behavior by instructors, and the creation of a moral milieu that envelops the students. Ethics was to suffuse the entire curriculum and was to be "practiced" by students at every turn. Actual examples were to be discussed, drawn from history, literature, poetry in order to communicate that sense of ethics in the whole of a person's life, not limited to nursing alone. On top of this, there were to be private conferences, and students encouraged to find examples themselves.

Much more could be said, of course, but what we have in these 1915–1919 requirements is a learned, coherent, and comprehensive ethics education drawn from a range of impeccable sources, and to be implemented nationwide. The course teaches that personal and professional life is one life and that ethics covers every nook and cranny of life. The course covers general applied ethical theory, but then applies it to the nurse. There is nothing ancillary about this ethics: it is not an icing on the cake—it is part of the cake itself.

By Way of Comparison: The AACN Essential for Ethics Education, 2021

Today, the American Association of Colleges of Nursing (AACN) establishes core competencies for nursing education, published in their document *The Essentials: Core Competencies for Professional Nursing Education* (2021).[63] Their curricular requirements for ethics are:

> Core to professional nursing practice, ethics refers to principles that guide a person's behavior. Ethics is closely tied to moral philosophy involving the study of or examination of morality through a variety of different approaches (Tubbs, 2009). There are commonly accepted principles in bioethics that include autonomy, beneficence, non-maleficence, and justice (ANA 2015; ACNM, 2015; AANA, 2018; ICN, 2012). The study of ethics as it relates to nursing practice has led to the exploration of other relevant concepts, including moral distress, moral hazard, moral community, and moral or critical resilience.[64]

Commentary

Within the AACN *Essentials* document, ethics is one of the eight *concepts* that is to be represented across the ten *domains* of the AACN *Essentials* document. The eight *concepts* are:

- Clinical judgments
- Communication
- Compassionate care

- Diversity, equity, and inclusivity
- Ethics
- Evidence-based practice
- Health policy
- Social determinants of health

Taking *concept* in terms of natural language (and not a philosophical statement), this list is an untidy amalgamation of processes, concepts, skills, goals, and factors, of which ethics is one *concept* among equals, a likely consequence of *competency-based standards*. In addition, a competency-based standards approach precludes concern for clinical wisdom (phronesis), which receives no attention.

To focus on the ethics component, ethics is seen as core to nursing practice, as it should be, though it is not heavily weighted in the *Essentials*. The declaration that "ethics refers to principles that guide a person's behavior" is problematic, especially its focus on the particularistic principles of autonomy, beneficence, nonmaleficence, and justice, reflecting the influence of Beauchamp and Childress' *Principles of Biomedical Ethics*,[65] which is not undergirded by a theory of ethics but rather rooted in an alleged "common morality." Since the publication of its first edition (1979; now, in its eighth edition), this excellent text has been challenged as to its principlism per se, but also its suitability for nursing, as nursing moved toward an ethics shaped by feminist ethics and an ethics of care. The *Essentials* implicitly endorses bioethics, and it must be granted that the four principles remain the *lingua franca* of institutional ethics committees and bioethics in medicine. The document also mentions *moral distress, moral hazard, moral community* and *moral resilience*, all of which are drawn from conflictual concerns raised by nurses. Here, the *Essentials* focuses on structural problems related to the inequality and subordinate status of the nurse, not on the recipient of nursing care.

Ethics in nursing is substantially more, and substantially other than, problems, conflicts, and competencies, and certainly more than principles of biomedical ethics as the four principles. A larger part of ethics in nursing has to do with the realization of the notions of good intrinsic to practice, practical wisdom, and moral character as it emerges in the nurse–patient relationship. It is this aspect of ethics-in-a-practice-discipline, that is what it means to be a *good nurse*, where the realization of those goods entails skillful practice interfused with morally good practice. To say this another way, skilled nursing entails the actualization of the notions of good intrinsic to nursing, embedded in the tradition, narrative, and practice of nursing, and in so doing co-realizes the moral basis of the profession. Morally good nursing is skilled nursing and skilled nursing is morally good nursing; one does not exist without or separate from the other.

This kind of practice is dependent upon the moral formation of the nurse, specifically the *instantiation*[66] of nursing values, goods, ideals, ends, and aspirations as part of the nurse's personal identity. In ethics, a nurse is not one who *does* nursing, but one who *is* a nurse. The *is-ness*, then, makes nursing a *profession* in the sense of what one *professes*, as a part of one's self, as opposed to a task or occupation. Identity issues into ethical comportment. In nursing education, this requires the amalgamation of ethics and nursing, forming an alloy: *good nursing*, in both a moral and skilled sense. Ethics must not be adjunctive or an add-on to nursing curriculum, it must be central.

As will be discussed elsewhere, ethics in nursing is relationally based; thus, its ethics is enacted in ways that preserve and foster relationships, and is responsive to the specific person(s) and contextual features. It is person-centered, engaging both the person of the patient and the person of the nurse. Ethics must not be reduced to principles, to decision making, to conflict management, to restoring the good that has been lost. Relationally based ethics is intrinsically a preventive ethics. It represents the vast majority of nursing practice. Bioethics, in its predominant American form, does not serve to further notions of *good* that inhere to nursing practice. Instead, it serves best when relationships break down, in situations where conflicts arise, and relationships are fractured or frangible—as in moral distress—where it is a "best of bad choices" situation, or for dramatic headlines.

These ethics core competencies do, elsewhere in the document, indicate an expectation that nurses will be familiar with the ANA *Code of Ethics* (the *Code*; 2015), but, though it is the central ethical document of the profession, it is not a part of the ethics essentials and neither the *Code* nor ethics receive pride of place as in the NLNE requirements. The document states that "diversity, equity, inclusion, and ethics must be emphasized and valued."[67] Throughout the document, *diversity, equity, and inclusion* greatly overshadow ethics, and ethics receives relatively little attention. It is tragic that the deep moral failures that *diversity, equity, and inclusion* represent are not addressed. Reconciliation, if there is to be reconciliation, requires authentic confession, contrition, and *metanoia* (turning around) before there can be forgiveness and reconciliation. Superficial or simplistic measures hoping for cheap forgiveness are themselves moral failures,[68] as *diversity—equity—inclusion* has become a catchphrase without actual *metanoia*.

Conceptually, this is ethically problematic. Social ethics, which early modern nursing ardently embraced, engages in *social criticism and social change*; it is concerned about a range of issues, principally around social justice, dignity, respect, fairness, the common good, freedom, and more, issues relating to diversity, equity, and inclusion. In particular, social ethics is concerned about the social balance of *power structures* (including structures of oppression and disadvantagement) over *meaning and value structures* (ideals, values, ethics).[69] Power structures are related to all forms of social power including law, regulation, money, institutions, etc.; in short, all those structures that can implement (or force) actions toward the accomplishment of desired ends. Meaning and value structures are those social structures that constrain the means that are used, and direct actions toward morally acceptable ends. A simple example would be the power structures of law, treaties, and the military industrial complex that enables warfare, and the ethical structures (international conventions) that limit the initiation, conduct, and ends of warfare. Both are needed—power structures, to get things done—and meaning and value structures that rein in and direct or redirect power and prevent its abuse. Inequity, injustice, exclusion, unfairness, disrespect, and so forth are examples of power structures that have not been bound and constrained or corrected by meaning and value structures.

Rooted in a sound ethics education and painful sociopolitical experience, our nursing forebears understood that issues of diversity, equity, and inclusion were not stand-alone issues. They were part and parcel of the domain of social ethics, to be subsumed under ethics. In the AACN essentials, equity, diversity, and inclusion are free floating, with no foundation. It is important to note that the way in which *bioethics* addresses social justice has had principally to do with the allocation and cost of care, and not specifically structures of oppression (though there are hints that change is coming).

As the NLNE requirements observe, ethics education must be leveled from basic to more advanced. So too, the AACN *Essentials* has leveled behavioral expectations for ethics. Section 9.1 calls for a demonstration of "an ethical comportment in one's practice reflective of nursing's mission to society." It is at this point that the *Essentials* could have brought in diversity, equity, and inclusion. There is, then, a recognition that nursing does have a mission to society which, again, is at the heart of an earlier social ethics in nursing.

The additional behavioral expectations are, at entry level, demonstrated by

9.1a Apply principles of professional nursing ethics and human rights in patient care and professional situations; 9.1b Reflect on one's actions and their consequences; 9.1c Demonstrate ethical behaviors in practice; 9.1d Change behavior based on self and situational awareness; 9.1e Report unethical behaviors when observed; 9.1f Safeguard privacy, confidentiality, and autonomy in all interactions; 9.1g Advocate for the individual's right to self-determination.[70]

At the advanced level of nursing education the expectations are

9.1h Analyze current policies and practices in the context of an ethical framework; 9.1i Model ethical behaviors in practice and leadership roles; 9.1j Suggest solutions when unethical behaviors are observed; 9.1k Assume accountability for working to resolve ethical dilemmas.[71]

These are not measurable behavioral objectives, nor are they designed as such. Neither does the content of the ethics *concept* fully support the realization of the objectives. In relation to ethics, the *Essentials* would be well served by drawing upon a wider base of ethics sources and more heavily upon the ANA *Code of Ethics for Nurses*.

Crafting Ethics Requirements for Nursing Education

The NLNE requirements offer us much to consider. First, they have a respected, widely adopted, coherent, consistent, and thoroughgoing philosophical basis. Pragmatism was the prevailing philosophy in the US in the late 1800s and into the 1900s when the World Wars broke out. It ebbed and flowed and today it is being renewed both in a feminist pragmatism and in radical Black feminist pragmatism. Perhaps Pragmatism offers something for nursing today. Second, consistent with the notion of nurse-as-identity, instantiated with notions of good resident and abiding in the nursing tradition, narrative, and practice, requires a holistic ethics that encompasses the whole of the person. This is not an ethics that is loculated as a professional ethics. Instead, it recognizes that the nurse is a whole person; both personal and professional are one. Anything else is to fragment identity. Third, ethics must encompass the whole of nursing practice from social engagement through clinical practice and every nursing role between. Early nursing ethics was ardently a social ethics that was interrelated with clinical practice, thus nursing addressed health disparities, both through the activism of the profession collectively, and through individual nurse participation in the duties of democracy.

Fourth, ethics in nursing education must engage in identity formation, which will be considered in a subsequent chapter. Fifth, the NLNE requirements address the relationship between culture and ideals or ethics, that is, how society and ethics interact, and how group and individual moralities interact; these are largely issues that bioethics as a field does not address and yet they are keenly relevant to multicultural societies. While bioethics focuses on decision making, nursing ethics has focused on relational ethics, the place of the self in ethics, practical reasoning, and wisdom. This would be a sixth area to incorporate in ethics education. Seventh, the development of moral fiber is of concern—of the ability of the person to stand up for that which is the moral good and one's own moral integrity. It can be addressed in nursing ethics education, properly developed. With a more granular reading, there are additional recommendations that can be drawn from the NLNE requirements. The recommendations are not for didactic curriculum only; they are recommendations for the three apprenticeships (as articulated by Patricia Benner), and for every aspect of the nursing curriculum.

Contemporary nursing has yet to establish requirements for nursing ethics education that meets the needs of nurses and nursing practice in their fullness. In this, our predecessors have a great deal to offer us today.

Appendix I: 1915 NLNE Ethics Requirements Supporting Textbooks for Faculty

The NLNE Ethics Requirements contains a list of textbooks for faculty reference in teaching, but give only the author and title. The full citation for each of the textbooks is provided below, rearranged into alphabetical order within US and UK lists. As all of the textbooks predate US copyright strictures, they fall into the public domain. Several of these are available digitally, in full text, online from a range of sources that digitize works in the public domain. Source examples include Google Books, Hathi Trust, Project Gutenberg, WorldCat, and the Library of Congress.

US

Cabot, E.L. *Every Day Ethics*. New York: Holt, 1906.
Cabot, Richard. *What Men Live By*. Boston: Houghton Mifflin, 1906.
Dewey, John and James A. Tufts. *Ethics*. New York: Henry Holt, 1908.
Emerson, Ralph Waldo. *Essays*. Boston: Phillips, Sampson and Company, 1857.
James, William. *Talks to Teachers on Psychology and to Students on Some of Life's Ideals*. New York: Henry Holt and Company, 1899.
Parsons, Sara E. *Nursing Problems and Obligations*. Whitcomb & Barrows, 1916.
Robb, Isabel. *Nursing Ethics: For Hospital and Private Use*. New York: Koeckert, 1900.

UK

Mackenzie, John S. *Manual of Ethics*. London: Hinds, Noble & Eldridge, 1901.
McCunn, John. *Making of Character*. London: Macmillan, 1900.
McDougall, William. *An Introduction to Social Psychology*. London: Luce & Co., 1908. (US/UK)
Nightingale, Florence. *Notes on Nursing: What It Is, and What It Is Not*. London: Harrison, 1859.
Nightingale, Florence. *Talks to Pupil Nurses: A Selection of Addresses to Probationers and Nurses.* London: Macmillan, Harrison, 1914.
Osler, William. *Æquanimitas: With Addresses to Medical Students, Nurses and Practitioners of Medicine*. Philadelphia: The Blakiston Company, 1904.

Notes

1 Ann Taylor Allen, "Introduction: An Entangled History," in Ann T. Allen, *The Transatlantic Kindergarten: Education and Women's Movements in Germany and the United States* (Oxford: Oxford University Press, 2017), 1–9.
2 Amatai Etzioni, *The Semi-professions and Their Organization: Teachers, Nurses, Social Workers* (New York: Collier-Macmillan, 1969).
3 Aeleah Soine, "'The Relation of the Nurse to the Working World': Professionalization, Citizenship, and Class in Germany, Great Britain, and the United States before World War I," *Nursing History Review* 18 (2010): 51–80.
4 Schools in the US and Canada modified Nightingale's model in relation to control and authority over the school (e.g., independent and free-standing versus hospital control) or financial basis (again, independent or by the hospital).
5 Juanita De Barros, Steven Palmer, and David Wright (eds.), *Health and Medicine in the Circum-Caribbean, 1800–1968* (New York: Routledge, 2009).
6 Diocese of Jamaica and the Cayman Islands, "Enos Nuttall: Spiritual Leader and More." https://www.anglicandioceseja.org/?p=5866
7 Matthew Mulcahy, *Hubs of Empire: The Southeastern Lowcountry and British Caribbean* (Baltimore, MD: Johns Hopkins University Press, 2014).

8 Janet Wilson James, Review of *Writing and Rewriting Nursing History: A Review Essay*, By Stella Bingham, Mary Breckinridge, M. Louise Fitzpatrick, Jane E. Mottus, Barbara Melosh, Celia Davies, Christopher J. Maggs, Bonnie Bullough, Vern L. Bullough, and Barrett Elcano, *Bulletin of the History of Medicine* 58, no. 4 (1984): 568–584.

9 Homi K. Bhabha, "The Commitment to Theory," *New Formations* 5 (Summer 1988): 5–23.

10 Gayatri Chakravorty Spivak, "Can the Subaltern Speak?" in C. Nelson and L. Grossberg (eds.), *Marxism and the Interpretation of Culture* (Basingstoke: Macmillan Education, 1988), 271–313.

11 Gayatri C. Spivak, *In Other Worlds* (London: Methuen, 1987), 166–167.

12 Homi K. Bhabha, *The Location of Culture* (London: Routledge, 1994).

13 Warwick Anderson, "Where Is the Postcolonial History of Medicine?" *Bulletin of the History of Medicine* 72, no. 3 (1998): 528.

14 Steen Bille Jørgensen and Hans-Jürgen Lüsebrink, "Introduction: Reframing the Cultural Transfer Approach," In *Cultural Transfer Reconsidered* (Leiden: Brill, 2021), 1–22.

15 Raul Ramos, "Reframing Borderland Studies: Placing Silenced Subjects at the Center," *American Journal of Ethnic History* 29, no. 3 (2010): 79–83.

16 Michael Werner and Bénédicte Zimmermann, "Penser l'histoire croisée: entre empirie et réflexivité," *Annales. Histoire, Sciences Sociales* (2003/1, 58e année), 7–36.

17 Guillaume Lachenal, Médecine, comparaisons et échanges inter-impériaux dans le mandat camerounais: Une histoire croisée 1 franco-allemande de la mission Jamot. *Canadian Bulletin of Medical History* 30, no. 2 (Fall 2013): 23–45.

18 Ian Tyrrell, Transnational Nation, *United States History in Global Perspective since 1789* (Basingstoke, UK: Palgrave Macmillan, 2007).

19 Itiye Akira, "Transnational History" (Review), *Contemporary European History* 13, no. 2 (May, 2004): 211–222.

20 Patrick O'Brian, "Historiographical Traditions and Modern Imperatives for the Restoration of Global History," *Journal of Global History* 1, no. 1 (2006): 3–39. DOI:10.1017/S1740022806000027

21 Eliga H. Gould, "Entangled Histories, Entangled Worlds: The English-Speaking Atlantic as a Spanish Periphery," *American Historical Review* 112, no. 3 (2007): 764–786.

22 Matthew Mulcahy, *Hubs of Empire: The Southeastern Lowcountry and British Caribbean.* (Baltimore, MD: Johns Hopkins University Press, 2014), 3.

23 Angelo Torre, "A 'Spatial Turn' in History? Landscapes, Visions, Resources," *Annales. Histoire, Sciences Sociales* 63, no. 5 (2008): 1127–1144.

24 Patricia D'Antonio, "Thinking about Place: Researching and Reading the Global History of Nursing," *Texto Contexto-Enferm* 18, no. 4 (October/December 2009): 766–772.

25 John A. Agnew and James S. Duncan (eds.), *The Power of Place: Bringing Together Geographical and Sociological Imaginations* (London: Routledge, 1989).

26 Edward Said, *Orientalism* (New York: Pantheon Books, 1978).

27 John Billings and Henry Hurd, *Hospitals Dispensaries and Nursing: Papers and Discussion in the International Congress of Charities, Correction and Philanthropy, Section III, Chicago, June 12th to 17th, 1893* (Baltimore: Johns Hopkins Press, 1894), 35. See also Isabel Robb, "Educational Standards for Nurses," in *Educational Standards for Nurses: With Other Addresses on Nursing Subjects* (New York: E.C. Koeckert, 1907), 9–29.

28 Chris Leonards and Nico Randeraad, "Transnational Experts in Social Reform, 1840–1880," *International Review of Social History* 55, no. 2 (August 2010): 215–239.

29 US publications prior to 1923 are designated in the public domain and do not require copyright permission.

30 This appears to be a misquote, but not taken from Dewey & Tufts. The authors of the requirements do not distinguish between *wisdom* (Greek, *sophia*) and *prudence*, or *practical wisdom* (Greek, *phronesis*). Aquinas termed *prudence* the *auriga virtutum* (Latin for *charioteer of all virtues*). *Prudence* has also been variously termed the father or mother of all virtues. *Wisdom* was not.

31 National League for Nursing Education, Committee on Education. *Standard Curriculum for Schools of Nursing (1915–1918)* (Baltimore, MD: Waverly Press, 1917). Subsequently retitled *A Curriculum Guide for Schools of Nursing*.

32 Diane Hamilton, "Constructing the Mind of Nursing," in Ellen D. Baer, Patricia D'Antonio, Sylvia Rinker, and Joan E. Lynaugh (eds.), *Enduring Issues in American Nursing* (New York: Springer, 2002), 240–261.

33 Susan Reverby, "A Legitimate Relationship: Nursing, Hospitals and Science in the Century," in Ellen D. Baer, Patricia D'Antonio, Sylvia Rinker, Joan E. Lynaugh (eds.), *Enduring Issues in American Nursing* (New York: Springer, 2002), 262–281.

34 Annie W. Goodrich, *The Social and Ethical Significance of Nursing: A Series of Addresses*. (New York: Macmillan, 1932).

35 John Dewey, *Reconstruction in Philosophy* (New York: Henry Holt and Company, 1920).

36 John Dewey, *Experience and Nature* (London: Allen & Unwin, 1929).

37 John Dewey, The *Quest for Certainty* (London: G. Allen and Unwin, 1929).

38 John Dewey, "American Education and Culture," *The New Republic* (July 1, 1916).

39 John Dewey, "Individuality, Equality, and Superiority," *The New Republic* (Dec. 13, 1922).

40 Goodrich, *Social*, 294. Quote from John Dewey. "Significance of the School of Education," *Elementary School Teacher*, 4 (1904): 441–453.

41 Cheryl Misak and Huw Price (eds.) *The Practical Turn: Pragmatism in the Long Twentieth Century* (Oxford: Oxford University Press, 2018).

42 Cornel West, *The American Evasion of Philosophy: A Genealogy of Pragmatism* (Madison, WI: University of Wisconsin Press, 1989).

43 Cheryl Misak and Robert B. Talisse, "Pragmatism Endures," *Aeon* (Nov. 18, 2019). https://aeon.co/essays/pragmatism-is-one-of-the-most-successful-idioms-in-philosophy

44 Richard Bernstein, "The Resurgence of Pragmatism," *Social Research* 59, no. 4 (Winter 1992): 813–40.

45 More will be said about Pragmatism in other chapters.

46 William James, *Pragmatism: A New Name for Some Old Ways of Thinking* (New York: Longmans, Green, and Co., 1907), 51.

47 John Dewey and James Tufts, *Ethics* (New York: Henry Holt and Company, 1908).

48 William James, *Talks to Teachers: On Psychology: and to Students on Some of Life's Ideals* (New York: Henry Holt and Company, 1912).

49 William James, *The Principles of Psychology* 2 (New York: Henry Holt and Co., 1890), 383 ff.

50 William Osler, *Æquanimitas: With Addresses to Medical Students, Nurses and Practitioners of Medicine* (Philadelphia: The Blakiston Company, 1904).

51 Richard Chabot, *What Men Live By: Work, Play, Love, Worship* (Boston: Houghton Mifflin Company, 1914).

52 John Mackenzie, *A Manual of Ethics* (London: W.B. Clive, 1897).

53 National League for Nursing Education, Committee on Education. *Standard Curriculum for Schools of Nursing (1915–1918)* (Baltimore, MD: Waverly Press, 1917).

54 Lawrence Kohlberg, *Essays on Moral Development, Vol. I: The Philosophy of Moral Development* (San Francisco: Harper & Row, 1981). See also Lawrence Kohlberg (1958), "The Development of Modes of Thinking and Choices in Years 10 to 16," PhD Dissertation, University of Chicago.

55 Carol Gilligan, *In a Different Voice: Psychological Theory and Women's Development* (Cambridge, MA: Harvard University Press, 1982).

56 Lawrence Kohlberg, *Essays on Moral Development: Vol. II. The Psychology of Moral Development: The Nature and Validity of Moral Stages* (San Francisco, CA: Harper & Row, 1984).

57 American Nurses Association, *Code of Ethics for Nurses with Interpretive Statements* (Silver Spring, MD: ANA, 2015).

58 Canadian Nurses Association, *Code of Ethics for Registered Nurses* (Ottawa: CNA, 2017).

59 Royal College of Nursing, *RCN Code of Conduct* (London: RCN, 2019).
60 Nursing and Midwifery Council, *The Code: Professional Standards of Practice and Behaviour for Nurses, Midwives and Nursing Associates* (London: NMC, 2018).
61 Patricia Benner, "Curricular and Pedagogical Implications for the Carnegie Study, Educating Nurses: A Call for Radical Transformation," *Asian Nursing Research* (Korean Society of Nursing Science) 9, no. 1 (2015): 1–6.
62 Amy Haddad, *An Otherwise Healthy Woman* (Lincoln, NE: The Backwaters Press, 2022).
63 American Association of Colleges of Nursing [AACN], *The Essentials: Core Competencies for Professional Nursing Education* (2021). https://www.aacnnursing.org/AACN-Essentials
64 American Association of Colleges of Nursing, *The Essentials: Core Competencies for Professional Nursing Education* (2021), 13.
65 Tom Beauchamp and James Childress, *Principles of Biomedical Ethics* (New York: Oxford University Press, 1979).
66 To instantiate is to internalize and become an embodied representative of the *good nurse*, good in both a clinical and moral sense as defined by the tradition, narrative, and community of practice. Instantiation is a process from novice to expert.
67 American Association of Colleges of Nursing, *The Essentials*, 33.
68 Marsha D.M. Fowler, "Cheap Forgiveness," *Nursology* (4 April 2023). https://nursology.net/2023/04/04/cheap-forgiveness/
69 Marsha D.M. Fowler, "Nursing and Social Ethics," in N.A. Chaska (ed.), *The Nursing Profession: Turning Points* (St. Louis, MO: C.V. Mosby, 1989), 24–30.
70 AACN, 50.
71 Ibid.

2

AN ARCHAEOLOGY OF THE NURSING ETHICS LITERATURE

Digging Up Textbooks

Years of plowing had scattered small bits of metal across a field in Hammerwich, Staffordshire. They were found by a metal detectorist who recovered 244 gold objects, in five days, in the freshly plowed soil. An excavation was begun and led to the discovery of the Staffordshire Hoard, the largest hoard of Anglo-Saxon gold and metal work ever discovered. The pieces are exquisite, with filigree, garnet cloisonné, zoomorphic designs, inlay, glasswork, and more.[1] Despite their largely military use, they are early medieval Mercian works of breathtaking beauty—and value. It is infrequent that an ethics scholar can unearth a gleaming trove of golden resources, but such is the early nursing ethics literature, our own Staffordshire Hoard. Like the Staffordshire Hoard, our cache of treasure has yet to be fully excavated, catalogued, and analyzed, but it is both exquisite and of incalculable value. Further, it is also beyond the capacity of any single scholar to do all the archaeological work necessary. As much as is possible, the nature, geolocation, and depth of this treasure are laid out herein, for nursing ethics scholars to come.

The Literature: *Ethics in Nursing* (and) *Nursing Ethics*

From the 1880s to 1965, the nursing ethics literature includes hundreds of journal articles, columns, commencement addresses, ICN speeches, codes of ethics, pledges, textbooks, and more. And yet it is a largely unexplored, even untouched, literature. In some cases, it is simply dismissed as "primarily feminine etiquette."[2] That is a deeply mistaken appraisal, for it is a sturdy, philosophically informed literature communicated through experience; as well as through the style of the late Victorian rhetoric, vocabulary, circumlocution, and prolixity of this period literature. The list includes books in French that were used by Québécois nurses. While the majority of the almost 100 textbooks and editions devoted to nursing ethics are

DOI: 10.4324/9781003262107-3

written by nurses for nurses, and more specifically by women for women, there are some written by non-nurses for nurses, all but one of whom were men. For our purposes here, *nursing ethics* refers to books on ethics by nurses for nurses. Books termed *ethics in nursing* refers to books written by non-nurses for nurses. These non-nurses included Roman Catholic priests, a protestant pastor, and a female psychologist. In this "review of the literature," it is easiest, perhaps, to begin with the non-nurse-authored books before proceeding to those written by nurses.

The Ethics in Nursing Literature: Non-Nurse Authors

The Edgy Psychologist

Approximately a third of the books were written by non-nurses, and are qualitatively different in content and character from those written by nurses. The majority of these authors are Roman Catholic priests. There are also physician authors, and Beatrice Edgell the sole psychologist and female non-nurse author, who is an outlier in this canon.

Beatrice Edgell (1871–1948) was a renowned psychologist, researcher, and university professor, the first woman to receive a PhD in psychology and the first female professor of psychology in the UK.[3] She held a degree in philosophy as well. Edgell served as an examiner in psychology for the Royal College of Nursing, and thus had more than passing contact with nurses and nursing students. Her book expands upon a series of lectures given to nursing students, and incorporates social workers. As one might expect, the book draws heavily upon psychology, beginning with reflexes, moving successively in a finely crafted, sequential, psychological chain of instincts, values and ends, meaning, intelligent action, intelligent analysis, intentional action, desire, volition, motive, intention with purpose, and resolve. Along the way, she disagrees with John Stuart Mill's understanding of pain and pleasure as being a "confusion of ideas" and an "inadequate psychological analysis."[4] In this chain, moral formation receives a contribution from each successive link, culminating in *habitudes* that produce character, meaning *moral character* or *virtue*. Edgell writes:

> In considering character we may claim generally that the higher the character the greater the value of the service which nurse or social worker can render through her own personality. Where there is vocation the nurse or worker will give of her best, and this best is something for which professional skill and knowledge is not enough. In the thoroughly trained nurse or worker we may take efficiency for granted. Character supplies that something more which makes the nurse or worker a power for good in the service to which she is devoted.[5]

Her description is that of a *good nurse* (or social worker) whose sense of vocation, that is, devotion to the profession and an embrace of nursing identity, combined with professional skill and knowledge, gives the nurse "a power for good." In effect, Edgell is saying that character must be combined with professional knowledge and skill to be productive of the good intrinsic to nursing.

Edgell continues with her discussion of virtue and the nurse, focusing on courage and wisdom. Contemporary nursing ethics tends to think of moral courage as a recent "invention." It is not. It is found throughout the early nursing ethics literature. Note that Edgell links virtue, courage, wisdom, knowledge, and *phronesis*. In some ways, her work is a harbinger of the work of Patricia Benner, almost a hundred years later.[6] Edgell writes:

> If one looks at the list of excellences set forth by Plato and Aristotle one can recognize two virtues where a full and abundant measure is required by the nurse or social worker... what is intended here is the fixed habitude of moral courage. It is the courage that is prepared to face whatever may come in following out the work one finds to do. The social worker or the nurse who is working outside the walls of the hospital is confronted with many situations that call for the greatest moral courage. She may have to tackle 'difficult' people, she may have to track down and show up bold abuses. In much of her work, she may meet with resistance and will need both courage and patience to overcome opposition. With the cultivation of courage should go the cultivation of wisdom. Wisdom is hard to define. It is not knowledge, although it presupposes knowledge; it is rather ability to apply knowledge in the right way and at the right time. It implies knowledge of persons as well as knowledge of some branch of science or general learning. Inasmuch as it is ability to recognize when and how to use knowledge, wisdom requires experience.... To size up a person or a situation, to realize what can or cannot be done, when it is useful and when it is useless to speak, demands judgment, and such judgment is based on much past experience. Mere experience will teach nothing unless there is reflection thereon, comparison of this and that, a noting of consequences and circumstances.... The professional training of the nurse arms her for many of the situations she will meet both within and without a hospital.... The more she has reflected on what she has learned both in training and through her own experience, the more likely is she to deal wisely with new and unprecedented events. Both nurse and [social] worker need to be clear about general principles, to have ideals, a sense of the direction which they wish to go. If they have taken their general bearings well, they will be more able to judge correctly the significance of any particular episode. Wisdom will ensure a sense of proportion, and under the shadow thereof a sense of humor may flourish.[7]

Edgell is an appropriate author with whom to begin. She was not a nurse but had deep associations with nursing students and educators. However, as a British scholar working in nursing ethics, Edgell serves to identify the direction ethics will take in the UK, with a focus on character. The US literature has, as well, a focus on character, but it uses a vocabulary of *ethics* throughout its literature, whereas the British does so but a bit less. The US literature, under the rubric of *ethics*, also becomes more specific in its designation of moral duties than does the British literature. Eventually, after World War II, nursing ethics in the US will stray from its focus on character, moving (or perhaps drifting) with American society toward the specification of moral duties divorced from attention to moral character. As is obvious from these quotes, Edgell was an Aristotelian in her ethics; she was also the president of the UK Aristotelian Society. While American Pragmatism gains only a small toehold in British philosophy,[8] Edgell does draw from and cites the American Pragmatist and psychologist William James in her book. Edgell, James, and Dewey share a common interest in psychology, and it plays a part in the ethics of each.

Physician Trespassers

The lecture "Nursing Ethics" by T. Percy C. Kirkpatrick, MD is important as an early Irish contribution to the literature. It is a bit homespun, lacking in rigor, and neither systematic nor informed by moral philosophy, and fails to comprehend the abilities of nurses—or their role. He defines "'Nursing Ethics' as the rules governing the duties of nurses to the public, to each other, and to themselves, in regard to the exercise of their profession."[9] He praises Florence Nightingale "who united with the highest moral principles a careful training in the special duties of the nurse."[10] He does touch upon professional secrets, but otherwise calls for devotion, progress in knowledge, hospitality (in the older sense) toward patients, sympathy for the sick and poor, and obedience and loyal service to superior officers. He has one caution of interest:

> There is one danger that dogs the path of the private nurse, and against which she must constantly be on her guard: the intimate relations that exist between her, her patient and the members of her patient's family, may be a source of great temptation—a temptation in no way due to word or action of hers, but so subtle in its onset is almost to be overwhelming before it is recognized. Such temptation must be resisted at all costs. Be careful how you try your strength against such temptation. Flight from it is no dishonor, and is much more safe.[11]

This is an early awareness of *lust* in the workplace, though in today's vernacular it would be termed sexual harassment. Sexual harassment would have been *ungentlemanly* but not actionable and, in private duty (nursing in the patient's home), the nurse would have had no recourse other than to leave the case.

Arrah B. Evarts is also a physician. His contribution to nursing ethics does not fare well under review by nurse M. Louise Beaty in the *American Journal of Nursing (AJN)* (1937).[12] It demonstrates some of the same defects of Kirkpatrick's work. Both he and Kirkpatrick underestimate nurses, and their abilities, and present a poorly informed, reductionistic, and watery ethics. To be fair, they are physicians and may not have more than a primitive understanding of moral philosophy, but both seem to have a low estimation of the capacities of nurses. Beaty (getting Evarts' gender wrong) writes, "usually characterizing nursing education as training, Dr. Evarts gives her reasons for adding another volume to those already in print."[13] "The first [chapter] is devoted to a rather superficial discussion of the definition and meaning of ethics" with "8 chapters [that] constitute a series of preachments" and "this is just another of the old-style treatises on 'Ethics for Nurses' and there seems to be little justification for adding it to the list."[14] In between these comments, she excoriates the errors he commits.

The difficulty with physicians writing on ethics for nurses is that their *ought* for nurses is self-serving, and not what nurses would see as the *ought* for their own practice. This distinction can be seen clearly by comparing E. Margaret Fox's first chapter (see Chapter 3) with that of Edwin Healy.

Priestly Denunciation of Others' Views

Thomas Verner Moore regards the nursing ethics textbooks as works of moral suggestions and moral advice, but not works of ethics. He reserves that designation for the ethics in nursing textbooks written by priest-theologians, representing natural law ethics. In his unwillingness to accept other approaches to ethics, he even dismisses John Dewey's *Ethics*,[15] as ethics.[16] A deeper read of the nursing ethics textbooks would uncover the practice and tradition-based ethics, and prevent their dismissal as moral advice, counsel, or suggestions, instead of as ethics. Beyond this, Moore finds the "ethics of conditionate morality," that is consequentialist theories such as Mill's Utilitarianism (specifically), to be inadequate; and any "ethics of absolute morality" (duty-based ethics, such as Kant's emphasis upon reason, specifically) as also inadequate.[17] Priest Spalding (1920) outright refers to the "false theory of Dewey, Aikens and Robb." He differs with Dewey on the source of *rights*; says of nurse Charlotte Aikens' book that "very little in the book can be classified under ethics," and refers to nurse Isabel Robb's book as "practical advice and common sense," while misidentifying her as Elizabeth Hampton Robb not Isabel.[18]

The Clergy Authors on Ethics in Nursing

The remaining textbooks on ethics in nursing are largely written by Roman Catholic priests, the majority of whom are Jesuit theologians. There is one lone Baptist (Protestant) theologian among them. The number of books by Roman Catholic priests reflects their long tradition of consideration of the moral aspects of medicine, as well as their Church's centuries-long involvement with the provision of care for the ill and indigent through nursing orders, and in the past century the development of many Catholic schools of nursing. These books fall into two large categories: (a) books that focus on morally contested medical procedures such as abortion, sterilization, and euthanasia, and (b) those focused more broadly on the life of the good Catholic woman and nurse (and including those same medical issues). The difference of focus and the breadth of what is encompassed distinguished the two categories. Among the clergy-authored textbooks, there are outliers. Healy, for example, structures the content of his book using the Ten Commandments.[19] Some of the clergy books look less to medical procedures and more to the spiritual or religious life of the nurse.

The Lone Protestant Clergyperson

Samuel Southard, a Baptist pastor and theologian is the sole Protestant author in the group. His book *Religion and Nursing*[20] is unlike the other works: he intersperses illustrative patient–nurse conversations throughout the narrative. As would be expected in a Baptist work, he begins with a chapter on the Bible and biblical interpretation, followed by a chapter on theology, or more specifically constructive theology. He has a chapter on the spiritual significance of illness, on suffering, guilt and forgiveness, depression and doubt, and dying and bereavement. Though there is ethics throughout, there are chapters focused on ethics that are relationally based. He also points to resources that would be useful for a nurse in understanding patients from other Christian traditions. Southard provides the foundation for nurses to provide spiritual care in relation to health, illness, dying, and bereavement, as well as guidance for the nurse's own spiritual life. It is both an excellent book and a sound representative of a Protestant tradition.

The more procedurally focused books dwell upon the rationale for prohibiting contraception, abortion, sterilization, artificial insemination, immoral operations, and collaterally, masturbation. Though these books are directed toward nurses it is unclear how they actually relate to nurses, as these are medical procedures and the role or responsibilities of the nurse receive little attention. These works are, presumably, intended simply to teach nurses that these procedures are morally wrong and why and not specifically to equip the nurse for ethical practice. The extent of the discussion relative to nursing is that "the Catholic nurse may never counsel or praise any operation or medical treatment that is immoral. Patients sometimes consult the nurse on questions of this nature and are willing to follow her advice."[21] Without helping with the procedure itself, the nurse may help prepare a patient for an immoral procedure or operation as such involvement is "remote" (i.e., not directly complicit).

The Priests: Father Knows Best

The priest-authored books that look more fully at the life of the nurse vary widely in their level of intrusiveness. Some call the nurse to remember the spiritual nature of her vocation and to represent that in the care of patients. Others make assumptions about the naivete of the nursing student and are more granular in their exhortation. McAllister is a good example. He cautions against provocative dancing; he divides kissing into "nonsensual kissing, sensual kissing, and passionate kissing," condemns petting, and warns against going to parties in cars and the "practice of parking." He writes that

> there is no reason for doubting the startling figures of a study made some years ago, that of the girls who went to parties in cars, a great majority of them went in for petting. And that of these at least half allowed outrageously improper liberties and that those who began by petting some 15 to 25 per cent went the limit.[22]

However, nursing study can be dangerous in itself. He writes:

> Duty sometimes *obliges* the person to think about things ordinarily dangerous to chastity. Medical students and nurses, to have the professional knowledge they need, must give considerable thought to matters of sex and processes of human reproduction. To say that they can do this without the slightest danger is being blandly unpsychological. There is danger, but it is a lawful risk... Even so, and especially in the beginning, they should guard against *morbid curiosity* and be cautious lest their studies become *causes of venereal pleasure*.[23]

The point here is not that sexual mores have changed since the 1950s. They have. Instead, what this points to is that these, and the nursing ethics textbooks as well, regarded the nursing student as vulnerable, naive, and inexperienced and the school of nursing as a place of moral formation.

A Priest and a Nun Walk into a Book...

Amongst the priest-authored books, there is one unusual collaboration—between Dom (signifying a monk) Thomas Verner Moore and Sr. Rose Hélène Vaughan of the Sisters of St. Joseph. Moore was the dissertation advisor for Vaughan's master's degree dissertation (thesis). He asked her to explore the actual incidence of moral problems among nurses to help inform him as he wrote his book of ethics in nursing. Her dissertation will receive greater attention at another point (Chapter 3), but she did gather "2,265 moral problems, 67 problems of etiquette and 110 questions as to the proper course of action in certain situations."[24] Her work does not seem to have influenced the content of his book which is a standard treatise on Roman Catholic natural law ethics. He did, however, use her work to incorporate a brief enumerated list of "Principles" and a set of 2–5-sentence "Problems for Discussion" as cases taken from Vaughan's work at the conclusion of a number of his chapters. Many of the "principles" are rather diffuse and abstruse and it is not clear that they would sufficiently guide a nurse; others are more directive. For example, these principles in the section on "Personal Obligations of the Moral Life":

1. Moral goodness is like a bridge. All virtue must be present or it is no longer goodness, as a bridge does not bridge a river if a single span is lacking.

2. Moral principles must be so developed in their application to the ordinary problems of life that proper conduct in and of the usual situations follows, as it were, with reflex spontaneity and is never a matter of question and argument.
3. It is a personal duty of prime importance for every man to extend further and further his realm of self-evident moral principles.
4. Life is a campaign that must be planned with prudence.[25]

Here is a sample of the case examples he takes from Vaughan's dissertation:

- I have a slight sore throat today and feel miserable. I suppose I should report it as I am working around patients, but maybe it will pass off and I do hate to lose the time.[26]
- My patient was in a dying condition. Her brother came to see her but did not know her condition because it had been serious for several weeks. Should I have told him of his sister's condition even though he didn't ask me? I happen to be the only nurse in the department at the time he called.[27]
- If a certain instrument must be boiled several minutes and an interne asked you to remove the article in less time, how could you arrange this so as to be honest with yourself and at the same time not tell the intern he is wrong?[28]
- What can a student nurse do in the situation of being forced into a profession by her parents?[29]

Moore includes a chapter at the end of the book on the history of medical ethics, and a much shorter chapter on the history of nursing ethics. It is noteworthy and commendable that, in the preface to the book, Moore acknowledges Vaughan's contribution, and retains that acknowledgment in successive editions.

Despite Moore's attempt to address nurses through the principles and case problems, it is simply an add-on to his standard theological ethics and does not tackle nursing values or concerns. That remains for the nurse authors to do in their books.

Overview of Nursing Ethics Textbooks

The titles of the *nursing ethics* textbooks varied over the years. Some were titled "Nursing Ethics," or a variation thereof, while others were titled "Professional Obligations," "Professional Problems," "Professional Relationships," or "Professional Adjustments." Around 1940, the change from *ethics* to *adjustments* in the titles reflected a curricular change where non-clinical topics were combined into one course. The textbooks for that course were usually two volumes, and *Professional Adjustments I* was always the ethics volume, and always the first of the two volumes. In addition to dedicated ethics textbooks, ethics content is also customarily found in textbooks that cover history, issues, and trends. As previously noted, many of the early general clinical textbooks contained a first chapter on nursing ethics.

The nursing ethics textbooks were uniformly written by leaders in nursing. Some were presidents of ANA, leaders in the NLNE, progenitors of the ICN. The others

were superintendents of schools and hospitals. All these leaders had first-hand experience of direct patient care, and many were active in social reform, including
the suffrage movement, or in pressing for nursing legislation that would advance
nursing education and practice. Ethics was thought too important to be left in the
hands of junior nursing faculty.

The task of this chapter is to give an overview of the nursing ethics textbooks.
The next chapter will introduce additional, non-textbook literature. It is necessary to
introduce the literature and to provide an overview before a deeper analysis of nursing
ethics can commence. This deeper and more comprehensive analysis will follow anon.

A Roll-Call of Nurse-Authors in Nursing Ethics

Starting with Robb

Isabel Robb's book *Nursing Ethics: For Hospital and Private Use* (1900)[30] is the
oldest extant book. There may be books that predate it, books from small, religiously based, publishing houses, with a limited print run and limited circulation,
but to date none have been found. Robb's book, due to her untimely death, went to
multiple reprintings but no additional editions. Of all the older works, this remains
the best known and widely unread nursing ethics textbook today. Robb's book is
about nursing ethics in hospital and in private duty (in the patient's home) practice.
In the title, *private* refers to private duty nursing, not to personal ethics.

Robb, like the other authors we will consider, views ethics education as essential to nursing education and that it should commence at the start. She gives it equal
weight to the science of nursing. She writes:

> We will consider another form of education that should go hand in hand from the
> very beginning with the practical training and teaching, and that must be attended
> to just as diligently as any part of her technique, if the pupil hopes to finally be-
> come an all-round nurse of a high order, who's perceptive faculties are so finely
> trained as to know by intuition, as it were, what conduces to her patient's comfort.
> The cultivation of certain habits of body and mind should begin with the first put-
> ting on of her uniform for the acquisition of a habit of any kind necessitates time
> and persistent effort. The systematic study of the subjects dealing with the ethical
> side of nursing work should be regarded as most important, until the principles
> involved have become the mainspring which controls her every action.[31]

She then goes on to discuss the ethics operative at every level of nurse preparation from the probationer through the graduate nurse. It is important, however, to
provide some initial examples that offset the claim (priests Moore and Spalding,
above) that this literature is moral advice and not ethics. That judgment appears
to stem from the nurse-author use of clinical narratives and a personal, speaking
style of writing to impart the moral point, rather than to state an abstract principle.
Early nursing ethics is a virtue ethics, which one can see embedded in this quote,

but more on virtue ethics later. It is hoped that this and the following example will counter the dismissal of this literature as primarily feminine etiquette. Robb writes:

[the nurse] must not under any circumstances talk about one patient to another. To confide to another the disease from which one patient is suffering, whether he is likely to recover and the like, is a sin of which a nurse should never be guilty; to tell the names of any new arrivals in the ward, to discuss the various visitors and their sayings and doings, would be equally reprehensible. In fact, absolutely nothing should be passed from one patient to another through the nurses. If a death has occurred, it is not to be mentioned... Patients and their friends soon recognize a nurse who makes it a principle never to talk about such affairs, and although they may be disappointed at not having their curiosity gratified, their respect for, and confidence in, the nurse and the institution increases. An inquisitive patient once gave me it as her opinion that the nurses were "like so many clams," for after being ten days in the hospital, she had never been able to find out, from any one of them, who was her next door neighbor, or what was the matter with any of the patients. This was just as it should have been...[32]

She is, of course, speaking of what bioethics will term *privacy* and *confidentiality*, wrapped around her interaction with a patient who wanted information on other patients. We have the norm, and some of its parameters, bundled into her own experience. If one were to draw out a principle, it would more likely be stated as simply "nothing should be passed from one patient to another through the nurses." Nursing of the period termed this *professional secrets*, which differs from *privacy* and *confidentiality*. There are, however, additional discussions of information sharing in the book that further delineate the expectations for safeguarding patient information—and the nurse–patient relationship.

In another example of ethics enfolded within clinical examples, with regard to a night nurse, Robb writes:

At the same time all her observations should be made so quietly that her presence will never disturb her patients. To be able to slip frequently into and out of the room, to note the condition and to take the pulse of the sleeping patient without awakening him, means the perfection of nursing. She should never forget, towards the early morning, to see that additional coverings are put over patients, who may feel the extra chilliness of those hours, and that hot cans are kept in readiness for anyone who needs them. All such attentions are included in true nursing; just the perfunctory carrying out a specified orders will not suffice. During my own training one of the first true lessons, I ever received in nursing ethics came to me very forcibly upon hearing the patients say of the night nurse, "Oh, Miss — is a good night nurse, she takes such good care of her patients; if any one of them wants a drink, she never brings it without first letting the water run until it is nice and cold, and she does everything in just such a way.[33]

This is not, of course, about warm blankets and cool water. Where one looks more deeply, concrete cases give way to contextual notions of good internal to nursing, skilled know-how, clinical discernment, relationship, vulnerability, and more. As Alastair MacIntyre notes, members of a practice discipline engage in a practice formed by the knowledge, skills, and notions of good internal to their practice.[34] (This will be fleshed out in Chapter 9.)

As an aside, and to pick up an earlier point about nursing's entangled history, Robb notes that "in 1873 Sister Helen, a Nightingale Sister or Trained Nurse, came over to America and started the New York Training School of Nurses in connection with the Bellevue Hospital in the city of New York."[35] Robb herself was a Canadian transplanted to the US. Aikens (1867–1949), too, was Canadian born. Is Robb Canadian or American? Aikens? Given that some nurses were transplants, some books were published simultaneously in more than one country, and exchanges of nursing leaders across great bodies of water occurred, it is not always easy to discern which is whose.

Charlotte Aikens: An Enduring Legacy

While Robb's book is the best known, Charlotte Albina Aikens' book *Studies in Ethics for Nurses* was the most enduring, going to five editions and many additional reprintings between 1916 and 1943.[36] In her first edition, she identifies her reference sources as:[37,38]

Browne, Principles of Ethics
Ely, Social Law of Service
Courtney, Constructive Ethics
Dewey, Outlines of a Critical Theory of Ethics
Griggs, The Ethics of Personal Life
Robb, Nursing Ethics

In the third edition and thereafter, she adds Dewey and Tufts' *Ethics*, and the footnotes in the book indicate additional sources.[39] Her books have a more academic tone than a number of others, in that she does not use first person narrative to communicate clinical examples, embedding them in the text. Instead, remarkably, she illustrates each chapter at the end with a set of questions, or "practical illustrations of ethical problems encountered in daily routine."[40] Her questions reflect upon the content of the chapter that precedes it. For example:

- Can you trace the relation between ethics and health as it relates to nurses and nursing?[41]
- What tests might a nurse apply to her conduct to be sure that it is right?[42]
- What ethical principle does a nurse violate when she gives to others information that has come to her because of her work as a nurse?[43]

- Show that in performing one's duty one may have a curious mixture of motives.[44]
- Mention at least a dozen "comfort methods" which a night nurse might use, which are not likely to be in the standing orders.[45]

Take note of the comfort methods question as independent nursing practice, knowledge, and the good intrinsic to nursing practice. As the editions evolve, later editions have fewer questions and more clinical illustrations. Aikens is candid about the illustrations. She writes:

> The illustrations and practical problems used in the book are drawn from life, and each teacher can add to them or substitute from her own experience. The author makes no apology for revealing certain ethical failures, believing that only by the frank recognition of existing weaknesses can the weak points be strengthened; only by bringing the results of ethical failures into an open forum for discussion can conditions be improved. The only way by which the common ethical failures complained of today in nurses can ever be corrected, is by instilling in the heart of every nurse a desire to be true to her own best self; by giving each individual nurse higher standards of life and conduct, and showing how she may reach those standards.[46]

While there are cases strewn throughout the book, Chapter XV contains an additional 57 cases for discussion. Like the ethics of most of these books, they are comprehensive, and not limited to professional practice. Thus, there are problems or cases related to personal as well as professional life.

Early ethics educators, informed by William James and John Dewey on teaching methods, eschewed straight lecture for a mixed methods approach including discussion, quiet reflection on ethical problems in practice and matters of conduct, written responses, real illustrations from practice, and other forms of engagement. Aikens writes:

> The plan of the book calls for a combination of the recitation and discussion method of class teaching... serious reflection on concrete problems in which ethical principles are involved... [not in] lectures in which the nurse is simply a passive agent who is expected to absorb a certain amount of ethical instruction she is listening to.... The requiring at intervals of written personal opinions on the method of which should be pursued in certain situations in which nurses are obliged to decide ethical questions is a valuable method in the teaching of ethics. Nurses should be trained to think things through to a logical conclusion and to be able to give reasons why they reached the decisions at which they arrived.[47]

Over the five editions, the essential structure remains consistent though she adds content.

In the third edition, she adds the chapter "The Evolution of Nursing." In the fourth edition, she adds the chapter "The Hospital and the Nurse as Social Factors in the Community." The fifth edition is the most changed, with the addition of an introductory chapter and several new sections.

> In the preparation of the fifth edition the entire contents of the book have been rearranged to conform to the [NLN] Curriculum Guide for Schools of Nursing.... Many chapters have been expanded and rewritten. In the new chapter on Truth-telling and Its Difficulties, and in the new discussions of Prejudice, Sex Matters, Social Freedom and Good Citizenship, and other topics, important phases of common ethical problems have been given fresh emphasis.[48]

The sections are brief. For example, the chapter on truth-telling and its difficulties is eight pages of content, another three pages of 13 actual situations, and a page of issues and questions for discussion and review. Despite its brevity the chapter is remarkably comprehensive and nuanced. Indeed, the book is widely inclusive of the ethics of the whole of a nurse's life.

Those Who Followed Thereafter

Parson's *Nursing Problems and Obligations* (1926) lacks the rigor and comprehensiveness of Aikens' book, largely because it is a compilation of speeches she gave annually to nursing students at Massachusetts General Hospital in Boston. The speeches were "somewhat amplified" to be put into book form, but they retain the character of spoken rather than written text; that is, as something meant to be heard rather than read.[49] She, like other authors, divides the contents along the lines of levels of students to nurses, from probationer to graduates. The first edition contains deliberately blank pages, perhaps to fill out the sewn-in book signatures. No changes were made to the body of the text across editions. However, in the third edition, the original inclusion of blank pages allowed Parsons to add a "Topics of Conversation" section and a brief set of "Cases for Discussion" to each chapter without changing the pagination of the main text across editions. The cases she adds are not unlike those of Aikens:

> Obstetric case in country. Patient shows every symptom of septicemia and is constantly growing worse. Nurse believes an expert should be called in consultation; thinks patient requires curettage, but physician makes no move for consultation or operation. What would you do in such a case?
>
> Nurse has patient with morphine habit. Nurse can see no physical necessity for indulgence. Patient becoming more and more degraded. Physician continues to prescribe drugs. What should nurse do?[50]

This is not a text to rival Aikens in content, rigor, or academic style. It is a gentle and engaging introduction to ethics, suitable for entry-level students (probationers).

We can turn now to a very different book, rife with classist sentiments and prejudices, and problematic in its approach. Gertrude Harding's book *Higher Aspects of Nursing* takes

> The object of the following chapters on *"Temptations"* is to define, identify, classify and illustrate as many of the most common temptations of the nurse's life as possible; and to do this in such a manner that each and every nurse will be able to recognize the various temptations, whenever and wherever she meets them, and thus be prepared to overcome them.[51]

She begins with several observations. First, that "all nurses intermingle in the hospitals. Those whose motives are the noblest and most unselfish live and work side by side with those who are actuated by motives and impulses the meanest, most sordid, and selfish."[52] Apparently these mean, sordid, and selfish nurses have a subtle, cunning, clever, and adroit ability to lead the noblest and unselfish nurses astray; theirs is a potent corrosive and erosive power. Harding writes that:

> From personal experience it has been noted that, in the majority of cases, women enter upon their training as nurses innocently and comparatively ignorant of human nature in its many different phases. The average novitiate enters upon her studies with a very limited idea of the many and various temptations and difficulties she will have to meet and face alone, as an individual, in her chosen profession. Not realizing these temptations she enters upon her training almost wholly unprepared for sidestepping the many pitfalls she inevitably will find in her pathway.... Because of certain degrading influences and tendencies unavoidably surrounding her in the training school such high ideals of individual character and of the nursing profession as she may have possessed before entering have been, to some extent vitiated or destroyed.[53]

The pages that follow include chapters on unworthy motives, the demoralizing influence of physicians, intolerance, indolence, emotionalism, gossip, dishonesty, officiousness, and more. She has a startling, and odd, chapter on "discordant magnetism" that asserts:

> Every human being is a dynamo of vital energy. This vital energy radiates from the center of his being. Every individual has an abundance of such vital force and energy, which constantly is radiating outward from his essential self. This vital force, or energy, is called *"Human Magnetism."* This human magnetism constantly forms an atmosphere about the individual, in which he lives, moves, and has his being. He is never without this environment *during his waking moments.* From the very beginning of his physical life he is radiating, during his waking moments, his own vital force which we designate *"Magnetism."*[54]

She goes on to describe how this magnetism is the source of our attraction or aversion toward other persons, physicians, and patients. While Harding attempts to give a vision of the higher aspects of nursing, those attempts are overwhelmed by the corrosive temptations she explicates. It is like a belly crawl through the mud. That said, she is not wrong that there are those who enter nursing from baser motives.

As the last of the books of the 1920s, Charlotte Talley's book *Ethics: A Textbook for Nurses*[55] is actually a textbook on ethics per se, with application to the whole of life, and only three pages of application to nursing. Nursing ethics, prior to its colonization by bioethics, is almost universally a whole life ethics and not limited to professional life. Talley gives a survey of the origin and development of ethics, then embarks upon specific topics such as individualism, ethical judgment, will and habit, values, virtues and more. In each section she covers a wide range of philosophical and religious literature including philosophers Socrates, Plato, Aristotle, Epictetus, Seneca, Hobbs, Spencer, Spinoza, Hegel, Kant, Bentham and James Mill, J.S. Mill, Carlyle, Comte, Kropotkin, Schopenhauer, Dewey, James, Emerson, Royce, and more; and a range of literary writers including Goethe, Browning, Eliot, Whitman, Kipling, and more; and various religious figures including Confucius, Jesus, Swedenborg, the Puritans, and the Neoplatonists. Much of this nursing ethics literature is informed by religion, specifically Christianity, and Talley's book is no exception. In the second edition, Talley includes a separately paginated, lengthy section, perhaps a separate book, *Lesson Plans in Ethics for Schools of Nursing.*[56] The outlines are based on the NLNE Standard Curriculum for Nursing Schools and include questions and case examples. In her preface to that section she writes:

> Modern education endeavors to establish contact with the life experience of the student at the beginning of a course, regardless of whether the logical organization of the subject is interfered with or not, and topics are sometimes introduced with apparent irrelevance. In teaching ethics this contact is readily established by beginning the discussion of ethical problems which have some connection with the intellectual or social or professional life of the student at the first lesson. The acquisition on the part of students of a large number of facts relating to ethics is not so important as is their power to judge moral questions wisely and to act upon their decisions.[57]

While not all authors are equally erudite, Talley's book, like others, makes clear that *nursing ethics* is informed by a wide range of philosophers, across the whole field of philosophical ethics, read from primary sources; and that it is a whole life ethics, philosophically informed. Nursing ethics is not a narrow professional practice-based ethics that draws from a narrow range of philosophers, with reliance upon secondary sources.

In the first edition of *Ethics: Talks to Nurses*[58] Gladwin, like others, takes note of nursing history and prominent nursing figures as exemplars of nursing and the place it could have in the world. As with the NLNE ethics education requirements where nursing ethics follows nursing history, the two subjects are interlinked. Gladwin's book is a compilation of talks and, like Parsons, represents oral transmission and is not as intricate as texts meant to be conveyed in writing. Its style is conversational with stories drawn from life and literature. Her book takes up issues and concerns shared by other authors, but does not cover new ground. By the time she develops the second edition, the book has an additional 84 pages—it is significantly enlarged, revised, and rewritten, and has become better and an actual textbook.

Gladwin's second edition begins with a statement that, again, indicates a whole life perspective common to nursing ethics:

> The purpose of this book is to help the undergraduate or graduate, to answer the questions which arise regarding her duty, not only when she works in hospital, home, settlement, or industry, but also when she rests or plays. She is stimulated to find answers to her problems, by gaining a better comprehension of her relations with others, those who preceded her, those of her own generation with whom she lives and works, and those who are to come after her.[59]

She adds a new first chapter in the second edition that chronicles important persons and movements in the history of ethics, beginning with the Greeks and concluding with Thomas à Kempis. She dates "modern ethics" from Kant. There is also a new second chapter, "Modern Ethics." This is a noteworthy chapter that chronicles important persons and movements in nursing and health care that wrought social change. She discusses, briefly, changes in "treatment of the insane," workers' hours, hospital reforms, public health nursing, settlement work, the Red Cross, military nursing and more, noting that "*Ethics* and the *History of Nursing* are closely allied."[60] She adds the chapter "Health" that is focused on the health of the nurse, broadly understood—as a moral duty to self. In addition, she adds extensive review questions at the end of each chapter. These questions call for thoughtful responses and not simply directing a regurgitation of chapter content. The extensive footnotes are to philosophical, literary, historical, and other sources. This is a worthy book, different from but qualitatively comparable to Aikens' books.

The Nuns

We now turn to a group of books written by Roman Catholic religious sisters (nuns) who were nurses: Sr. John Gabriel (Ryan), *Professional Problems: A Textbook for Nurses*, Mother Catharine De Jésus-Christ, *At the Bedside of the Sick: Precepts and Counsels for Hospital Nurses*, Sr. Mary Isidore Lennon, *Professional Adjustments*; and Sr. Mary Miranda Plachata, *Spiritualize Your Nursing*. Given that they span 30 years, it might, perhaps, be unwise to consider these books together based on the religious profession of these women; two of the books predate World War II, and two follow the end of the war, which puts them in significantly different world contexts. Sr. Rose Hélène Vaughan's dissertation will be considered separately in Chapter 3. These books were written for nursing students, not specifically for other nuns entering nursing.

Sr. Gabriel's book is a book of case studies organized by student level or area of practice (e.g., public health). It differs from all previous works containing case studies for discussion, in that every case study presented is followed by a normative discussion that is fairly directive. Mother Catherine's book, *At the Bedside of the Sick: Precepts and Counsels for Hospital Nurses (Au Chevet de la Souffrance)*,[61] first published in French and then republished in English, is a series of lectures originally intended for the Sisters of St. Joseph of Cluny, Paris, but becomes a brief textbook. Mother Catherine was the vice president of the *Association Nationale des Infirmières Diplômées de l'État Français*. Her book gives a nod to Natural Law Ethics, but focuses on virtue with each chapter devoted to one or two virtues. On the surface the virtues she names appear to be in the realm of etiquette (e.g., tact, politeness, cheerfulness); however, the pages are remarkably nuanced and pithy treatments of virtue ethics. Sr. Mary Isadore Lennon's book covers the whole life of the nurse including the nurse's spiritual (religious) life. It includes a brief chapter on "The Nurse's Duty to Society" that contains some remarkable assertions such as "she lends her assistance in times of emergency and gives active support to the advancement of scientific medicines and uses her influence to protect the community from non-scientific exploitation."[62] Her book contains examination questions (matching, true and false, etc.) for each chapter. Sr. Mary Miranda Plachata's book, intended to be a series of meditations, is an untidy collection of ethics (e.g., patient secrets), devotions, prayers, clinical cases, biblical direction, ecclesial codes, and more, with no discernible principle of organization. This unorganized content is, nevertheless, thoughtful and interesting and would be an encouragement to persons of faith.

There is a stark difference between the books written by these nuns for nursing students and the books written by the Catholic priests for nursing students and nurses. The nuns do not discuss the medical interventions that the priests dwell upon: abortion, sterilization, euthanasia, contraception, etc. Lennon's book includes the "Ethical and Religious Directives for Catholic Hospitals," which mentions these procedures, and some state laws that govern abortion, but this material receives minimal or no discussion.

Goodrich's Difficult Read

The Social and Ethical Significance of Nursing: A Series of Addresses,[63] by Annie Warburton Goodrich, is another of the books that is a compilation of addresses. It is not a textbook of ethics. Though a worthy read, her writing style makes for a difficult read. MacDougall's review gives a generous spin to Goodrich's rhetorical style:

Nurses everywhere will hasten to read this book which is a compilation of a series of addresses made by the author, who is one of the most brilliant nurses in America, over a period of more than a decade. These addresses deal with the nurse in her relation to ethics, education, the hospital, the community, the university, and the world. Nurses will travel long distances to hear Miss Goodrich talk, and all their powers of concentration are called into play in listening, because her language is not that of the ordinary expository writer but that of the most finished literary scholar who draws from a wide range of literature for quotations to prove her points. She leaves her listeners and her readers with minds in the clouds and seeing some of the visions she sees of what the social and ethical significance of nursing has been, is now, and can be in the future. She is a highly inspirational speaker and writer, and might be called the nursing world's least mortal mind.[64]

The reviewer is over-generous. While erudite, and filled with learned allusions, her writing is abstruse and at points impenetrable, and not congenial for the modern reader or, based on the review in its own day, readers then. Still, Goodrich was (rightly) a luminary in nursing whom it would have been unthinkable to criticize. Goodrich's book is heavily influenced by the philosophy of Pragmatism and the aims of the Progressive Era. As noted above, Moore discounts her book as not having anything to do with ethics, which goes too far. It does in part address ethics, through the lens of Pragmatism, with an emphasis on social ethics.

An Unfortunate Professional Adjustment

Harrison's book *Ethics in Nursing* is problematic. It is not informed by any knowledge or readings in ethics and makes no reference to any. In fact, there are no citations at all. It is largely an uninformed lay-person's firmly relativistic take on ethics, and even defines *ethics* in error. She rejects all prior works in nursing ethics as dated and inadequate. In dismissing those books, she writes "my aim is [to] point out the true meaning of ethics, then to show how a code for any given people evolves, and later to give the students some of the necessary help toward solving the many problems she will meet."[65] Harrison accomplishes none of this. The examples she gives are of her own invention and are "straw-man arguments" to make her points. There is little ethics in the book, and what there is, is inaccurate, misleading, and mistaken. She eschews clinical examples as inappropriate in teaching. As to her relativism, for example, she writes:

> The factors governing the working out of a [societal] code of ethics vary widely from age to age and from place to place, and differ according to species, race and people. Down at the very bottom of things, a code of ethics depends on the instincts of the body of individuals concerned.[66]

While it is clear that the author has grappled with issues and has given what she has written a great deal of thought, this work is not learned, and it is elementally racist, classist, and misinformed.

In the late 1930s and early 1940s, the NLN shifts in curricular requirements resulted in combining smaller content areas, such as issues, trends, roles, fields of nursing, professional associations, and ethics into a single course called *Professional Adjustments*, ostensibly about the adjustments a person must make in becoming a nurse and entering the profession as a graduate. For several reasons, this effectively dislodges ethics from its preeminence. In this shift, there are usually two-volume works, "Professional Adjustments I" (generally on ethics and fields of nursing) and "Professional Adjustments II" (usually on issues, trends, organizations, etc.), though, as with Spaulding (see below), it may be one large volume. This becomes a period of muddlement for ethics largely because the professional adjustments faculty are more interested and knowledgeable in issues and trends than in ethics. While some of the ethics topics appear in these books, they tend to be shorn of the ethical discourse that would otherwise surround them. In addition, integrating content in education customarily results in the loss of content, in this case, the loss of explicit ethical discourse.

Lena Dixon Dietz's first and second editions are *Professional Problems in Nursing*, but by the third edition it becomes *Professional Adjustments I*. The content does differ but both titles deal with the adaptation of the student to the professional expectations and behaviors demanded of nurses. The books still contain a whole-life perspective, though less vigorously so. The ethics content, per se, is much diminished in both volumes. As with previous authors, Dietz cites Dewey and Tufts' *Ethics*. It is important to remember, though, that Aikens' and Robb's nursing ethics books (and others) are still being published at this time, so there are dedicated ethics textbooks that remain available.

Eugenia Spaulding, like Dietz, falls into that "professional adjustments" transition period. Her books on professional adjustments become explicitly "issues and trends" books by 1950.[67] Her book, the usual two volumes combined into one, is a good example of what happens when ethics is integrated into other content (and then lost), and when an author has less interest in ethics than in issues. For example, she discusses nursing as a profession, which was and remains a social and political battle for nursing, but which has profound ethical parameters. She fails to discuss these parameters. In her chapter "Nursing in the Present Social and Economic Situation," she takes four pages to list monumental social issues and changes, which have profound ethical implications, for which she provides no ethical discussion whatsoever. This is how her book differs from prior ethics books that discuss the same issues, but from the perspective of ethics. In her extensive list, Spaulding includes:

- conditions of modern industry with the introduction of machinery, scientific management and loss of interest in the personality of the worker;
- trends towards sponsorship of housing projects by the government;
- the changing attitude in relation to international relations;
- the increased interdependence which has brought about a great amount of disorganization and economic, political and social affairs;

- emphasis on the need of more definite planning in order to meet present demands of society;
- widened gap between the rich and the poor;
- the experimentation with birth control education which has raised many problems for the nurse as well as the family and the nation;
- the decadence of rural government and the increase in rural health problems;
- urbanism, or movement of population to the periphery of the city, and its resulting health problems;
- the spread of the eight-hour day and its effect professionally and socially on
  nurses in the various fields;
- increased interest in women's organizations in nursing education and better
  sickness and health programs.[68]

All of these topics had received extensive attention in the ethical discourse of the profession, but not in Spaulding's book. Her interest is in whether or not nursing is a profession, not in the ethical analysis of the social context of nursing and its status as a profession. Her chapter on nursing as a profession is particularly remarkable for its lack of conceptual rigor, clarity, incisiveness, or original think-ing, and the weaknesses of her arguments (e.g., nursing is a profession because several organizations and agencies have termed it as such).[69] This is surprising given her qualifications and academic credentials. The issue of nursing as a pro-fession does, incidentally, make its way into the ANA "Tentative Code of Ethics" in 1940.[70]

Different in purpose, Ella Rothweiler's *Davis' Cumulative Continued Study Units on Ethics* is a comprehensive nursing ethics, but more pedantic, directive, and gendered than many earlier works. It is not a nursing ethics book per se: it is a pithy "continued study unit" that represents the publisher's intent to publish separately bound, evolving material, of up to 64 pages each, to supplement an eth-ics course textbook. This ostensibly allowed the publisher to be more nimble and provide new material without a new edition of a textbook. Some of her remarks are simply lovely: "the study of a specific disease may be called a 'case study,' but we must not for that reason think of the patient as a 'case.' If we do, we soon lose interest in the patient as an individual, and in the real profession of nursing."[71]

For an example of an educated but philosophically poorly informed work, we turn to Goodall's *Ethics: The Inner Realities*. She believes that, since she is com-municating "truths" that are long established and well accepted, there is no need for citations.

> The subject matter herein is composed of those truths that appeared equally lu-
> cid and sure to the early Greeks, the medieval monks, and many of our late and
> present masters in the field of humanics. It has therefore not seemed necessary
> to burden the text with quotations in support of these truths.[72]

Humanics is "the subject or study of human affairs or relations, esp. of the human element of a problem or situation as opposed to the mechanical."[73] This should be distinguished from *the humanities*, "the branch of learning concerned with human culture; the academic subjects [such] as history, literature, ancient and modern languages, law, philosophy, art, and music."[74]

The fact that Goodall's book is not philosophically informed does not mean, however, that the text should be rejected out of hand. She writes from a position of immersion in nursing tradition and culture, and experience both at the bedside and in hospital administration (in Chicago, Brooklyn, and Washington state). The book is of value because is it unadornedly based in the lived nursing experience of the author, though it must be read recognizing the positionality of the author (white, female, Christian, middle class, in a position of authority). The book is directed toward entry-level students and has questions and discussion points at the conclusion of each chapter. It is pedantic with moments of sensitivity, such as her recognition of homesickness among students. It also contains more troubling content, such as her section on friendships among nurses.

Goodall identifies 19 character traits (virtues) around which she organizes the content of the book. They are: fortitude, courage, purity, perseverance, ambition, loyalty, usefulness, truthfulness, courtesy, patience, temperance, fidelity, determination, hopefulness, self-control, self-reliance, self-respect, consecration, and humor.[75] Though moral courage is treated as a contemporary concern *de novo*, this is, as noted above, a long-standing concern in the nursing literature. With respect to courage, Goodall is particularly concerned about moral courage (as opposed to physical courage), and addresses it in some detail.[76] Goodall sees her book as within the professional adjustments family, if not the category itself: "the interpretation and application of nursing ethics may well be called professional adjustment."[77]

Helen Hansen's *Professional Relationships of the Nurse*, one of the initial post-war books, begins with a panegyric on America and an emphasis upon citizenship. The nursing ethics literature has always emphasized the nurse's duties of citizenship (at a minimum to vote), and the nurse's civic engagement, but it was driven by issues of the enfranchisement of women and suffrage. Here, it is driven by wartime and (in the second edition) post-war sentiment. While Hansen covers topics that appear in the nursing ethics texts, she does so without reference to ethics. For example, the ethics textbooks spoke of the nurse's duties to herself and their ethical rationale, one duty of which was ongoing learning and reading. Hansen discusses "The Nurse and Her Reading." She writes:

> In this age of rush and radio there is a tendency to place in the background of one's daily life the enjoyment that is derived from reading and meditation upon what is read and yet, there has never before been such great need for breadth of vision, understanding of world events and philosophies, professional growth... The books and magazines that one reads serve as a mirror in which is reflected one's philosophy of life, ambitions, professional and civic interest. Emphasis

has already been placed upon the fact that a nurse needs a good cultural background in order to assume her professional responsibilities and be a citizen of the world. Because of this, the pre-nursing student is encouraged to devote a great deal of time to the study of English, history, civics, and foreign languages. Fortunate, indeed, are those who are able to read literature in the language in which it is written as a translation must, perforce, detract from the spirit of the author and often alter the original sentiment.[78]

Hansen then proceeds to discuss categories of books to read and makes specific recommendations for magazines and professional journals and topics. The readings, as in the ethics books, are both personal and professional; that is, they cover the whole of the nurse's life. The personal–professional divide has not yet taken hold in nursing ethics. As with reading and other topics, Hansen approaches the door to ethics but does not cross the threshold. Though she deals with professional relationships, she fails to embrace the ethics content of those relationships that are seen in the prior nursing ethics literature. Still, Aikens, Robb, and other ethics textbooks are in print and in use at this time, so all is not lost. In the second edition, she adjusts the content from wartime to a post-war context.

A Shining Star: Reclaiming Professional Adjustments

Co-authors Katherine Densford, a nurse and nursing school dean, and Everett Millard, a philosopher, manage in their book to reclaim a better understanding of professional adjustments as the formation of the student into a nursing identity with the *instantiation*[79] of the values, virtues, duties, and ideals of nursing. That is, they re-situate professional adjustments within the context of nursing ethics and correct the losses effected by Dietz, Spaulding, and Hansen. This is an extraordinary and commendable book for scholars in nursing ethics.

They begin their *Ethics for Modern Nurses: Professional Adjustments, I*[80] with this statement:

> When a student enters a School of Nursing, she has many problems. Among them are two of prime importance. One concerns her initial adjustment to the environment. The other is inherent in the first period, it has to do with the development of a philosophy of life—the formulation and application of principles of conduct. *Ethics for Modern Nurses* is designed to deal with both of these problems.[81]

Theirs is explicitly a whole-life ethics that is "not limited to ethics of nursing in any narrow sense." The book

> discusses the moral principles involved in purposeful, satisfying, useful living. By examining several fundamentally different philosophies of conduct, the student comes to understand more clearly her own moral choices as well as those of

others. This fosters tolerance. At the same time, sympathetic understanding and tolerance are not to be confused with indifference, but positive aid is given to those who wish to apply modern, common sense ethical methods to the solution of personal, professional, and social problems.[82]

Each chapter concludes with sections of study questions, questions for thought and discussion, and books to read. The adjustments section of the book touches upon ethics while emphasizing adjustments, but the second half of the book is focused on ethics. The ethics section is extraordinarily competent, rigorous, and relevant; written with great clarity, and nursing and health are woven into its fabric. It calls the student to thoughtful reflection at a college level and is wholly unlike the pedantic, concrete, simplistic edge found in Spaulding.

While multiple sections are worth calling out, we can pause to take note of but two: the chapters "Living Democratically" and "Democratic Ideals." As a reminder, the book (1946) predates the UN Universal Declaration of Human Rights (December 1948) by more than two years. In these chapters, the authors touch upon a range of issues. "Living Democratically" addresses: the right to work, just wages; the right to adequate food, clothing, shelter, and medical care; the right to security; the right to live in a society of free enterprise; the right to come and go and to speak or remain silent; the right to education; the right to rest; and the right to equality before the law. These authors address racial, social, political, economic, health, and international inequality. When they tackle racism, they pull no punches:

> If we believe that life should be a race,... an elementary sense of justice forces us to admit that it should be a fair race, with no one having a head start or suffering any handicap in so far as it is in our power to prevent injustices. Probably the most deep-seated kind of unfairness is racial prejudice.[83]

They then discuss racial inequality, disparities in "incomes of Negros and Whites," and "Medical Care of Negroes and Whites," including disparities in educational opportunity.

> It would be easy to be democratic in a completely democratic world. The believer in equality, however, is confronted by a world that is democratic only in spots. A nurse, for example, may find that the hospital for which she works as one of the 1,577 hospitals (out of 6,300 In the United States) that do not accept Negro patients. Or, perhaps, the hospital discriminates against Jews or members of some other religion. Or, she may be employed in a clinic where it is traditional to make poor people conscious of their poverty.[84]

While the language, concepts, and analysis of social contexts is now dated and does not have the benefit of critical theories developed later, this book is a good reflection of the breadth, depth, and capaciousness of nursing ethics. Its extensivity is greater than that of what will come to be bioethics. In addition, it still has something to say to nurses in ethics today.

A Farrago of Final Works

Florence Kempf's *The Person as a Nurse: Professional Adjustments* apparently originated as a series of lectures to students and thus has a "conversational style."[85] It is an odd book. The first chapter on the selection of students for nursing is something like the minutes of an admissions committee evaluation of candidates, including personal and family information and test scores of the candidates, and the individual committee member's contributions to the discussion as to the student's attributes, strengths, and liabilities, and the committee's decision-making process. The chapter-end includes words to define and suggested readings. The chapters that follow have a mix of narrative style, outlines, enumerated points, lists, and a significant number of illustrative case studies (rather like expanded lecture notes), with exercises and readings at the end of each chapter. It does contain normative content on character (virtue) and ideals, thus does contain ethics, at points more overtly than at others. The author is articulate and well read, and the bibliographies (suggested readings) are sound, but the book does not seem to have any organizing framework. It does in fact read like an expanded set of lectures, but it also appears to be course content that incorporates material that did not fit into other courses so is an amorphous amalgam of topics. It covers such things as how to get admitted to nursing school, world religions, personality, democracy, the values of a mature woman, student governance, and more. There is some excellent content, but one must weed through the chaos to find it.

English nurse Evelyn Pearce focuses her book uniquely.[86] While Pearce's book *Nurse and Patient: An Ethical Consideration of Human Relations* is in the family of books on professional adjustments, it differs in that it focuses on, in three sections, the patient, the nurse, and then patients and nurses as people. Pearce reflects the political situation of the day. Both of the book's editions are: post-World War II, post-Universal Declaration of Human Rights,[87] after the foundation of the World Medical Association and the Declaration of Helsinki, and declaration of Geneva, but prior to the foundation of the World Health Organization.[88] Note that there is a separate American edition of this book (1954). The World Wars have influenced the content of her book especially in its inclusion of content on "the dignity of man" and on human rights.[89] Hereinafter, books on nursing history and ethics will include content on human rights.

Margaret Sanner's book *Trends and Professional Adjustments in Nursing*[90] (1962) represents the continuing devolution of ethics, but even more, the devolution of professional adjustments, and perhaps even the humanities within nursing education. Despite the title, there is no material on professional adjustments, and nothing whatsoever on ethics. She defines *duty* in specifically legal, contractual, terms and does not accord it ethical meaning.[91] The book is an inadequate history of nursing, from "the beginnings of civilization," through to the establishment of the United Nations. She does not mention human rights. Following her history, drawn only from secondary sources, her final section of the book discusses fields of nursing and nursing organizations. The completely misfit last chapter is on the "management of money," the sole nod to the earlier books on ethics that included management of one's finances as part of duties-to-self. This is an extremely weak book on many counts, but it is comparatively interesting as it provides evidence of the successive devolution of ethics, the devolution of professional adjustments, the devolution of a nuanced and high level of scholarship, and the devolution of the conceptual demands upon nursing students. This book compares most unfavorably with that of Densford, and falls closer to that of Spaulding.

Ethics for Nurses, by UK nurse Hillary Way, is a series of articles she prepared for *The Nursing Times. The Times* describes it as "a series of articles on our duty to others and our duty to ourselves, with special reference to nursing and hospital life, written particularly for student nurses."[92] It includes sections on "A Sense of Duty," "Duty to Ourselves," "The Nurse's Virtues," "Duty to Others," "Authority and Discipline," and "Unwritten Laws of Nursing." It is not a rigorous or systematic exposition, nor does it quite cohere.

Hayes, Hayes, and Kelly's 1964 book *Moral Principles of Nursing*[93] should have, perhaps, been included among the clergy-authored books, but it is included here as one of the authors, Kelly, was a nurse. However, the content of the book is overwhelmingly that of the concerns of Roman Catholic priests for the issues of abortion, euthanasia, sterilization, other procedures, and administration of the sacraments. Kelly's contribution appears to be that of the chapters on nursing as a profession and vocation, the ideal nurse, and a collection of prayers covering a wide range of topics that render the book a bit different from those authored only by priests. This is a devoutly religious book for nurses within the Roman Catholic faith tradition.

Canadian nurse Thelma Pelley's professional adjustments book *Nursing: Its History, Trends, Philosophy, Ethics and Ethos*[94] covers topics similar to those of its American counterparts. In some respects, it is more comprehensive in that it ties nursing and its progress to nursing history—an approach from which the US nursing authors could have benefitted. Despite having ethics in its title, attention to ethics is scant. Its usefulness resides, in part, in having a Canadian voice on the professionalization and development of nursing, and the challenges that it encountered, some of which endure.

Conclusion

There is unevenness of quality among these works, and indeed relevance to nursing as the clergy-written works show. Many, if not most, of these works reflect an older vocabulary and writing style, and even dated concepts such as those associated with gendered social norms. Still, many of these works are philosophically informed from a breadth of ethics literature. They draw upon all the major philosophical works referenced in the bioethics literature (Kant, Mill, Aristotle, etc.) and significantly more. Their ethics is also rooted in nursing history, practice, and experience. They also demonstrate a breadth of concern for the structure and shape of society, as will be developed further by and by.

The nursing ethics literature does not end with its textbooks. There is more literature to consider to the end of laying a foundation for a deeper analysis of nursing ethics, essential to a new synthesis for nursing ethics' future. Of the books discussed here, the key works, for different reasons, are those of Robb, Aikens, Edgell, Goodrich, and Densford and Millard. The first chapters' contributions to the literature, Vaughan's dissertation, and Lavinia Dock's *Hygiene and Morality* will be discussed at another point. A course in nursing ethics should include these works, as should nursing ethics libraries. Several of the works published prior to 1923 are available in digital format through a variety of sources, as they fall into the US public domain. A number of the works published in 1923 and later are available in print-on-demand format through online booksellers. These books are not "primarily feminine etiquette." They emerge from women's struggle for a place in society, for authority, for the vote, and for the foundation of an educated, scientific, paid, extra-domestic, profession for women-as-nurses in a resistant society in need of a further developed nursing.

Appendix II: Full Working List of Early Works on Nursing Ethics and Ethics in Nursing, 1900–1960s, Listed Chronologically by First Edition[95]

This list includes *nursing ethics* books, i.e., books on ethics by nurses for nurses. It also includes those books termed *ethics in nursing* that are written by non-nurses for nurses. The full list includes both nursing ethics and ethics in nursing books, and includes a few clinical textbooks ("medical-surgical textbooks") that contain a first chapter devoted to ethics. A couple of the works are booklets, and two are physician lectures to nurses on ethics. Before the use of bibliographic citations became standard, there are allusions in the early ethics literature of works prior to 1900, though those works remain to be identified. This is a working list in the hope that additional works will be found by future scholars in nursing ethics. Certainly, there are additional "first chapters" that remain to be incorporated into this list.

Camp, Harriet C. [RN]. *Making Good on Private Duty: Practical Hints to Graduate Nurses.* Philadelphia: J.B. Lippincott, 1889. Reprinted 1912 under Harriet Camp Lounsbery. (Also known as: *The Nurse's Calling: Practical Hints to Graduate Nurses*). (First chapter)

Lewis, Percy C. [MD]. *The Theory and Practice of Nursing: A Text-Book for Nurses.* London: Scientific Press, 1893. (First chapter)

Fox, E. Margaret. *First Lines in Nursing.* London: Scientific Press, 1914. (First chapter)

Robb, Isabel Adams Hampton. *Nursing Ethics: For Hospital and Private Use.* New York: E.C. Koeckert, 1900. Reprinted without revision in 1912, 1916, 1920.

Maxwell, Anna Caroline and Pope, Amy Elizabeth. *Practical Nursing: A Text-Book for Nurses*. New York: G.P. Putnam's sons, 1907. (First chapter)

Dock, Lavinia Lloyd [RN]. *Hygiene and Morality*. 1910.

Goodnow, Minnie. *First Year Nursing: A Text-book for Pupils in their First Year of Hospital Work*. Philadelphia: W.B. Saunders, 1912. (First chapter)

Aikens, Charlotte Albina. *Studies in Ethics for Nurses*. Philadelphia: W.B. Saunders, 1916. Reprinted annually 1916–1922; 2nd ed. 1923; rev. 1928, 1931; 3rd ed. 1935; 4th ed. 1937; 5th ed. 1943.

Parsons, Sara E. [RN]. *Nursing Problems and Obligations*. Boston: Whitcomb and Barrows, 1916. Also, 1919, 1922.

Kirkpatrick, Thomas Percy Claude. *Nursing Ethics: A Lecture*. Dublin, Eire: The University Press, 1917. (Irish)

Harding, Gertrude [RN]. *Higher Aspects of Nursing*. Philadelphia: W.B. Saunders, 1919.

Spalding, Henry Stanislaus [The Rev.; SJ]. *Talks to Nurses: The Ethics of Nursing*. New York: Benziger Brothers, 1920.

Bourke, M.P. [The Rev., AM, LL.B.]. *Some Medical and Ethical Problems Solved*. Milwaukee, WI: the Bruce Publishing Co, 1921. 1937. (Pamphlet)

Finney, Patrick A. *Moral Problems in Hospital Practice*. St. Louis: B. Herder Book Co., 1922.

Harmer, Bertha [RN]. *Text-Book of the Principles and Practice of Nursing*. New York: Macmillan, 1922. (First chapter)

Murphy, Richard J. [The Rev.]. *The Catholic Nurse: Her Spirit and Her Duties*. Milwaukee: Bruce, 1923.

Brogan, James M. [The Rev.; SJ]. *Ethical Principles for the Character of a Nurse*. Milwaukee: Bruce, 1924.

Talley, Charlotte. [RN]. *Ethics: A Textbook for Nurses*. New York: Putnam's, 1925; 2nd ed. 1928.

Chaptal de Chanteloup, Léonie [RN; 1873–1937]. *Morale Professionnelle de l'infirmière*. Paris: A. Poinat, 1926. And 1932.

Garesché, Edward Francis [The Rev.; SJ]. *A Vade Mecum for Nurses and Social Workers*. Milwaukee: Bruce, 1926.

Talley, Charlotte E. [RN]. *Lesson Plans in Ethics for Nurses*. New York: G.P. Putnam's, 1927.

Garesché, Edward Francis [The Rev.; SJ]. *Couriers of Mercy: Friendly Talks to Nurses*. Milwaukee, WI: Bruce, 1928.

Garesché, Edward Francis [The Rev.; SJ]. *Ethics and the Art of Conduct for Nurses*. Philadelphia: W.B. Saunders, 1929. Also 1944; 358 pages.

Edgell, Beatrice [PhD; Psychologist]. *Ethical Problems: An Introduction to Ethics for Hospital Nurses and Social Workers*. London: Methuen and Company, 1929.

Russell, Frederick J. *Ethics in General and Special. For Schools of Nursing*. Emmitsburg, MD: Sisters of Charity, 1929.

Gladwin, Mary Elizabeth. *Ethics: Talks to Nurses*. Philadelphia: F.A. Davis, 1st ed. 1930.

Jamieson, Elizabeth Marion [BA, RN] and Sewell, Elizabeth. *Ethics Notebook for Nurses*. Philadelphia: J.B. Lippincott, 1931. 22 pages. Also 1933, 1935, 1940, 1944.

Gabriel (Ryan), Sr. John [AB, RN]. *Professional Problems: A Textbook for Nurses*. Philadelphia: W.B. Saunders, 1932.

Goodrich, Annie Warburton [RN; 1866–1954]. *The Social and Ethical Significance of Nursing: A Series of Addresses*. New York: Macmillan, 1932.

Harrison, Gene [AB, RN]. *Ethics in Nursing.* St. Louis: C.V. Mosby, 1932.

Génin, L. Aux [The Rev.]. *Précis de Morale Professionnelle: Aux Infirmières.* Paris: L'Institut des Franciscaines Missionnaires de Marie, 1934. Also 1944.

Dietz, Lena Dixon [RN]. *Professional Problems in Nursing.* Philadelphia: F.A. Davis, 1935.

Moore, Thomas Verner [The Rev.; PhD; 1877–1969]. *Principles of Ethics.* Philadelphia: J.B. Lippincott, 1935. Also 1937, 1939, 1943.

Vaughan, Sr. Rose Hélène [MA, RN]. *The Actual Incidence of Moral Problems in Nursing: A Preliminary Study in Empirical Ethics.* Washington, DC: Catholic University Press, 1935. Master's Dissertation.

Evarts, Arrah B. [MD]. *Ethics of Nursing.* Minneapolis, MN: Burgess, 1935. Lecture.

Gladwin, Mary Elizabeth. *Ethics: A Textbook for Nurses.* Philadelphia: F.A. Davis, 2nd ed. 1937; 3rd ed. 1938.

Rothweiler, Ella L. [MA, RN]. *Davis' Cumulative Continued Study Units on Ethics.* Philadelphia: F.A. Davis, 1938.

De Jésus-Christ, Catherine [Mother; b. 1869]. *At the Bedside of the Sick: Precepts and Counsels for Hospital Nurses.* E.F. Peeler, trans. [*Au Chevet de la Souffrance*]. London: Burns, Oats & Washbourne, 1938.

Spaulding, Eugenia K. [RN]. *Professional Adjustments in Nursing, Being Professional Adjustments II.* Philadelphia: J.B. Lippincott, 1939.

Dietz, Lena Dixon [RN; 1890–1964]. *Professional Adjustments, I.* Philadelphia: F.A. Davis, 1940.

La Rochelle, Stanislaus A., Fink, C.T. *Precis der morale medicale pour infumieres, medicins, et pretres.* Quebec: L'Action cathololique. Poupore, M.E., Trans.: *Handbook of Medical Ethics for Nurses, Physicians, and Priests.* Newman Book Shop, 1940. 1948. (Canadian)

Spaulding, Eugenia Kennedy [AM, DHL, RN]. *Professional Adjustments in Nursing for Senior Students and Graduates.* Philadelphia: JB Lippincott, 1941. 2nd ed. 1942; 3rd ed. 1946. (Went to eight editions then was taken over by Lucille Notter)

Goodall, Phyllis A. [RN]. *Ethics: The Inner Realities.* Philadelphia: F.A. Davis, 1942. Also 1943.

Hansen, Helen F. [MA, RN]. *Professional Relationships of the Nurse.* Philadelphia: W.B. Saunders, 1942. 2nd ed. 1948.

Healy, Edwin [The Rev.; SJ]. *Moral Guidance: A Textbook in Principles of Conduct for Colleges and Universities.* Chicago: Lloyola University Press, 1943. With chapter XVII specific to nursing.

Harrison, Gene [AB, RN]. *Professional Adjustments, I.* St. Louis: C.V. Mosby, 1941.

Densford, Katherine Jane [MA, RN, DSc] and Everett, Millard S. [PhD]. *Ethics for Modern Nurses: Professional Adjustments, I.* Philadelphia: W.B. Saunders, 1946.

Lennon, Sister Mary Isidore [RSM, BS, MA, RN]. *Professional Adjustments.* St. Louis: C.V. Mosby, 1946.

Connell, Francis J. [The Rev.; SSR]. *Morals in Politics and Professions: A Guide for Catholics in Public Life.* Westminster, MD: Newman Bookshop, 1946. Chapter XI specific to nursing.

Rumble, L. [The Rev. Dr.] and Charles M. Carty. *Quizzes on Hospital Ethics for Nurses, Doctors, Priests, and Sisters.* 1946. (Booklet)

McFadden, Charles J. [The Rev., PhD]. *Medical Ethics for Nurses.* Philadelphia: F.A. Davis, 1946. Also 1949.

Price, Alice Louise. [RN]. *Professional Adjustments, I.* Philadelphia: W.B. Saunders, 1946.

Johnson, Brian D. [MD]. *The Catholic Nurse.* London: Burns Oats & Washbourne, 1950.

McAllister, Joseph Bernard [The Rev. Monsignor; SS]. *Ethics with Special Application to Medical and Nursing Professions.* Philadelphia: W.B. Saunders, 1948. 2nd ed. 1955.

Gounley, Martin E. *Digest of Ethics for Nurses.* Paterson: St. Anthony Guild, 1949.

Spaulding, Eugenia Kennedy [AM, DHL, RN]. *Professional Nursing. Trends and Adjustments.* Philadelphia: J.B. Lippincott, 1950.

Kempf, Florence C. [BS, MA, RN]. *The Person as a Nurse: Professional Adjustments.* NY: Macmillan, 1950. Also 1953. 2nd ed., 1957.

Pearce, Evelyn C. [SRN, RFN, SCM, MCSP, Teacher's Cert.]. *The Nurse and the Patient: An Ethical Consideration of Human Relations.* London: Faber and Faber, 1953. (UK)

Hayes, Edward J. [The Rev.] et al. *Moral Handbook of Nursing: A Compendium of Principles, Spiritual Aids, and Concise Answers Regarding Catholic Personnel, Patients and Problems.* New York: Macmillan, 1956.

Southard, Samuel [The Rev.]. *Religion and Nursing.* Nashville, TN: Broadman Press, 1959.

Sanner, Margaret Clementine. *Trends and professional adjustments in nursing.* W.B. Saunders, 1962.

Way, Hillary [RN]. *Ethics for Nurses.* London: Macmillan, 1962. (UK: reprinted from *Nursing Times*)

Plachata, Sr. Mary Miranda [CSSF, RN]. *Spiritualize Your Nursing.* No place: Felician Sisters, 1963.

Pelley, Thelma. [RN]. *Nursing: Its History, Trends, Philosophy, Ethics and Ethos.* Philadelphia: W.B. Saunders, 1964.

Hayes, Edward J. [The Rev.], Hayes, Paul J. [The Rev.], and Kelly, Dorothy Ellen [RN]. *Moral Principles of Nursing.* New York: Macmillan, 1964.

Pole, K.F.M. *Handbook for the Catholic Nurse.* London: Robert Hale, 1964.

Leclerq, Jacques. *The Apostolic Spirituality of the Nursing Sister.* Staten Island, New York: Alba House, 1967. *La Soeur Hospitalière.* Tournai, Belgium, 1966. (For nuns in nursing orders)

Notes on Authors

Where known, the dates, degrees, religious and professional credentials are given for the authors. Some nurse authors may predate the legislation for nursing registration and may not have used the "RN" designation. Some clergy authors are only designated "The Rev." with no affiliation given in the text.

With the exception of Beatrice Edgell (PhD), the female authors are "trained nurses," though some predate the inception of registration. The majority of male authors are Roman Catholic priests, though there is a Protestant pastor. Moore's work is unique in that it was in part a collaborative effort with Sr. Rose Hélène Vaughan, based on her master's degree dissertation.

Note on Publication Dates

In some instances, the work was copyrighted late in one year but not printed until early the next year so that the copyright and first printing dates may differ.

Note on Publication Location and Text Conventions

There was a good bit of interaction among nursing leaders in the anglophone world, and a good number of textbooks were published or used in multiple countries. In a few instances, the works were reprinted for another country, changing only spelling and punctuation (and a few bits of vocabulary) in order to conform to the conventions of the other countries.

Notes on Book Titles

In some instances, the book title on the frontispiece differs from that on the spine of the book, as a matter of space.

Notes

1 BBC Two, "Saxon Hoard: A Golden Discovery," broadcast January 26, 2012. http://www.bbc.co.uk/programmes/b01bf4h6
2 Sara T. Fry, "The Role of Caring in Nursing Ethics," *Hypatia* 4, no. 2 (Summer 1989), 88–103.
3 Elizabeth R. Valentine, *Beatrice Edgell: Pioneer Woman Psychologist* (Charlottesville, VA: University of Virginia, 2006).
4 Beatrice Edgell, *Ethical Problems: An Introduction to Ethics for Hospital Nurses and Social Workers* (London: Methuen and Company, 1929).
5 Ibid., 140.
6 The reader is referred to Benner's chapter (9) for further development of the concepts of virtue, wisdom, and *phronesis*.
7 Edgell, *Ethical Problems*, 140–141.
8 Cheryl Misak and Huw Price, *The Practical Turn: Pragmatism in Britain in the Long Twentieth Century* (Oxford: The British Academy, 2017).
9 Thomas Percy Claude Kirkpatrick, *Nursing Ethics: A Lecture* (Dublin, Eire: The University Press, 1917).
10 Ibid., 12.
11 Ibid., 36–37.
12 M. Louise Beaty, "Ethics of Nursing. Book Review by Arrah B. Evarts, MD," *American Journal of Nursing* 37, no. 11 (1937): 1301–1302.
13 Ibid., 1301.
14 Ibid., 1302.
15 John Dewey and James Tufts, *Ethics* (New York: Henry Holt and Company, 1908).
16 Thomas Verner Moore [The Rev.; PhD; 1877–1969], *Principles of Ethics* (Philadelphia: J.B. Lippincott, 1935), 365.
17 Thomas Verner Moore, *A Historical Introduction to Ethics* (New York: American Book Company, 1915).
18 Henry Stanislaus Spalding [The Rev.; SJ; 1865–1934], *Talks to Nurses: The Ethics of Nursing* (New York: Benziger Brothers, 1920), 13–15.
19 Edwin Healy [The Rev.; SJ], *Moral Guidance: A Textbook in Principles of Conduct for Colleges and Universities* (Chicago: Lloyola University Press, 1943).
20 Samuel Southard, *Religion and Nursing* (Nashville, TN: Broadman Press, 1959).
21 Francis J. Connell [The Rev.; SSR], *Morals in Politics and Professions: A Guide for Catholics in Public Life* (Westminster, MD: Newman Bookshop, 1946), 139.

22 Joseph Bernard McAllister [The Rev. Monsignor; SS], *Ethics with Special Application to Medical and Nursing Professions* (Philadelphia: W.B. Saunders, 1948), 231–234.

23 Ibid., 28–29; italics in original.

24 Thomas Verner Moore, *Principles of Ethics* (Philadelphia: J.B. Lippincott, 1935), v.

25 Ibid., 67.

26 Ibid., 71.

27 Ibid., 87.

28 Ibid., 88.

29 Ibid., 239.

30 Isabel Adams Hampton Robb, *Nursing Ethics: For Hospital and Private Use* (New York: E.C. Koeckert, 1900).

31 Ibid., 71–72.

32 Ibid., 149.

33 Ibid., 134.

34 Alaisdair MacIntyre, *After Virtue* (Notre Dame, France: University of Notre Dame Press, 1981).

35 Robb, *Nursing Ethics*, 27.

36 Charlotte Albina Aikens, *Studies in Ethics for Nurses* (Philadelphia: W.B. Saunders, 1916).

37 Richard Ely, *The Law of Social Service* (New York: Eaton & Mains, 1896); W.L. Courtney, *Constructive Ethics: A Review of Modern Moral Philosophy in Its Three Stages of Interpretation, Criticism, and Reconstruction* (London: Chapman Hall, 1895); Edward Howard Griggs, *The Ethics of Personal Life: A Handbook of Six Lectures* (New York: P.W. Huebsch Publisher, 1906); Isabel Adams Hampton Robb, *Nursing Ethics: For Hospital and Private Use* (New York: E.C. Koeckert, 1900); John Dewey, *Outlines of A Critical Theory of Ethics* (Ann Arbor, MI: Register Publishing Company, 1891); Browne's book could not be identified. In the 5th edition she adds: John Dewey and James Tufts. *Ethics* (New York: Henry Holt and Company, 1908).

38 She does not give full citations.

39 John Dewey and James Tufts, *Ethics* (New York: Henry Holt and Company, 1908).

40 Charlotte Albina Aikens, *Studies in Ethics for Nurses*, 2nd ed. (Philadelphia: W.B. Saunders, 1923).

41 Aikens, *Studies*, 2nd ed., 56.

42 Ibid., 63.

43 Ibid., 64.

44 Ibid., 72.

45 Ibid., 134.

46 Ibid., 9.

47 Aikens, *Studies*, 1916, 8.

48 Aikens, *Studies*, 5th ed., vii.

49 Sara E. Parsons, *Nursing Problems and Obligations* (Boston: Whitcomb and Barrows, 1916).

50 Ibid., 106.

51 Gertrude Harding, *Higher Aspects of Nursing* (Philadelphia: W.B. Saunders, 1919).

52 Ibid., 8.

53 Ibid., 18.

54 Ibid., 48; italics in original.

55 Charlotte Talley, *Ethics: A Textbook for Nurses* (New York: Putnam's, 1925).

56 Charlotte E. Talley, *Lesson Plans in Ethics for Nurses* (New York: G.P. Putnam's, 1927).

57 Ibid., 3–4.

58 Mary Elizabeth Gladwin, *Ethics: Talks to Nurses* (Philadelphia: F.A. Davis, 1st ed. 1930).

59 Ibid., 2nd ed., 1937, 9.

60 Ibid., 54.

61 Mother Catherine De Jésus-Christ, *At the Bedside of the Sick: Precepts and Counsels for Hospital Nurses*. E.F. Peeler, trans. [*Au Chevet de la Souffrance*] (London: Burns, Oates & Washbourne, 1938).

62 Sister Mary Isidore Lennon, *Professional Adjustments* (St. Louis: C.V. Mosby, 1946), 242.

63 Annie Warburton Goodrich, *The Social and Ethical Significance of Nursing: A Series of Addresses* (New York: Macmillan, 1932).

64 E.F. MacDougall, "The Social and Ethical Significance of Nursing. Review," *American Journal of Public Health Nations Health* 22, no. 7 (July 1932): 787.

65 Gene Harrison, *Ethics in Nursing* (St. Louis: C.V. Mosby, 1932), 14.

66 Ibid., 37.

67 Eugenia Kennedy Spaulding, *Professional Nursing: Trends and Adjustments* (Philadelphia: J.B. Lippincott, 1950).

68 Eugenia Kennedy Spaulding, *Professional Adjustments in Nursing for Senior Students and Graduates* (Philadelphia: J.B. Lippincott, 1941), 66–69.

69 Ibid., 96–97.

70 American Nurses Association, "A Tentative Code," *American Journal of Nursing* 40, no. 9 (1940): 977–980.

71 Ella L. Rothweiler, *Davis' Cumulative Continued Study Units on Ethics* (Philadelphia: F.A. Davis, 1938), 25.

72 Phyllis A. Goodall, *Ethics: The Inner Realities* (Philadelphia: F.A. Davis, 1942), x.

73 "humanics, n." OED Online (Oxford University Press, September 2022). https://www.oed.com/view/Entry/89268?redirectedFrom=humanics& (accessed October 20, 2022).

74 "humanity, n." OED Online (Oxford University Press, September 2022). https://www.oed.com/view/Entry/89280?redirectedFrom=humanities& (accessed October 20, 2022).

75 Goodall, *Ethics* 1942, 33–34.

76 Ibid., 39–43.

77 Ibid., 28.

78 Helen F. Hansen, *Professional Relationships of the Nurse* (Philadelphia: W.B. Saunders, 1942), 25.

79 To instantiate is to internalize and become an embodied representative of the *good nurse*, good in both a clinical and moral sense as defined by the tradition, narrative, and community of practice. Instantiation is a process from novice to expert.

80 Katherine Jane Densford and Millard S. Everett, *Ethics for Modern Nurses: Professional Adjustments, I* (Philadelphia: W.B. Saunders, 1946).

81 Ibid., v.

82 Ibid., v.

83 Ibid., 210.

84 Ibid., 215.

85 Florence C. Kempf, *The Person as a Nurse: Professional Adjustments* (New York: Macmillan, 1950), v.

86 Evelyn C. Pearce, *Nurse and Patient: An Ethical Consideration of Human Relations* (London: Faber and Faber, 1953).

87 United Nations. Universal Declaration of Human Rights (New York: UN, 1948). https://www.un.org/en/udhrbook/pdf/udhr_booklet_en_web.pdf

88 https://www.csce.gov/sites/helsinkicommission.house.gov/files/Helsinki%20Final%-20Act.pdf

89 Pearce, *Nurse and Patient: An Ethical Consideration of Human Relations*, 143–156.

90 Margaret Clementine Sanner, *Trends and Professional Adjustments in Nursing* (Philadelphia: W.B. Saunders, 1962).

91 Ibid., 276.

92 Hillary Way, *Ethics for Nurses* (London: Macmillan, 1962), title page, unnumbered.

93 Edward J. Hayes, Paul J. Hayes, and Dorothy Ellen Kelly, *Moral Principles of Nursing* (New York: Macmillan, 1964).
94 Thelma Pelley, *Nursing: Its History, Trends, Philosophy, Ethics and Ethos* (Philadelphia: W.B. Saunders, 1964).
95 Modified from Marsha D. Fowler, *Ethics and Nursing, 1893–1984: The Ideal of Service, The Reality of History* (Los Angeles: University of Southern California, 1984).

3

THE NURSING ETHICS LITERATURE

More to Read

While textbooks provide a foundational source for nursing ethics, there is much more to read. Other sources include the first dissertation on ethical problems in nursing practice, "first chapters" of early medical-surgical textbooks, ICN and ANA speeches, journal articles, commencement addresses, ethics committees' minutes, state board ethics requirements, and more. While many of these represent the same textbook authors, others bring in new persons and different voices, not just those of nursing's leaders. The content of these works often coordinates with the textbooks, but also raises different issues or has an expanded topical focus. Together with the nursing ethics textbooks, these sources fill out a broader picture of nursing ethics that will then require deeper analysis as to the nature of the ethics being propounded. Many of these works are difficult to obtain. Though some commentary is provided, the purpose of this chapter is to provide a select set of the earliest shorter texts, now in the public domain, for the reader to have at hand. Among these works, pride of place belongs to Sister Rose Hélène Vaughan.

The First Dissertation on Ethical Problems in Nursing Practice, 1935

Sister Rose Hélène Vaughan, born Hazel Lillian Paugh, was born in 1899. She died in 1962 following heart surgery related to a myocardial infarction. In the intervening years, she made a remarkable and unparalleled contribution to nursing ethics. Following the death of her husband, James Vaughan, from tuberculosis, she converted to Roman Catholicism. She entered the Convent of the Sisters of St. Joseph of Carondelet—and subsequently entered nursing school. After taking a bachelor's degree, she matriculated at Catholic University of America to take a master's degree in nursing. She was interested in nursing ethics. Her dissertation

DOI: 10.4324/9781003262107-4

(though actually a master's thesis) advisor was Fr. Thomas Verner Moore. Moore was a polymath, priest, monk, psychologist, psychiatrist, and medical army captain during World War I. As Vaughan's advisor, he suggested that she explore ethical issues that nurses encounter in clinical practice, which he could use to inform his textbook on nursing ethics. Written by a nurse, this dissertation would become the first extant empirical study on ethical problems in nursing.[1]

The purpose of her study "was to obtain, by means of diaries, the actual incidence of moral problems occurring among nurses. It is hoped that the knowledge obtained through the study will ultimately form the basis of a course of Ethics for Nurses."[2] She asked a group of nurses (students, graduates, lay, and religious) to keep journals of moral problems that arose in their personal and professional lives, for a period of three months. A total of 95 nurses returned journals, 18 of whom kept the journals for the full three months. The diaries "yielded 2265 moral problems, 67 problems of etiquette, and 110 questions."

> As the material came in, each of the problems was copied verbatim on cards which were filed according to Lehmkuhl's classification of moral problems[3] with some slight modifications. Lehmkuhl's "duties to the state" was omitted and, for our purpose, "duties to the patient", "duties to the hospital", and "duties to the profession" supplied. Problems of finance and personality, while not exactly ethical problems, were felt to be sufficiently distinctive, because of their consequent moral potentialities, to permit of special classification. This classification yielded a sum of 33 groups of moral problems.[4]

In her analysis, she divided the problems "into three general classes: moral problems, cultural problems, and questions which do not seem to imply problems. The morally-involved problems, ... exceed out of all proportion the balance of the material."[5]

Her categories, based in part on Lehmkuhl, reflect an underlying Roman Catholic theology, and some of the categories would be viewed differently today. The prime example of this is her category of *lust*; the examples that she gives are what would, today, be termed *sexual harassment* and generally involved unwanted, unsolicited, and unwelcome touching of female nurses by male patients, family members, or physicians.

These charts from her dissertation tabulate the results of her data:

TABLE 3.1 Frequency of moral problems in nursing

Rank	Moral Problems in Order of Frequency	Incidence	Total Incidence	Per Cent of Problems	No. of Problems overlapping	No. of Nurses	Per Cent of Nurses
1	Concerning Cooperation		527	23.2		85	88
	Between Nurses and Doctors	145		6.4		47	49.4

TABLE 3.1 Continued

Rank	Moral Problems in Order of Frequency	Incidence	Total Incidence	Per Cent of Problems	No. of Problems overlapping	No. of Nurses	Per Cent of Nurses
	Among Nurses in General	132		5.8		42	44
	With and Among Supervisors	104		4.5		51	54
	In General	51		2.2		34	36
	Between Nurses and Patients' Relatives	33		1.4		18	18.9
	In Giving Medicine and Treatment	32		1.4		18	18.9
	In Matters of Asepsis	30		1.3		18	18.9
2	Duties to the Nursing School		194	8.5	3	68	71.6
3	Lying		181	8		57	60
	In General	80		3.5	5	30	31.5
	Dishonest Charting	51		2.2	16	26	27.3
	In Answer to Forbidden Questions	50		2.2		27	28.5
4	Duties to Patients		163	7.1	42	50	52.6
5	External Duties to One's Neighbor			7	26	59	62.1
6	Lust		159	6.4	4	50	52.6
	Sexual Problems in General	98	145	4.3		41	43
	Relations with Internes	32		1.4		19	20
	Homosexuality	8		0.3		5	5.2
	Vulgar and Profane Language	7		0.3		6	6.3
7	Temperance		140	6.1		67	70.5
	Smoking	88		3.8		34	35.7
	Drinking	52		2.2		35	36.8
8	Duties to the Profession		133	5.8	3	53	55.7
9	Injuring Reputation	90		3.9	3	43	44.2
10	Duties to the Hospital	88		3.8	19	35	36.8
11	Anger	57		2.5		17	17.8
12	Acquisition of Knowledge	56		2.4	11	25	26.3

(*Continued*)

TABLE 3.1 Continued

Rank	Moral Problems in Order of Frequency	Incidence	Total Incidence	Per Cent of Problems	No. of Problems overlapping	No. of Nurses	Per Cent of Nurses
13	Justice		54	2.4	2	36	37.8
14	Stealing		50	2.2	20	31	32.6
15	Care of Spiritual Life		32	1.4	1	19	20
16	Impatience		31	1.3	3	17	17.8
17	Duties Concerning Life and Person of Others		31	1.3		14	14.7
	Abortions	11		0.4		7	7.3
	Sterilization	8		0.3		6	6.3
	Birth Control	6		0.2		5	5.2
	Miscellaneous	6		0.2		5	16.8
18	Concerning the Sacraments		28	1.2		16	17.8
19	Acting Negligently		28	1.2	17	17	20
20	Care of Body and Life		28	1.2	1	19	21
21	Prudence		25	1.1		20	15.7
22	Scandal		21	0.9	3	14	9.4
23	Duties to Parent and Child		14	0.6		9	6.3
24	Envy		14	0.6		6	5
25	Personality		13	0.5		11	11
26	Virtue of Religion		11	0.4		8	8.4
27	Restitution		9	0.3		9	9.4
28	Internal Charity to One's Neighbor		9	0.3		4	4.2
29	Laws of the Church		8	0.3		6	6.3
30	Reverence to God and Sacred Things		7	0.3		7	7.3
31	Pride		7	0.3		6	6.3
32	Finances		7	0.3	2	6	6.3
33	Injuring Property		6	0.2		5	5.2
	Total		2366				
	Correction for Overlapping		101				
	Grand Total		2265				

Source: Sr. Rose Hélène Vaughan, *The Actual Incidence of Moral Problems in Nursing: A Preliminary Study in Empirical Ethics* (used with permission of Georgetown University)

The largest category of ethical incident was that of cooperation with others and within that cooperation with physicians, then with nursing colleagues and nursing supervisors. She summarizes each category and then gives case examples. For nurse–physician cooperation, she writes that "the greater number of these involved questions of the propriety of the nurses making suggestions to the doctor regarding his orders, questions of loyalty to the physician, and doubts in matters of making hospital rounds with the doctor."[6] The examples reflect behavioral expectations, the hospital etiquette of yesteryear, such as nurses carrying the physician's charts on morning rounds. And yet, other examples are a strong reminder of Leonard Stein's "The Doctor–Nurse Game."[7,8,9] Some examples reflect social norms and expectations for women of the era. Still, a number of the examples are of issues that persist in nursing today. Vaughan includes hundreds of examples in her dissertation that we need not repeat here; they have been previously noted in the discussion of Moore's textbook (Chapter 2). Vaughan's dissertation is commended to those nursing ethics scholars who wish to examine the ethical problems that nurses of the period encountered in personal and professional life, and to note, especially, the issues that persist.[10]

First Chapters

Many of the earliest clinical nursing textbooks, that is medical-surgical nursing textbooks from the later 1800s, contained a first chapter on the duties of the nurse or the character of the nurse. These first chapters were about ethics although the term *ethics* may or may not have been used in these chapters, even though that was the subject matter. This is also true of many early journal articles. For the most part, the term *ethics* was more frequently used in the US literature than in the UK literature, even where both were dealing with an *ethics of character*, that is, with *virtue ethics*, though the term is not by any means absent from the UK literature

First Chapter: E. Margaret Fox, 1914

E. Margaret Fox's first chapter in *First Lines in Nursing* (1914) is an excellent example of "first chapters."[11] She addresses both character (virtue), and duties, as well as etiquette under the rubric of *Nursing Ethics*. These words are the centerpiece to her approach to virtue:

Therefore, as conduct is the outcome of character, so character is more important in a nurse than mere cleverness. How necessary is it, then, that such attributes as reverence, gentleness, discretion, and uprightness should enter into every nurse's character, and be continually cultivated by the earnest practice of good habits and patient continuance in well-doing.[12]

For Fox, *the good* precedes *the right*; that is, *character enables the realization of duties*. She addresses a number of duties, such as maintaining hospital discipline, for which she uses the vehicle of etiquette. There are class and gender norms that suffuse the text, yet note that hospital order upends class order. The duties she addresses are set within the context of her nursing experience, but she notes that principles of conduct underlie the concrete examples that she presents.

> Experience in the work, knowledge of human nature, and observation of the failures or successes of others have resulted in all authorities on nursing matters being in unity as to certain principles of conduct applicable to nurses in hospital and elsewhere. These principles are best described as "Nursing Ethics," and on them are based all rules relating to hospital etiquette and manners; all regulations concerning a nurse's conduct, mode of dress, even methods of study. To go through each one would take too long; *tracing a few of them to their source may be helpful, as it may serve to show the underlying reasons for the various relations* in which all workers in hospitals are expected to stand towards one another.[13]

This is where some interpreters have gone wrong in reading this literature, as if its concrete clinical specifications were its "ethics," rather than reading more deeply for the intended virtues, values, duties, and ideals. The ethics resides, deliberately, in the subtext of the student textbook.

Here that subtext contains concern for moral character, professional boundaries, and what will remain a steady concern in the nursing ethics literature, the notion of moral duties to self. This customarily begins with a concern for the health of the nurse, but goes on to include rest, recreation, personal and professional reading, ongoing learning, avoiding fatigue and overstrain, and more. This subtext is only overtly about well-fitting shoes with India rubber pads, the antiseptic lotions and chilblains that cause chapped hands, or woolen stockings or open-air exercise; it is more fundamentally about caring for one's self as a moral duty, both for the sake of fulfilling professional responsibilities well, but also for the sake of the nurse herself.

E. Margaret Fox was an English nurse, and her book was published in the UK for a British nursing audience, but it was also released in the US and reviewed in US nursing journals. This is her first chapter.

FIRST LINES IN NURSING, CHAPTER I: THE ETHICS OF NURSING AND THE CARE OF THE NURSE'S OWN HEALTH.

In this short series I want to cover with you as far as possible the ground of your first year in hospital; to indicate and explain what will be expected from you in the way of conduct and work as well as professional and intellectual attainments; to make easy for you the difficult task of adapting yourselves to an entirely new environment; and to show you how you may use the limitless opportunities you will meet with for learning your work to the best advantage.

In no way will these articles usurp the place of the lectures from the surgeons and physicians that you will attend later on; they are not going to attempt to teach you either anatomy, medicine, or surgery, but I hope you will find that what you learn now will prepare and make ready the way for more and yet more detailed instruction, so that at the end of your course you will feel you have every right to the coveted "Certificate of Training" and can each of you be truly described as a "really competent nurse."

This first year in hospital is the most important of all. It is the basis of the whole of your future work. The professional habits you form now, the views you learn to take of people and things around you, the "tone" you cultivate, the friendships you make will all influence, consciously or unconsciously, your program as you go farther on, and assure your success or your undoing.

Some of you have not yet completed your three months' trial, yet already you have made a lasting impression on those with whom you have been working, and the patients you have helped to nurse. This is true, whether you are sufficiently humble-minded to think yourself of little importance, or conceited enough to imagine you are the centre of your tiny circle. I want you to magnify your office. In many of the relationships of life, people are inclined to take themselves too seriously; with regard to the profession of nursing, you can hardly do so. In no other field of work, save that of medicine, are you brought into such a succession of close and delicate intimacies with others. You are admitted where the patient's nearest and dearest relatives are excluded; you are told what is never breathed even in confidence to wife, mother, or son; your hasty, lightly-expressed opinion may depress or exalt some yearning spirit in a manner out of all proportion to your knowledge or experience. It is also true that what seems to you a trifling error may prove a fatal mistake, dragging after it a never-ending train of tragic consequences. Is it not, then, important that you should at once begin to realise the responsibilities you have taken upon yourselves in becoming nurses? This sense of responsibility should influence all you say and do, for your words and actions will show what you are.

Therefore, as conduct is the outcome of character, so character is more important in a nurse than mere cleverness. How necessary is it, then, that such attributes as reverence, gentleness, discretion, and uprightness should enter into every nurse's character, and be continually cultivated by the earnest practice of good habits and patient continuance in well-doing.

Experience in the work, knowledge of human nature, and observation of the failures or successes of others have resulted in all authorities on nursing matters being in unity as to certain principles of conduct applicable to nurses in hospital and elsewhere. These principles are best described as "Nursing Ethics," and on them are based all rules relating to hospital etiquette and manners; all regulations concerning a nurse's conduct, mode of dress, even methods of study. To go through each one would take too long; tracing a few of them to their source may be helpful, as it may serve to show the underlying reasons for the various relations in which all workers in hospitals are expected to stand towards one another.

Take, for instance, the rules concerning the etiquette to be observed by the nurses in a ward towards a member of the medical staff. They may not sit down, talk, or move about unnecessarily, make any noise, or allow the patients to do so while he is present. They must not address him unless he speaks first to them, and then only as "sir," never as "Mr. So-and-so." If directly asked a question, they may answer, but must never express an opinion of a patient's condition unless desired to do so. They must open and close the door for the doctor's in-coming and out-going, see that he has water to wash his hands, and wait on him quietly and unobtrusively.

The same etiquette, slightly modified, is also required towards resident medical officers and all grades of medical students. This seems very strange and even ridiculous to some new-comers, being a complete upheaval of all preconceived notions respecting the relations between modern man and woman. The daughter of a duchess, if she becomes a probationer, has to treat the surgeon, even though he should be the son of the local pork butcher, with the same deference, for the reason that in hospital her relations towards him are not social, but professional. He is her "superior officer," and must be recognised as such.

The barrier thus raised by common consent between doctors and nurses is really helpful to a probationer from the very commencement of her training. It helps her to maintain a certain official attitude; to be self-controlled and re-served. It tends to order and decorum in the ward, and impresses the patients with a sense of discipline. Lounging while receiving orders, laughing and joking on ordinary subjects, all tend to undesirable familiarity, and make it hard for a nurse to discuss with the doctor in a professional manner and without self-consciousness the everyday duties of her work, to remember the directions given her, and to carry them out in such a way as to win the confidence and respect of her patients.

Take, again, the rules concerning the relationship of nurses and patients. Kindness is enjoined, but not familiarity; cheerfulness, but not levity. Gossiping with them is absolutely prohibited, so also is discussion of the doctors and their treatment, or any expression of opinion on the patient's disease or operation. Nurses often unwittingly offend in this manner. They cannot be too careful of what they say. Never criticise the doctor's treatment of a patient in the hearing of that patient or his friends. Even apparently unconscious people hear often great deal more than they are supposed to, and many a patient has before now come into possession of all the details of his operation through the heedless conversation of two nurses while making his bed, who imagined he was still unconscious. Sooner or later, such indiscretions are sure to come home to roost, and a nurse once convicted of them is ever after a suspected person, liable to be considered the originator of all sorts of scandal, whether she is really guilty or not.

The etiquette to be observed by probationers towards their matron is much the same as that accorded to the headmistress of a school by her pupils, and in this matter, you will be guided by the ordinary rules of good manners.

The ward sisters, also, are entitled to respect as being trained nurses and heads of your various departments of work; it is your duty to obey their orders in a willing and pleasant manner.

Nursing ethics lay great stress on loyalty, which includes the idea of obedience to rules and orders without grumbling; of upholding your hospital whenever it is attacked by outsiders; feeling responsible for bringing credit on it by your own personal demeanour, tidiness, punctuality, intelligence, and trustworthiness; and helping and standing by one another in all that makes for truth and equity.

Nurses who begin their training by being as jealous for the honour of their hospital as for that of their own home begin well and in the right spirit. Such an attitude of mind banishes effectually discontent and grumbling, gossip and scandal-mongering, redounds to the nurse's own benefit, and maintains the dignity and honour of the profession she has entered.

The point next in importance to character in a nurse is that of health. No matter how suitable you may be in other respects, if your health is not sound you cannot succeed as a nurse. That is why you are required to answer so many searching questions, and to produce a recent medical certificate before you are accepted as a probationer. Nursing invariably finds out the weak spot in your armour sooner or later, and usually the first year in hospital is the most trying one as regards health. Although all of you have the undoubted advantage of beginning your work when perfectly well and strong, you must not depend too much on the fact of having a good constitution and excellent health, but must also do your utmost to keep well. Nursing is a great strain on mind and body. Nerves and muscles alike have much demanded from them, and become fatigued; their recuperative power is weakened, and unless adequate rest is forthcoming they will rebel. Given a sound organism, then the maintenance of health is largely in your own hands, and now in the early months of your training you must begin to form the habit of keeping well.

You all know in a general sort of way that fresh air and exercise, good food and cleanliness are necessary to health, and that if these are neglected the strongest person in the world will in time succumb to illness, but when it comes to putting your knowledge into practice I am afraid many of you are inconsistent. You certainly live in an airy building, kept constantly clean in a way that few private dwellings are kept; but if you shut the windows and ventilators in your bedroom at night, sleep with your head smothered in bedclothes, and go to bed wearing the same undervest that you wore during the day; if you neglect the daily walk in the open air, or the daily bath because you were so "tired"; if you go out in thin shoes on a wet "day off," wearing a thin blouse, and discarding the warm, high-necked underclothing in spite of a keen east wind; if you eat sweets, cakes and pastry between meals, and instead of plain, wholesome food, fall back on stray cups of tea, how can you be surprised if your once splendid health begins to flag, and you develop first one and then another common ailment, not serious perhaps in itself, but just sufficiently debilitating to make you feel all the time tired, slack and out of sorts?

Most probationers enter hospital with a determination to keep well, if possible, to go out as often as they are allowed, and to keep up some favourite occupation when off duty, so as not to become what so many nurses are accused of being—narrow-minded, with no thought of anything but their work, and unable to converse on any other subject. These are altogether laudable resolutions but, alas! they are not often kept for long, and the reason for breaking them nearly always lies at the door of that first most common enemy of the probationer—over-fatigue.

Now, although it is the favourite idea of the lay public that this fatigue is owing entirely to overwork, it is not really anything of the sort. Overstrain, if you like, but that is largely caused by the mental and physical efforts to accommodate yourself to your new surroundings, and will pass off as you become accustomed to them; it is due to the struggle to remember so many new things at once—to the number of unnecessary steps taken by the newcomer in her ignorance—the needless expenditure of strength and energy over tasks that in a little while become familiar with practice, and, therefore, far less exacting. You all remember how tired you felt after the first day or two, when the excitement of novelty began to wear off; more tired than ever you do now, even after a specially heavy day because you are becoming more used to the work.

The form this early fatigue takes is usually that of tired and aching or swollen feet from the unaccustomed standing and running about, so because of this the off-duty outdoor exercise is shirked. Now your feet being a most important asset in your physical stock-in-trade must not be neglected. First see that your shoes are well fitting, being neither too loose nor too tight. They should be soft and flexible, with soles not too thin, and moderately low heels with India rubber pads. A perfectly new pair should not be put on for the first day's work in hospital and be worn all day. They are sure to make the feet ache. It is best to have two pairs in use, changing into slightly older ones towards the end of the day. Wash the feet daily, night and morning, and if they are inclined to perspire, dust between the toes with boracic powder, and rub the soles with methylated spirit. See that your stockings fit well and are free from lumpy darns. Wear no garters nor tight bands of any kind. On coming off duty remove the shoes and lie down flat for half an hour, with the feet slightly above the level of the body. This will rest them, and make it possible afterwards to change into walking shoes and go outdoors for an hour. Persistent aching must be reported, as you may be threatened with flat foot. A remedy for this in its early stages is to raise one's self on tip-toe several times, once or twice a day, and to rest as much as possible. Any varicose veins in the leg or continued swelling of the ankles at night must also be reported.

Another trouble is apt to arise from the hands. In cold weather and from constant use of antiseptic lotions some nurses suffer greatly from chilblains and chapped hands. To prevent them is not easy, but the hands should not be put into cold water if it can be avoided, and must be well dried after washing. A little pure glycerine rubbed in after drying, and every night before going to bed, helps to keep them from chapping; cotton gloves should be worn for sleeping in, and woollen ones when outdoors. Hands subject to chilblains should not be held too near the fire when cold, and must be kept as warm as possible. Plenty of milk, butter and fatty food should be taken, and perhaps cod-liver oil will be needed as well. If the chilblains are on the feet, woollen stockings should be worn, and the general circulation needs improving. Open-air exercise is beneficial if the person is warmly clothed.

Coughs, colds and sore throats are also among the minor ills of winter time. Proper food and sufficiently warm underclothing, plenty of fresh air and cold baths, with avoidance of hot, crowded places, will often serve to prevent such ailments. A habit of breathing through the nose rather than the mouth will also render you less susceptible to the infection.

Sore throat is less often the result of cold than of enlarged tonsils, or some septic infection. It is one of those things that a nurse must always report to her ward sister or matron, as it may mean diphtheria, with consequent danger to others as well as herself if she is allowed to go about her daily work as usual. Other ailments that must likewise be reported without delay are a rash of any kind, a rise of temperature, and a poisoned finger. This last, if taken in time, may save weeks of treatment, but if not, may mean the loss of a finger and a dangerous illness. A prick with a safety pin is usually the beginning of this trouble, and soon after a throbbing pain is felt at the end of the finger, when a boracic fomentation should be at once applied, and the matter reported.

Toothache, indigestion, and constipation are all troubles that are apt to lie in wait for the nurse in her first year; sometimes also anæmia with other irregularities, which need not cause anxiety, provided the general health is not affected.

Many of these ailments may be prevented by right living and regular habits, and the tendency to some of them will diminish as you grow older, but they must not be neglected, nor treated by attempting to drug yourselves. This practice cannot be too strongly condemned, and is strictly forbidden in all training schools.

First Chapter: Bertha Harmer, 1922

Bertha Harmer (1885–1934) was born in Canada and received her diploma in nursing education in Canada. She earned both the bachelor's and master's degrees in nursing in the United States. In 1928, after working and studying in the US for 13 years she returned to Canada to teach at McGill University. In 1922 she published her textbook, *Text-Book of the Principles and Practice of Nursing.*[14] It was a well-received book that went to three editions (1922, 1928, 1934) during her lifetime and, after her death, was continued by Virginia Henderson (US) for another two editions (1939, 1955). Here we have more entangled history, more entangled literature.

The Ideal of Service

Harmer is not the only nurse author to view *service* as the guiding ideal of nursing. It is a continuing perspective from the mid-1800s into the 1960s. It may credibly be asked if *service* is a better metaphor for nursing than the contemporary *caring*.[15] Perhaps caring should be viewed as a local metaphor, for us for now. However, her notion that "nursing is rooted in the needs of humanity and is founded on the ideal of service" challenges nursing to interrogate its received options.[16] It is important to notice that Harmer links nursing to preventive health, social services, and the heath of the public, an expansive view of nursing's purview. Given social structures that obstruct, Harmer has, perhaps, an outsized view of what education for health can accomplish in society. She does recognize that some impediments to the health of individuals can be ameliorated through social services. Her section on the responsibility of the nurse to the person who is sick is lovely. She writes:

> nursing springs from the ideals of service, love and brotherhood—of service to those in trouble, sorrow, sickness or pain and in the time of death. There is no person (except possibly the physician and the clergyman) who touches so closely on the inner life of the people. The nurse is with them when all the conventions of life seem trivial, when all the barriers and reserves are broken down and the innermost cherished and secret thoughts, hopes, and fears stand revealed. *Sympathy*, *kindness* and *unselfishness* are needed but also something more—something deeper and more helpful, more loving and spiritual which may support the patient with a feeling of strength, security, and comfort.[17]

There is a recognition of the vulnerability of the patient, the intimacy that resides within the nurse–patient relationship, and the intangibles, aesthetics, and good intrinsic to nursing resident within that relationship in expert nursing. So as not to overwork the commentary on this first chapter, it is presented here for closer examination.

THE PRINCIPLES AND PRACTICE OF NURSING, CHAPTER I: INTRODUCTION. THE OBJECT OF NURSING, WHAT IT IS, AND WHAT IT INCLUDES

Let us begin by considering what the object of nursing is, so that we may have a goal to strive for, a guiding purpose by which we measure what we are and what we do and a central controlling idea by which we see the bearing and relation of all our studies and experience and which serves to link them together so that we may remember and utilize them. For, if we have a definite object in view, we are naturally interested in whatever leads us toward it and in what we are interested we eagerly pay attention, deriving both pleasure and profit and learning, not without effort—for nursing demands our highest efforts—but with the effort which brings a glow of satisfaction for work well done. "The imagination of great men feeds upon difficulties and exercises itself upon overcoming them."

Nursing is rooted in the needs of humanity and is founded on the ideal of service. Its object is not only to cure the sick and heal the wounded but to bring health and ease, rest and comfort to mind and body, to shelter, nourish, and protect and to minister to all those who are helpless or handicapped, young, aged or immature.

Its object is to prevent disease and to preserve health. Nursing is therefore linked with every social agency which strives for the prevention of disease and the preservation of health. The nurse finds herself not only concerned with the care of the individual but with the health of a people. Her influence is spreading far and wide and deep into the hearts and problems of the people. We find her, not only in positions such as Inspector of Training Schools, Hospital Superintendent, Instructor, Supervisor or Dietitian and Laboratory Expert, but engaged in the boundless field of Public Health, Social Service, School Nursing, Infant Welfare, Industrial Nursing, Rural Nursing, and other fields. An eminent critic has said that the final test, as portrayed in the last Day of Judgment, is a social test—did ye visit the sick, the poor, the hungry? Nursing includes all of this.

What Nursing Includes.—Many years ago Florence Nightingale taught "that all disease, at some period or other of its course, is more or less a reparative process" and "that the symptoms or the sufferings generally considered to be inevitable and incident to the disease are very often not symptoms of the disease at all, but of something quite different—of the want of fresh air, or of light, or of warmth, or of quiet, or of cleanliness, or of punctuality, and care in the administration of diet, of each or of all of these,"—in other words,—in the want of good nursing, for nursing is concerned with and includes all of this.

To-day Dr. Hare, an eminent authority in the treatment of disease, in the directions given to his students, says: "In the treatment of all forms of disease the physician must never forget the following influential factors in the case, which are often of greater importance than the measures devoted to the treatment of the disease itself.

1. The maintenance of vital resistance by proper feeding.
2. The elimination of effete materials by the kidneys, bowels and skin.
3. The relief of annoying symptoms which sap the patient's vitality and often obscure the true state of the system.
4. That sufficient physical and mental rest and sleep are obtained if possible."
5. Nursing is concerned with and includes all of this.

It includes:—(1) The care of the patient's surroundings (which should be clean, attractive, quiet, orderly and comfortable) and of all things which add to his welfare and promote his recovery; (2) the personal care of the patient—bathing, feeding, making comfortable and attending to his personal wants, mental or physical; (3) assisting the physician—preparing for and assisting with examinations, treatments, operations and tests, and observing and reporting the condition of the patient and results of treatments, etc.; (4) the administration of special diets, drugs and treatments, etc. ordered; (5) teaching—in the hospital the older nurses teach the younger nurses and each nurse consciously or unconsciously by example teaches the patients, especially the children, the standards of personal hygiene. In all public health work, the whole problem is being attacked on an educational basis. Nursing here is teaching the individual proper habits of living relating to food, rest, exercise, recreation, sleep, and all the conditions which insure health of body and mind and increased resistance to disease; (6) informing the patients that, in the hospital, there is a Social Service Department which exists in order that patients, in need of its care, may consult with it and be relieved of financial difficulties and of worries regarding conditions in their homes. This department also makes provision for their convalescence and will give instruction regarding their future health and care. It will take care of all matters which might hinder their present recovery, restoration to, and preservation of health. Nurses should report to the Social Service Department all patients who are in need of its care.

THE SPIRIT, IDEALS AND POINT OF VIEW DESIRABLE
Responsibility of the Nurse in her Relation to the Sick.—As stated above, nursing springs from the ideals of service, love and brotherhood—of service to those in trouble, sorrow, sickness or pain and in the time of death. There is no person (except possibly the physician and the clergyman) who touches so closely the inner life of the people. The nurse is with them when all the conventions of life seem trivial, when all the barriers of reserve are broken down and the innermost cherished and secret thoughts, hopes, and fears stand revealed. *Sympathy, kindness* and *unselfishness* are needed but also something more—something deeper and more helpful, more loving and spiritual which may support the patient with a feeling of strength, security, and comfort.

Now, while all may have this spirit of sympathy, kindliness and helpfulness, even to the degree of self-sacrifice, at the beginning of training, it must be very carefully cherished and developed. If we neglect it and, day by day, in the rush, strain and fatigue, feel impatience and indifference, we may become incapable of feeling, and hardened. Nurses have sometimes, with justice, been accused of this. We must weed out such harmful thoughts and encourage kind thoughts and actions. No one becomes kind except by being kind, and no one can win this spirit of love and service unless they, day by day, do acts of kindness. In no field is there such light and warmth and inspiration, such a rich opportunity for fullness of development. Dr. Osler has said: "There is no higher mission in life than nursing God's poor. In so doing, a woman may not reach the ideal of her soul; she may fall short of the ideals of her head; but she will go far to satisfy those long-ings of the heart from which no woman can escape." It is distinctly a woman's work—the one profession in which women are admitted by all to excel men.

A cheerful, optimistic spirit is also very helpful both to the patient and the nurse. While the hospital is often a place of sadness, it is not one of gloom but often of rejoicing. It is our part not only to do the right things but to enjoy, to look and act as though we enjoyed. Gloom is most depressing to the mind and reacts very unfavorably on the patient's progress. Cheerfulness and optimism act as a tonic, or like sunlight—which is now recognized as one of the great healers. Cheerfulness must not be confused with frivolity or thoughtless mirth which disregards the sorrows of others. Sick people are very sensitive to the actions and presence of those around them. Happy persons bring new courage and give a new hold on life and this is valuable as the patient must help himself to live, so that his mental attitude is important. A nurse can do much to cultivate this spirit both in herself and her patients.

Reliability and **trustworthiness** in the care of patients and in carrying out in-structions, which inspires the confidence of patients, friends and superior officers.

Obedience and **willingness to be guided** by those responsible for the care of the patients and by those responsible for and striving for the interests and education of nurses.

The **Spartan spirit** which will not flinch from duty, which makes light of discomforts and dangers, and welcomes hard tasks; which is firm and unyield-ing in the face of duty but avoids an antagonistic attitude.

A professional spirit—a feeling of loyalty, not only to one's school but to the whole profession with a spirit of cooperation and desire to promote its in-terests as a whole.

A scientific spirit which promotes a love of truth and avoids exaggerations and vague, misleading statements or actions, which is not influenced by senti-mentality, which promotes a wholesome spirit of inquiry but never loses a feel-ing of wonder and reverence for the human body.

A critical attitude toward one's own work which may be measured by the following results:

(a) The speed and completeness of the patient's recovery.
(b) The comfort and satisfaction, freedom from suffering and worry for the patient and relatives.
(c) Economy of effort, time, and materials in nursing.
(d) The neatness and finished appearance of the work.

A spirit of appreciation of the work and all that it signifies. This includes (1) an *esthetic appreciation* in seeing a beautiful piece of finished work such as a beau-tifully made bed; (2) an appreciation of delight experienced in actually doing skilled work; (3) an *appreciation* of *human nature*, of the value of human life, of the greatness and weakness of humanity, of all its virtues and trials; (4) an *intellectual appreciation* in the sciences, etc., and study of diseases. Appreciation in all its phases must be developed. It makes one fall in love with, become absorbed in, and thoroughly enjoy one's work. But one must avoid the danger of developing one at the expense of the other. For instance, our delight in making a bed quickly and skilfully and our pleasure in seeing it beautifully finished, if overstressed may make us forget the patient in the bed so that he will be quite unable to appreciate it, however beautiful. Again, our intellectual pleasure in learning may cause us to regard the patient as a "case" forgetting that he is a human being. "The intellectual faculties of memory, judgment and criticism in studies—leave the learner cold—he knows, but it does not make any difference to him, he lacks sympathy and understanding."

It has been said that "a man's conscience is not the producer but the product of his career" and as ye sow ye shall reap; so that habits of sympathy, of kindness, and patience, or thoroughness, persistence, and punctuality have a real moral value.

A democratic spirit which leaves class and race prejudice behind. In a hospital it is the aim to give the same kind of care to men, women and children, to all colors and creeds, rich and poor, enemies and friends.

THE KIND OF QUALITIES AND TRAINING NEEDED
Health of mind and body which gives a wholesome, cheerful, sane outlook, steady nerves, a mind and body well under control with strength and endurance necessary to give the best care to the sick. Strength and vigor radiate from a healthy body and invigorate the weak.
Knowledge.—

1. Of oneself—one's strength and weakness and capacities.
2. Of the sciences—anatomy and physiology, bacteriology, chemistry, physics, psychology and sociology, etc.
3. The household sciences—housekeeping, household management, dietetics.
4. The methods used in the prevention of disease and the preservation of health—sanitation and personal hygiene, etc.
5. Disease and its treatments, etc.

Trained Faculties.—

1. Manual dexterity is essential. The hands must be deft, strong and capable, quick and light but steady, firm but gentle, sensitive to impressions, never nervous or hesitating, but with a sure touch.
2. Trained senses (the eye, ear, sense of smell, taste and touch)—quick, keen, accurate observation, alert for signs which note improvement or danger—all the windows and doors of the mind open and a mind trained and educated to respond immediately in the right way.

3. Nerves cool and steady, a mind quick in seeing and grasping things, re-sourceful, well-poised, quick-witted, undismayed by the unexpected, ready for emergencies.

4. Foresight, judgment, good sense and reasoning powers, decision, and fine discrimination.

5. A good memory, exact and reliable, which depends largely upon interest, attention, and training.

6. A real interest in people, a desire for their welfare and the faculty of making this felt; tact, cooperation, the ability to handle people and get along with them—if this is lacking, all the other virtues, capacities and knowledge may be of little value. Learn to understand and influence people.

7. A manner pleasing, discreet and courteous, soothing, not irritating, winning the confidence of friends and patients, firm and unyielding in duty without antagonizing.

8. Expression—ability to control one's emotions, the voice quiet and gentle, the expression of the face kindly, serene, impassive; ability to report, either in writing or orally, concise, clear, accurate statements unvarnished by sentiment.

9. Executive ability requiring foresight, the ability to organize, of getting things done on time, of subordinating nonessentials to essentials, of keeping a number of things in hand at once, running smoothly with no excitement or confusion—the ability of managing affairs and people.

PRACTICAL NURSING, ITS CORRELATION WITH THE CLASS-ROOM; ITS SUPERVISION

The time spent by the student on the wards in the care of her patients is the most valuable, the most memorable in her training. There is a wealth of priceless knowledge to be gained in the study of the patient. A nurse can gain knowledge regarding the patient himself, his history and social background, his symptoms, the tests used in diagnosis, his treatment and the results. This is a study fascinating and stimulating to the mind, the imagination and the sympathies, and is capable of developing a large-mindedness, a breadth of view and purpose not found in other fields. It is here that the nurse develops not only skill, but develops also in sympathy, judgment, self-control, and in all the other qualities so desirable and necessary in a nurse. It is here that the nurse learns to tackle and solve problems efficiently, for this ability like every other ability can only come through practice and training in doing. It is here that she becomes equipped to become a useful member of society for "education must proceed through the eyes and hands to the brain." Remember that a nurse is judged, not by what she knows but by what she does. As Ruskin says: "Education is not to make people know what they do not know, but to make them behave as they do not behave." If nurses would remember this, we would not hear complaints about the "overtrained" nurse or of the nurse "good in theory but hopeless on the wards." Everyone (children and grown folk) admires, respects, and has confidence in a person who can do things. It gives one influence and power and this power can only come from practice in doing.

In after years the part that stands out in the memory of the nurse is the unforgettable knowledge gained in her experience on the wards. She feels that she has a firm grasp, which can never be taken away from her, and which cannot be bought or found in books. Knowledge which is in books may be learned at any time, but the experience on the wards can never be repeated—every moment is precious.

All the time spent in the classroom, in the study of the sciences, etc., however interesting and instructive in themselves, is merely a preparation for the vital work on the wards. It throws light, supplies facts and underlying principles, and saves time. It makes the instruction more efficient, directs the attention, stimulates and excites the interest, organizes the knowledge gained on the wards so that all students may share alike, and it gives the student tools to work with. The wards are the workshops where these tools are brightened and sharpened by application and use. The only sure test of the knowledge gained in the classroom is in its application or use in the care of the patients. As Dr. Osler used to say: "To study the phenomena of disease without books is to sail an uncharted sea, while to read books without patients is not to go to sea at all."

Without the knowledge and the underlying principles studied in the classroom, to care for the patients on the ward is to "sail an uncharted sea," without a guide, helm or rudder. The practice is unsafe and the knowledge gained meager, haphazard, and unsound and there is no provision for initiative and growth or a basis for constructive work.

Supervision.—As the nursing is usually done by students, all of whom are in the process of learning, supervision of the work is absolutely essential if the care of the patient is to be satisfactory and if the student is to receive adequate instruction—for how can the blind lead the blind and how can they learn without a teacher? Even the best of us need to be spurred along at times and are glad to have standards kept before us which we are obliged to keep.

The hospital has accepted a sacred trust in the care of the patients who have confidence in and are entirely dependent upon the hospital, its doctors, and nurses. The reputation of the hospital and the welfare of the patients depend upon the quality of the nursing, and this depends to a large extent upon adequate supervision by qualified supervisors. Pupils are apt to misunderstand and to resent this supervision whereas they should demand it as their right. They should recognize that this constant checking up is what upholds the standards of the school which attracted them to it and gives them reason to be proud of it. It is stated that much of the success of any school system depends upon the quality of supervision, and that expert constructive supervision is the most potent force, acting as a pressure on everyone to become stronger, more useful and efficient.

Students frequently forget, misinterpret, or fail to apply what is taught in the classroom. The classroom teaching must therefore, be followed by inspection on the wards, for "Behold, a sower went forth to sow, and when he sowed, some seeds fell by the wayside, and the fowls came and devoured them up; some fell upon stony places where they had not much earth, and forthwith they sprung up, because they had no deepness of earth: and when the sun was up, they were scorched and because they had no root, they withered away. And some fell among thorns and the thorns sprung up and choked them. But others fell into good ground and brought forth fruit."

The value of the supervision given will depend quite as much upon the student nurse as upon the supervisor. Supervision to be successful can never be one-sided. No matter how well-informed and thoroughly equipped a supervisor may be to give advice, assistance, and instruction, and no matter how sympathetic and willing she may be to share her invaluable experience, her time and energy will be largely wasted, her results will be most disheartening, her efforts and good intentions will be entirely misunderstood and the student will profit very little if the student, herself, does not feel the need for guidance and instruction and look to the supervisor for it. Supervisors do not go about on the wards among the patients as inspectors or policemen to interfere, to find fault, to give orders, or to deprive the students of freedom, but as experts in the interests of both patients and students, ready to serve the patients dependent upon the nurses for their care, and to serve the students who have come to the hospital to be trained and educated in the difficult art and science of nursing.

THE FACILITIES AND CONDITIONS NECESSARY FOR TRAINING

There is only one place where nurses can learn to nurse and that is in the wards of a general hospital or in a hospital affiliated with other hospitals which round out their experience. All the knowledge necessary cannot, nor should not, be learned at once. The student goes through definite stages of learning, each of which prepares for the work which is to follow: (1) The probationary term, during which she becomes familiar with the hospital—its relation to the community, its various departments, their relation to each other and to the whole—and with the part she is to play in this great scheme of physical, mental and social betterment. During this period the student should become proficient in all that pertains to the care, comfort, and treatment of the convalescent, the chronically ill, and the patients not acutely ill. She may also assist in the care of the acutely ill and in this way gradually acquire the art which nothing but experience can teach; (2) the junior, and (perhaps) part of the intermediate year, during which she becomes proficient in the care and treatment of medical and surgical diseases, —the remaining part of her training being devoted to the special branches in nursing and to experience in that branch to which she seems particularly adapted. This book follows the student in her work through the probationary term, the junior, and part of the intermediate year only.

There are a significant number of first chapters that warrant attention. These are but two, but they communicate a more condensed perspective on nursing virtues, values, duties and ideals—nursing ethics—that also offer fresh, sometimes poetic, insights into the development of nursing ethics. We turn, now, to the first extant journal article on nursing ethics.

First Journal Article: Harriet Camp, *The Trained Nurse and Hospital Review*, 1899

It was not uncommon for authors of early journal articles, editorials, and columns to sign their contribution with initials only. Presumably nurses in that day would have known who the author was, but that is lost on us today, especially where the person is not otherwise listed within the journal (e.g., its managing committee or section heads). The article below was written by HCC, Harriet C. Camp, later Lounsbery. It is the first extant article on nursing ethics and was published in a six-part series, each part focusing on different "classes" of relationship of the nurses, such as nurse-to-patient or nurse-to-society.[18]

Though she is not the first to do so, this article is particularly noteworthy in that it articulates a relational nature for the structure of nursing ethics. Earlier works also structured nursing ethics by relationships, but she appears to be the first to lay out and discuss the relationships in sequence. The seven relationships that she identifies will be reshaped over the coming decades; nursing ethics retains the notion of relational content and structure, from which duties arise, as central to its ethics. Much of the remainder of the article series is similar to the two first chapters above, though it remains to be fleshed out in the succeeding five articles.

The Trained Nurse.
Consecrated to those who Minister to the Sick and Suffering.
VOL. II. NO. 5. BUFFALO, N. Y. MAY, 1889.
THE ETHICS OF NURSING.
TALKS OF A SUPERINTENDENT WITH HER GRADUATING CLASS.
For convenience sake, I will divide the duties of a nurse into seven classes: 1st. Those she owes to the patient. 2nd. Those she owes to the doctor. 3rd. Those owing the family, friends, and servants of the patient. 4th. To herself. 5th. To her own friends. 6th. To her own hospital or school. 7th. To other nurses.

First then, let us consider the duties you owe the patient. You may consider it very unnecessary for me to tell you about "the patient." You will say perhaps: "Have I had all this training, and must I yet be told how to treat a patient?" I answer that you have been taught how to watch the progress of disease, how to follow intelligently the doctor's orders, also certain manual arts, your proficiency in which is unquestionably most necessary, but there is much more comprehended in the meaning of the term "a good nurse" then this. How often do we hear stories of nurses who were—good—*but*—who were skillful—*but*—and after the *but* comes a long list of such faults as do not show so much in hospital life, where the routing and the many rules, and constant supervision make them less likely to become prominent. "She bangs the doors." "She breaks the fine china." "She wears heavy shoes," or "she talks too much," or "she is pretty and spends too much time over her front hair"—but why go on? You have heard all such tales, ad nauseum, and if you are wise, you will set up a sign-post against every one of these snares into which your sister nurses have fallen, and on this you will print in large clear letters: "Danger! Walking on this place forbidden." So much by way of apology for treating you once more to a lecture on "the patient."

The relation between nurse and patient should, from the first, be a more than amicable one. You have come to bestow the priceless blessing of unwearied, skillful care upon one who should thankfully receive it, and believe me, if you do not go to your patient with a feeling of devout thankfulness to God for allowing you to assume such a sacred trust as the care of a human life, you are in no condition to undertake the work. Your nursing should be, in a way, an exponent of your own spiritual state; looking at it in its highest aspect, an outward and visible sign of an inward and spiritual grace.

In the first place then, you must be in entire sympathy with the sick one—and here do not mistake me—by sympathy I do not mean sentimentalism. The two emotions are as far asunder as the poles. Sympathy then you must have, and if you do not intuitively feel it let me tell you what to do to rouse your dormant feelings. Try earnestly to put yourself in the patient's place. Has she had an operation of some kind, and you have all night been trying to keep her quiet on her back, and she has been begging you to Let her turn "ever so little?" When you go to lie down, and have perhaps a backache and feel tired, instead of settling yourself in the most comfortable position you can lie straight and square on your back and say to yourself, "Now, I can't turn over," and imagine you have by your side a nurse who will not let you turn. You will find out in the course of an hour that your patient has had a good excuse for all her complaints, and the next night you will know just where to slip your hand in the hollow of the back and under the shoulders, to give a little ease. The patient will profit by such exercise on the part of the nurse, and your sympathies will be quickened. Never forget that the patient is sick, and you are not. You can, you must indeed be firm in what you know is for your patient's best good, but you must never be dictatorial, or argumentative. It is hard I know to bear with all the foolish, unreasonable whims of sick people, but if you are true nurses, you will do it. There are, however, several consoling thoughts which have always helped me, and which I will tell you. In the first place always remember, as I said before, that the sick one *is* sick, and on that ground you can overlook much. In the second place remember that it will not last long. A few days or weeks will surely bring a change. She cannot in the nature of disease remain for long in the very trying stage, unless indeed she have some kind of mania, and of course if that is the case, you need pay no attention to her whims. If she says white is black, let it go. It does not make it so to have her say so, but if you argue the point, and bring all your wisdom to bear upon your demonstration, you may bring her pulse and temperature up to a point that will do her a real injury.

Tact, my dear girls, is worth everything to you, and by its use you will win your way to all hearts. Try then to feel as the patient does, and you will know by instinct how to treat her, and will, perhaps, be often rewarded for some little deed by the pleased surprise with which she will say: "How did you know I wanted it done?" You need not tell her how you knew, but you may be sure she will appreciate you all the more for your prescient thoughtfulness. Her pillows may be flat and hot, her hair uncomfortable, her under sheet wrinkled or untucked from the bottom, all these and a dozen more little things can be arranged so easily, and they conduce so much to the sick one's comfort when done, that you must ever have them and a hundred matters in your mind.

Be most careful also as to your patient's belongings, her top drawer, her various boxes, and her linen closet. You must keep all these things just as she did. You may think it a very foolish thing for her to have three piles of handkerchiefs each of a different age, or degree of fineness, but if that is her way, she will be better if she knows you will not lay a fine handkerchief over a more common one. So keep them as carefully divided as if they were two parts of a Seidlitz powder.

Hang her clothes up carefully whenever she goes back to bed, be it once or often during the day. Separate them and hang them up; don't pick all up together and put them over a chair. Put her shoes away, lay the stockings on a shelf or put them inside the shoes. Fold her pretty shawl or wrap and lay it in a drawer. Let her see that you know a good thing, and how you take care of it.

Put away fine china or glass breakables, if she is very ill, and you need space for necessary glasses or traps. It will be a pleasant way of beguiling the tedium of some long day in her convalescence to bring forth and arrange them in their accustomed places. Be careful of books, table-covers, and all the articles of luxury and beauty you will find in many of our city houses. Remember that these things belong to some one else, though you are for the present the custodian, and think how provoked you would feel if some stranger should come to your home, and even if she did nurse you back to health, she left many nicked plates, broken vases and handleless cups behind her. I think you would not want her to nurse you again.

I saw recently in an English magazine devoted to nursing a very clever article on "Talk." The writer, a nurse, thought subjects were scarce. She says: "We must not talk to the patient about her own complaint, that would make her morbid; or about the doctor, for that would be gossip; or the hospital, for hospitals are full of horrors: or the other nurses, for that might lead to talking scandal; or about other patients, for that would be a betrayal of confidence. Now what *are* we to talk about when a patient is well enough to talk, and your talking to her will not hurt her (but on this point be very sure before you air your eloquence). It is indeed quite a question, and the nurse must often use all her ingenuity to keep the patient to the right subjects, for even patients, though they hold it so reprehensible in a nurse to talk gossip, do not disdain to serve up their neighbors occasionally to the nurse, with some very highly seasoned scandal sauce, and here the honor of the nurse must come into play. Let her forget it if possible, as woe will betide the poor girl if in her next place she unwittingly lets out any of the secrets she has heard in these long talks. Try then to steer clear of the neighbors. If your patient be a cultivated person, and you yourself know anything about books, you have a never-failing topic. All the latest books, the famous books, the most entertaining books, and if you can read aloud and the patient likes to hear you, read to her, and it will do both good—only be sure not to tire her by reading too much at one time. Talk of interesting places you have visited and she will do the same, of pictures you have seen, and last but not least, you can talk about clothes. Generally the first serious piece of business a convalescent concerns herself about is the purchase and making of some new clothes. She wants something new and fresh, and if you can give her any new ideas on the subject or tell her of any pretty materials you have seen in the shop windows, you will prove as entertaining as if you talked on any of the forbidden topics, and many times more useful.

I would like in closing to say a word about reading the daily papers. If your patient is a woman she will want to know just what you would. Marriages and deaths and such reasonable topics will interest her, only be sure there are no deaths that will shock her, but if your patient be a man, it is harder to know what he will want, men being interested in such stupid subjects as politics, etc., which most women wisely skip when they read a paper. Commence on the first page and read slowly the headings of the news items, and when one strikes him as interesting he will tell you to read it. When you get through with the news you may turn to the editorial page and do the same there, unless it chance to be during an exciting presidential campaign. Do not, unless you know your patient very well, attempt to enlighten him on the subject of the stock market, for it is, I suppose, well nigh impossible for an ordinary woman to read it so that a man could understand her. If you know your patient very well, he can and probably will laugh long and heartily at your well-meant endeavor, but he will not know much more about stocks when you finish than when you began.

Brooklyn, April 11, 1889 H. C. C.

Lavinia's Rubbish Bin

While there is substantial additional literature that could be examined, we must comment on the notorious graduation speeches. It was customary for schools of nursing to invite a physician to give a speech to the nurses about to graduate. Though there could be exceptions, such speeches often evidenced a profound ignorance of nursing and flagrant patriarchal, even misogynist, sentiment. Where the topic of the speech was ethics, it generally imposed a physician's self-serving desired preferences for nurses' behavior, had little to do with ethics, and nothing to do with nursing ethics. Lavinia Dock offered her typically direct and excoriatingly delicious remarks on the topic of physician graduation addresses to nurses:

> We have had many talks and addresses from the doctors; serious lectures, these; often they are published and stand for future time. We must find something in them all, surely, to nourish our out-reaching aspirations!
>
> Oh these yearly recurring talks! One on every graduation day and every training school throughout the land. Let us be frank and admit plainly, once for all, that they are wearisome, perennial rubbish. These men who among themselves are so brilliant, so learned, so interesting, how can they—from which of their brain-cells do they produce the thin, unflavored mental pabulum which they gravely serve out to us? And we, as we sit on the platform full of enthusiasm, how gladly would we hear something to stimulate and inspire us as thinking beings!
>
> What do we really hear? Advice about squeaking shoes and rustling aprons, about washing up the dishes and not making work for the servants...[19]

She is correct—there are any number of rubbish physician commencement addresses that litter the nursing ethics literature. It is not limited, however, to commencement addresses. Any number of physician speeches to nurses at congresses and conferences bear the same defects. There are some addresses, however, that are worth retaining.

Saved in the Recycle Bin

For the benefit of nursing scholars and historians, and nurses to come, there are addresses that are worthy of recycling, at least for the purposes of research and scholarship. The annual meetings of national nursing associations and the congresses of the International Council of Nurses frequently featured papers on a topic in ethics. Fortunately, the NLN annual minutes are now openly available online in digital format through the NLN Archives collection at the Barbara Bates Center for the Study of the History of Nursing.[20] The following speeches can be read in their respective annual minutes volume:

TABLE 3.2 Speeches from the NLN annual minutes

Author	Title	Minutes Year
Lavinia L. Dock	What Is a Trained Nurse and What Are Nursing Ideals?	1894
Ava Allerton	How Far Are Training Schools Responsible for the Lack of Ethics among Nurses?	1898
Lillian Wald	Work of Women in Municipal Affairs	1899
Lucy Walker	How to Prepare Nurses for the Duties of the Alumnae	1900
Lavinia L. Dock	The Duty of This Society in Public Work	1903
Lavinia L. Dock	International Relationships	1905
Laura A. Beecroft	Ethics to be Observed between Training Schools	1910
Charlotte M. Perry	Nursing Ethics and Discipline	1913
Mrs. C.G. Stevenson	The Organization of Nurses for a Legislative Campaign	1914
S. Lillian Clayton	The Purpose and Place of Ethics in the Curriculum	1916
Adelaide Nutting	Some Ideals in Training School Work	1916
Mrs. Wm Falconer	The Relation of the Graduate Nurse to the Problem of Social Hygiene	1917
Committee	Report of the Committee on Ethical Standards	1922
Annie W. Goodrich	The Objective of the Nurse in a Democracy	1922
Carolyn E. Gray	Ideals of the Nursing Profession for Schools for Nurses	1922
Clara D. Noyes	Relation of Nursing Education to Community and National Welfare	1922
Clarke P. Bissett	The Present Trend of Ethics	1922
Stevenson Smith	The Present Trend of Ethics	1922
Louise H. Powell & S.L. Clayton	Report of the Committee on Ethical Standards	1923
Laura M. Grant	Teaching of Ethics and Ethical Problems	1927
Effie J. Taylor	Interprofessional Relationships from the Viewpoint of the Superintendent of Nurses	1929
Elizabeth C. Burgess	Effect on Nursing Education of American Traditions and Ideals	1931
D. Dean Urch	Through Better Selection of Students	1932
Roundtable	Roundtable Report: Effective Teaching of Ethics	1932
Wm J. Ellis	What Society Needs from Nursing	1935
Isabel M. Stewart	Preparing Nurses to Meet the Needs of a Changing Society	1936
Rufus C. Harris	The Obligations of Citizenship	1939
Mildred Fairchild	The Responsibility of the Professions in a Democracy	1940
F. Ernest Johnson	Character Education	1940
Mrs. Curtis Bok	Character Education	1940
Elizabeth S. Soule	Democratic Philosophies for a School of Nursing	1941
Committee	Society's Need for Nursing Service	1950

Online, open access to annual minutes:
https://www.nursing.upenn.edu/history/archives-collections/nln-collection/

Unwilling to try the readers' patience further, this selection of works is but an *amuse-bouche* from a 150-year banquet that is nursing ethics. Readers are encouraged to read the 400 ethics articles that can be found in the *AJN* between 1900 and 1970, a similar number of articles in both the *Nursing Record* (later, *British Journal of Nursing*) and *Nursing Times*, additional first chapters, codes of conduct, and more. This is a largely unexplored and neglected body of literature. There is more awaiting exploration than can possibly be analyzed comprehensively by any individual scholar. It will require the concerted efforts of multiple scholars and graduate/doctoral students to subdue this extensive body of literature.

Notes

1 Sr. Rose Hélène Vaughan, *The Actual Incidence of Moral Problems in Nursing: A Preliminary Study in Empirical Ethics* (Washington, DC: Catholic University of America, June 1935).
2 Ibid., 16.
3 Augustino Lehmkuhl, *Theologia Moralis* (2 vols. cpl./2 Bände): *Vol. I: Theologiam moralem generalem et ex speciali theologia morali tractatus de virtutibus et officiis vitae christianae; Vol. II: Theologiae moralis specialis partem secundam seu tractatus De subsidiis vitae christianae cum duabus appendicibus* (Friburgi Brisgoviae: Herder, 1910).
4 Vaughan, *Moral*, 19.
5 Ibid., 21.
6 Ibid., 25.
7 Leonard I. Stein, "The Doctor–Nurse Game," *American Journal of Nursing* 68, no. 1 (1968): 101–105.
8 Leonard I. Stein, "The Doctor–Nurse Game," *Archives of General Psychiatry* 16, no. 6 (1967): 699–703.
9 Leonard I. Stein, David T. Watts, & Timothy Howell, "The doctor–nurse game revisited," *New England Journal of Medicine* 322, no. 8 (1990): 546–549.
10 Vaughan's thesis is available on Interlibrary loan from Catholic University, Washington, DC and a few other libraries. It is available, but not widely so.
11 E. Margaret Fox, *First Lines in Nursing* (London: Scientific Press, 1914), 1–10.
12 Ibid., 2.
13 Ibid., 3; italics added.
14 Bertha Harmer, *Text-Book of the Principles and Practice of Nursing* (New York: Macmillan, 1922).
15 Marsha D. Fowler, *Nursing's Ethics, 1893–1983: The Ideal of Service, the Reality of History.* (Los Angeles: University of Southern California. 1984).
16 Harmer, *Principles*, 3.
17 Ibid., 5.
18 Harriet C. Camp [RN], *Making Good on Private Duty: Practical Hints to Graduate Nurses* (Philadelphia: J.B. Lippincott, 1889). Reprinted 1912 under Harriet Camp Lounsbery. (Also known as: *The Nurse's Calling: Practical Hints to Graduate Nurses*). First chapter.
19 Lavinia Dock, "The Graduation Talk" *The Trained Nurse and Hospital Review* XXV, no. 2 (August 1900), 126.
20 https://www.nursing.upenn.edu/history/archives-collections/nln-collection/

4

NURSING ETHICS AS SOCIAL ETHICS

Moral Courage on the March

Modern nursing forms in a period of wide social ferment which both shapes and informs our earliest nursing leaders in their activities and aims, and in their understanding of the role of nursing in relation to society. From early days, nursing leaders shared a concern for establishing the social purview of nursing, for nursing's social engagement for the improvement of the health of society, for the preparation of nursing graduates to be active participants in political processes, and for laying the groundwork for political action that would then authorize and protect nursing practice in all its roles and venues. In this way, nursing ethics as a social ethics is the broader and prior understanding of nursing ethics that then "authorizes," shapes, and guides practice ethics. Nursing's social ethics is far broader and encompassing than is the distributive justice-based ethics of bioethics. We, thus, will begin with nursing ethics as a social ethics, before separately addressing nursing's practice-based ethics (see Chapters 8, 9), undertaking an examination of a single exemplar, venereal disease, that demonstrates the reach of nursing's social analysis, social critique, recommendations for social change activism, curricular change, and practice implications.

To be more specific, bioethics looks more toward clinical practice than toward the social structures that affect health, though even then the focus is on social structures that create disease, not health. The principle of justice, as deployed in bioethics, largely focuses on distributive justice, in a European philosophical, political theory, and Rawlsian social contract sense. Its concerns are those of access to care, cost of care, allocation of resources, tiered health care, fragmented medical care, insurance affordability; and access and treatment of vulnerable groups such as the elderly, persons with disabilities, and persons of racial or ethnic heritage. In recent years this has also included concerns such as racial and gender inequalities in treatment, "greening" of hospitals, and triage in natural or human-made disasters.

DOI: 10.4324/9781003262107-5

Often, where there is a focus on social structures, it is limited to aspects of the health-care system itself, and not to the social structures that are antecedent to the system. Contemporary nursing, by limiting its ethical concerns to those identified by bioethics, with its focus on *distributive justice*, betrays our brilliant heritage. Nursing ethics, that is, the ethics generated by the nursing profession from 1800s to the mid-1960s, prior to the importation of bioethics, had a far more capacious social ethics and view of social justice.

Wide Social Ferment

In the second half of the 1800s, the early modern nursing leaders attempted to establish the educational, clinical, legislative, and regulatory components that would give shape and authority to the profession. Their activity is profoundly affected by the social location of women; the proto-feminism ("first-wave feminism") of these nursing leaders; the social and structural concerns of the Progressive Era (from the 1890s to the 1920s); and their efforts to establish nursing as a paid, educated, scientific, standardized, rigorous, professional occupation for women, working outside the home and outside domestic service. These factors converge to shape the ethics of the profession *ab initio* as a distinctly social ethics. Yet 125 years later, nursing's movement into the university, its embrace of bioethics, the ebbing of nursing humanities and philosophy, and the decline of theoretical thinking in nursing education (and thus of nursology) has caused its social ethics to languish and its ethics to become stunted. If nursing were to reclaim its plucky tradition of *nursing social ethics*, it would have a more robust, vital, powerful, and clearer vision of the good society, the good nurse, and good patient care—or the healthy society, the healthy nurse, and the healthy patient.[1]

Women Must Have Power

As a woman from a wealthy and well-connected family, Florence Nightingale had direct access to the men who held political power, several of whom would willingly further her reformist ends. Nursing leaders who followed her, in both the UK and US, were middle- or upper-middle-class white, Christian women who lacked the political access available to Nightingale. They were also hindered both by laws and social norms that left women and the emerging women's profession of nursing without formal social power or authority. More specifically they did not have the power to create the structures foundational to the architecture of an emerging women's profession. The acquisition of social power would require the enfranchisement of women, that is, women's suffrage. In addition to the vote, other legal disabilities also constrained women, such as a married woman's right to own property, even inherited property; a right to control her own money; to have child custody in a divorce; a right to engage a lawyer; to being a person before the law (i.e., the abolition of coverture laws); rights of access to education, employment; and more, with some differences depending upon the country.[2] There were, of course, social limitations that compounded and tightened the legal manacles. To have the political clout to form a profession of nursing, and to effect changes in the health of society, required the power to vote and to pressure legislators formally in order to create the legal structures foundational to nursing such as licensure, registration; control, formalization and standardization of education; title protection, and more. As Lavinia Dock noted in 1909:

> Women must have the power to make laws and enforce them; it was not enough to help to administer those made by a masculine, law-making body. Women must attain the capacity to legislate for the making and remaking of social conditions of work and labor, wages and salaries, education, home, business, and public life.[3]

Dock and other nursing leaders, in many countries, were active in the women's suffrage movement. Nurses wearing nursing uniforms would march in the nurses' section of the women's suffrage parade in Washington, DC in March 1913. They were joined by women and nurses from Canada, England, Australia, Norway and other counties. The parade was attacked, and 300 women were injured.[4,5] Lavinia Dock was arrested three times for public support of women's suffrage. Some nurse suffragists who picketed, or marched, were attacked, jailed, beaten, force-fed in prison, and more. Some died in jail. This was moral courage on the march, moral courage in action, moral courage that risked all.

There were legal battles, but there were also cultural battles. One cultural battle that stood as a barrier to women, and nurses, was the firm conception of the proper role of women and the *cult of true womanhood*.

Cycling Out of the Cult of True Womanhood

An educated, scientific, paid profession for women working outside the home was at odds with the prevailing social norms for women embedded in the *cult of true womanhood*. It can be encapsulated by four key characterological attributes: piety, purity, submission, and domesticity. Piety meant Christian religious piety.[6] An examination of the advertisements in nursing journals of the period, particularly for uniforms and nurses' bicycling caps shows a struggle between nursing as a profession and nurses as women. Bioethics tends to focus, understandably, on medical technology. However, there are other technologies beside those of medicine that have been important to women and nurses. The bicycle would seem out of place in this discussion, but it has a complex social history that intertwines class, gender, feminism, nursing, technology, and transport.

The bicycle, originally the high wheel cycle (or penny farthing) with a large wheel in front and a small wheel behind, required extreme balance and risked taking a header over the handlebars. It was thus a popular symbol of white, leisure-class masculinity in the 1880s. The tricycle developed as a safer option but was too slow, so a compromise was reached in the invention of the two-wheel cycle with same-sized wheels, called the *safety bicycle*, or simply the *safety*. The *safety* enabled two transitions: female riders, and the extension of the bicycle as a means of transport for the working class instead of leisure-class recreation. Here, technological innovation contributes to changes in gender roles, and transportation.[7] Anne-Katrin Ebert writes that:

> For women, cycling was both a discovery and a revelation. Thanks to the bicycle, they experienced wholly new freedom and independence in motion.... the significance of the bicycle for the emancipation of women was disputed. While some articles assessed cycling, as well as sports for women in general, as a result of women's emancipation struggles, others saw cycling itself as the origin of emancipation and praised the bicycle as the emancipator of women.[8]

The bicycle required another, even more symbolic, change—the development of a split skirt, long enough to still hide the ankles. More socially problematic was the rejection of a split skirt in favor of a garment reserved for males: trousers. Some women scandalously chose to wear bloomers, associated with first-wave feminists or suffragists.[9] Ebert continues:

> It seemed that at least one thing was true: the superficial appearance of a freer life for women had met with more resonance than ethical or rational reasons. It was however desirable that the women and girls, who now so freely and independently cycled on the streets, realized that they had to also dedicate their energy to the core of the matter and actively collaborate in the "actual women's movement". It was time that female cyclists, who moved so freely in the outside world, recognized that they owed it to themselves and their gender to invest at least part of the fresh, young and healthy strength gained during bicycle excursions into the fight for political rights and equality with men in the civil code.[10]

Bicycles were a marker of the transition from the *cult of true womanhood* to the much-vilified *New Woman*. Nurses, both as professionals and as women who rode bicycles, were thereby rendered the *New Woman*. Bicycles would become essential to district, public health, and visiting nursing. On the 1985 centenary of District Nursing Services, Australia issued a postage stamp depicting a district nurse in uniform—with a bicycle (and a split skirt, ankles covered). The acclaimed BBC television show *Call the Midwife* demonstrates the importance of bicycles to nursing. Nurses continue to ride bikes though now they are e-bikes! Bicycles, a technological innovation, changed women's lives, clothing, transport, identity, freedom, emancipation from the cult of true womanhood; removed the bicycle from the province of the bourgeoisie—and facilitated working nurses' access to patients.

The cult of true womanhood "held that white women were rightfully and naturally located in the private sphere of the household and not fit for public, political participation or labor in the waged economy."[11] As an important aside, further note that "the white middle-class leadership of the first wave [feminist] movement shaped the priorities of the movement, often excluding the concerns and participation of working-class women and women of color."[12] Issues of class, gender, race, and religious tradition played a part in early nursing and even into the present. Some of these issues are coming to be addressed with greater rigor as in, for instance, the project An Overdue Reckoning on Racism in Nursing,[13] and the creation of the National Commission to Address Racism in Nursing.[14] Most of the early nursing leaders in the anglophone nations were white, women, Christian, middle or upper middle class, predominantly unmarried, and educated (perhaps in the home; not necessarily schooled).[15] To construct the legal floor joists necessary to support nursing was one thing—to prepare society for women to be formally educated for a paid profession was entirely another as it was implicitly an assault upon True Womanhood.

Bread and Roses

Overcoming the legal and social barriers to nursing necessitated battling on two different fronts, with women in both camps. Some women actively resisted suffrage, others simply declined to be involved. In 1912, suffragist Rose Schneiderman addressed a group of wealthy women on behalf of the Woman Suffrage Party. She herself was a Jewish immigrant, to the US from Russia, who worked in the cloth hat trade for 14 years and was a leader in the Great Shirt Waist Strike of New York City (1904).[16] Minerva Brooks reports that

> We called it a wonderfully human talk and blessed her for frankly telling her hearers that the wage-earning woman scorned the rich woman's charity, scorned to receive her patronage. She said, "What the woman who labors wants is the right to live, not simply exist—the right to life as the rich woman has the right to life, and the sun and music and art. You have nothing that the humblest worker has not a right to have also. The worker must have bread, but she must have roses, too. Help you women of privilege, give her the ballot to fight with.[17]

Both society and nursing had a privileged class and a laboring class which, in nursing, separated the nursing leadership from the working nurse. The class division in society continues to be replicated in nursing, in part, by means of its educational structure and system.[18,19,20,21,22] However, not all women or nurses, then or now, support "equality for women."

The Progressive Era

Modern nursing's emergence, and the women's movement for enfranchisement and suffrage, are coincident and intertwined with the Progressive Era and its wide-ranging social reforms. It was an era of vigorous social activism concerned to address social ills that had resulted from industrialization, urbanization, and conurbation. While progressivism in the US and in the UK differed, both in terms of means and ends, they both sought to rectify social ills, to improve society, living and work conditions. These included problems of urbanization, industrialization, immigration, political corruption, alcoholism, worker exploitation, child labor, and business and political corruption. More granular issues included overcrowded and unsanitary housing and transmissible diseases, inadequate clean water, contaminated milk supplies, poor nutrition, lack of sanitation, lack of health education; tuberculosis, polio, typhus, and cholera. This was largely a middle-class movement that addressed myriad ills in larger domains of government policies, civil rights, worker rights, politics, and society. Societal reforms included the education of children and women, the scientization and professionalization of teaching and of the academic disciplines including medicine, social sciences, history, economics, education, political science, and the humanities.

Early nursing leaders were engaged in a breathtaking array of civic and social reforms. The letterheads of the personal correspondence among early nursing leaders hints at the extent of their engagement.[23] There are letters written on letterhead for the Red Cross, the Anti-Vivisection League, the Vaccination League, the Society for the Prevention of Cruelty to Animals, various women's suffrage organizations, and groups involved in the reform of child labor laws, women garment workers' unionization, workers' rights generally, and more.[24] Women's suffrage, women's rights, and social reform is a full plate of social activism, even before adding lashings of nursing.

Nurses' Education for Social Engagement

Ultimately, the early nursing leaders (who included organizational as well as educational leaders) were concerned to imbue a commitment to social engagement in nursing students through curricular requirements and moral formation. The 1916, California Bureau of Registration of Nurses curriculum requirements for ethics for schools of nursing mandated lectures and extensive readings on "Democracy and Social Ethics," "Modern Industry," "Housing Reform," "The Spirit of Youth and the City Streets," and other social-ethical concerns.[25,26] In 1917, the National League for Nursing Education published its "Standard Curriculum for Schools of Nursing" requiring ten hours of lecture on ethics in the second year, commensurate with the hours allotted other major topics (see Chapter 1). The mandated social-ethics lectures, in sequence, included major sections on "Social Virtues" and "Ethical Principles as Applied to Community Life."[27,28]

Apart from these mandated topics, additional ethics content was expected to be taught in units (courses) in five of six semesters of the curriculum. The ample ethics content, particularly social ethics, of this curriculum bears little resemblance to the paltry contemporary curricular content on ethics in basic nursing education.

The early content is grounded in basic personal and professional ethics but is overwhelmingly oriented toward social concerns. While there is sturdy content on moral reasoning, there is little in the way of the dilemmatic or ethical-conflict content of today's curriculum. Instead, there is an emphasis on the moral character of the nurse, the moral aspects of the several nursing relationships, including the moral obligations of the nurse-to-self relationship which receives little if any attention in bioethics. These emphases in nursing ethics would serve to prevent dilemmas and a need for problem- or dilemma-focused ethics.

Nurse-to-Society Relationship—Nursing Ethics' Relational Structure

Nursing ethics was, and remains, structured around classes of relationships. In 1889, Harriet Camp gave a series of speeches to her graduating class in a six-part series, "The Ethics of Nursing," published in *The Trained Nurse and Hospital Review*. She writes:

> For convenience sake I will divide the duties of a nurse into seven classes: 1st. Those she owes to the family. 2nd. Those she owes to the doctor. 3rd. Those owing the family, friends, and servants of the patient. 4th. To herself. 5th. To her own friends. 6th. To her own hospital or school. 7th. To other nurses.[29]

This configuration reflects the fact that nursing predominantly took place in the patient's home and that most of Camp's graduates would be giving nursing care in the home. Camp does not focus on the broader range of nursing, including district, visiting, or public health nursing. Going forward, nursing ethics would continue to be structured around the classes of relationship, though those relationships would be recombined and reconfigured over the years, most often into five relationships. The reconfigurations included (a) nurse to patient/family, (b) nurse to physician and other health professionals, (c) nurse to self, (d) nurse to profession and nurse-colleagues, and (e) nurse to society. Most of the nursing ethics textbooks dealt, intentionally, with all of these relationships, though there were some that focused exclusively on the nurse-to-patient relationship. The ethics of nursing articulated through these relationships suffused the theoretical and practical curricula and the clinical apprenticeship. The current American Nurses Association (ANA) *Code of Ethics for Nurses with Interpretive Statements, 2015* (the Code) retains the relational structure, though it reduces the relationships to three broad classes.[30] The ANA Code is a vestigial remnant of nursing ethics in an era now dominated by bioethics.

In terms of the nurse's relationship to society, students and graduates were formed into active civic engagement through lectures, conference papers, and more. The most basic level of the duties within the nurse-to-society relationship became the duty to vote (after suffrage was passed), or more specifically to be an informed voter. But even before suffrage was achieved, nursing leaders demonstrated a commitment to the rectification of social ills *as nurses*. However, the duty to vote, *as nurses*, even after suffrage was initially passed met with very specific legal obstacles.

Women, Legally Fettered

Legislation for suffrage was nothing short of a mess. It could be granted and then rescinded, could have restrictions such as voting in municipal but not national elections; and could have voting criteria for men and women that differed, to women's disadvantage. There were also hard racial divides with white women receiving the vote, but indigenous persons, male and female, would wait several decades to be enfranchised. In general, suffrage was granted in the UK in 1918 for women at the age of 30, but 21 for men. In 1928, equal suffrage was granted. In the US, some states granted suffrage, and some did not. Eventually, the 19th amendment to the US Constitution granted women's suffrage, in 1920, though in some states black Americans were denied access to the vote until it became protected in the civil rights movement of 1965. Canada passed women's suffrage for most of the country in 1917–1919, though First Nations persons would not receive the vote until 1960 when the requirement for ceding prior status was dropped. Australia passed women's suffrage for nonindigenous persons in 1902 and full suffrage in 1962. New Zealand stands out heroically as granting universal women's suffrage in 1893.

The conditions for individual women to be enfranchised presented a peculiar problem for British nurses. The condition for Local Government Franchise, upon which Parliamentary Franchise was based, was as follows:

A woman—provided she is of full age [30] and subject to no legal incapacity— who occupies as owner or tenant any land or premises in the local government electoral area for six months... Any woman lodger... who has occupied an unfurnished room or rooms for the same period will be deemed a tenant. Any woman... who inhabits any dwelling house by virtue of any office, service, or employment (namely, matron of a hospital, headmistress living in a school house, etc.), and the employer under whom she serves in such employment does not reside in the house, will be a tenant. Every eligible woman should go to her local Town Hall and see that her name is on the Occupiers' list.[31]

Under these criteria, the matron (similar to a clinical nurse manager in the US) qualified for the vote but nurses did not, as they did not have exclusive access to their rooms. While the nurses had a key to their own rooms, the matron had a key to all their rooms. Legally, "The control of nurses' rooms in English hospitals rests, it must be admitted, in the matron and not in the nurse."[32] One British nurse proposed:

If hospitals in this country would adopt the plan, which has been introduced with considerable success... in the United States, the difficulty... would be overcome... At those American hospitals the management of the nurses' homes or nurses' quarters is entirely in the hands of the nurses themselves... the matrons have nothing to do with them.[33]

Ultimately, both British[34] and American nurses were enfranchised. They could then set their course for social change and the development of nursing as a profession.

Lavinia Dock (1859–1956), an American, was a suffragist, nursing leader and social activist in both the US and UK. She was a co-founder, with Ethel Gordon Fenwick, of the International Council of Nurses (ICN), served as ICN secretary for 22 years and was instrumental in the founding years of the ANA and NLNE. In 1909, she expressed concern that younger nurses have forgotten or perhaps never known the struggles of their predecessors, and what it meant in enabling nurses to engage in social change. She writes, in the effusive rhetorical style typical of the period:

> I have felt greatly concerned about the nurses' attitude, because it shows that they had forgotten—or that the younger ones had never learned—that we owed our existence as an educated and respectable profession to the woman movement... The fact of this enormous debt, and that we would simply not exist, except as miserable Gamps and slaves, had it not been for the uprising of women (and I contend that the claim for the ballot cannot be separated from the general advance of women) makes the whole question... take on a very different aspect. For I feel that our younger members need to be told what has gone before... Oh, how much there is to be done that will never get done until women have power!... Child labor will not be ended in this country until women have the ballot. And I am perfectly certain that the question of venereal disease, resting as it does on the basis of prostitution, will never really be solved until that day, when women, realizing their sacred responsibility to the race, enact laws that will assist and encourage educational propaganda which must, of course go hand in hand with prevention... that has been made plain in Tuberculosis propaganda; but that is the glorious thing about education as to diseases is that it brings you straight and unerringly, and with no delay, down to the social causes which are contributory, and which need legislation for their removal. This strong light thrown on evil social conditions will show more urgent reasons for removing them than could be done by a century of argument.[35]

Like Dock, it is not inappropriate to express a similar concern that nurses today, unfamiliar with the history of women's suffrage and nursing history, and the costs of that history, have

> forgotten—or that the younger ones had never learned—that we owed our existence as an educated and respectable profession to the woman movement... The fact of this enormous debt, and that we would simply not exist... had it not been for the uprising of women.[36]

That uprising was not without its faults in that it most benefitted white women. And yet, the strength of uprising, with an equitable incorporation of persons of color, its ability to change society, its ability to improve the health of the nation, resides within nursing today—if nursing were collectively to exercise it.

While voting was the lowest level of expected civil engagement, it was foundational to protecting and developing the profession and practice of nursing, and ultimately to the power of nursing to work toward social change. Factors in the social construction of the conditions of illness and disease, and of health disparities, were vigorously denounced by the early nursing leaders. The amelioration of "evil social conditions" was seen as within nursing's duties to society and the expertise of nurses. The early nursing literature emphasizes that the nurse-to-society relationship includes the moral obligation to vote, stand for office if so skilled, and to advocate for the social changes that would provide for the health and well-being of all the residents of the nation. The *Nursing Record* (later the *British Journal of Nursing*) regularly reported on and reprinted excepted minutes of the actions of Parliament so that nurses would be politically informed, and also aware of nursing organizational participation in political action.

The editor of the *Nursing Times* (UK) asks "How shall I vote?" and indicates that the answer to this question requires nurses to ask "the kind of government we think desirable" to address the countless social problems.

> With regard to domestic affairs, as distinct from Imperial ones... there are many questions of housing (we shall want a healthy home for everyone, at a cost within the means of the wage earners); questions of equal pay for equal work; of divorce (is it fair that there should be inequality between men and women?); of infant life protection; of the motherhood of the nation; of the supply of pure milk; and so on.[37]

Not only were these thought to be questions women should tackle, but that nurses were particularly equipped to do so.

> "What will women do with the vote?," people are asking... We are members of one another; beyond the individual is the family or the profession; beyond the family or the profession is the community; beyond the community is the State; beyond the State is the nation; beyond the nation is the race. We want to use our newly acquired right of citizenship for the good of all these... such questions as education, housing, infant mortality and welfare come within the scope of women, and more especially of nurses, and all these are questions for Parliament. We remember rightly, on the historic occasion when a woman dared to appear on the floor of the House of Commons... the matter under discussion was flannelette for babies! And a question of the most vital importance to district nurses and midwives at this very moment is the adequate supply of milk for infants... Great questions—such as prohibition, conscription, foreign policy—are,

after all, only little questions writ large. Whether the supply of drink should be restricted, whether every man should be called into service... these are concerns of us all very closely indeed.... We look forward with high hopes that women will rise nobly to their grand opportunities for improving this old world, so that it may be a better and happier home...[38]

The expectation was expressed as a duty of individual nurses to strive for the social changes that would improve individual and national health. It was the collective responsibility of the professional association to act politically on behalf of both the society and the profession. Here, Dock acknowledges the ANA's "enormous *latent* power and influence which it possesses" over against her dismay regarding "the actual influence exerted and made manifest."[39] In Dock's estimation, admittedly quite demanding, the ANA had not lived up to its potential and promise:

> But to what extent is the [nursing] society an influence? To what extent does it affect the public? How much does it actually guide nursing education? What weight has it with hospital managers and staffs? What amount of force does it bring to bear on its own members in questions of education, ethics, etc.? An honest searching after true answers to all these questions will inevitably bring the admission that the society, in all these rather abstract but most important ways, has not done what it might do; has not made itself a moral force; is not a public conscience; takes no position on large public questions; is not feared by those of low standards; allows all manner of new conditions and developments in nursing affairs to arise, flourish, succeed, or fail without taking any notice whatever of them, apparently not even knowing about them. I am speaking—let me repeat—of the society as a body, not of individual members. Yet this society, as one body, would often be astonished at the actual extent and weight of its influence if its whole latent and at present unsuspected power were actually to be systematically exerted in an intelligent and energetic manner.[40]

She is not simply critical but proposes association changes that would enhance ANA's efficacy in society. She does acknowledge that the ANA formed a nurses' association, developed and offered a teacher's course to prepare nursing educators, and convened congresses, but that was not enough in terms of social criticism and social change.

The whole of society and indeed the world was, in the words of Benjamin Franklin, nursing's "hard nut to crack." Doing so was a social-ethical vision for nursing that subsequently waned as nursing left the hospital schools, entered the universities, gave up their libraries, ceded ethics to philosophers, and embraced bioethics. The social concern of bioethics does not have the compass of nursing ethics. This is, thus far, simply a thin overview of the social ethics of nursing as the core of nursing ethics. It is time to give it teeth with a specific, paradigmatic social issue: venereal disease. Though there is much written on this issue by a number of authors in early nursing journals, the work of three nurses, Irishwoman Albinia Broderick[41] (1861–1955), American Lavinia Dock, and Englishwoman Mary Burr are noteworthy for the purpose of examining nursing's social ethics.

The Social Evil

Here, we will use venereal disease as a single, stand-in, issue to represent nursing social ethics, that is, its engagement with social criticism and social change. To preserve the delicacies of social discourse, venereal diseases were referred to as *The Social Evil*. Venereal diseases were the scourge of societies around the globe, always worsening during wartime and worse around military bases. Antibiotics were in the distant future. Penicillin, which would become a strong line of defense, would not be available in a stable and easily produced form until 1943. Sir William Osler (1849–1919), a Canadian physician, and one of the co-founding professors of Johns Hopkins Hospital, called syphilis "the fourth killing disease, the other three being heart complaints, cancer, and tuberculosis."[42]

There was major concern about the transmission of venereal diseases between prostitutes and military men, prostitutes and civilian men, then men to their wives, wives to their unborn children, and patients to nurses. As venereal disease (then identified as syphilis, gonorrhoea, and soft chancre) ravaged society, it became a whole-society argument with various phalanxes including the military, nurses, physicians, church leaders, suffragists, and others. It largely boils down to two distinctively different approaches: *social morality* and *social hygiene*. In this period, *social* is a pristinated term for *sexual*. This is a Gordian knot that cannot be untied here, as multiple movements are intertwined in this period, including early feminism and suffrage, workers' rights, eugenics, birth control, sex education, prostitution, "white slavery," censorship and pornography, illegitimacy, utopianism, abolitionism, temperance, drug abuse, violence against women and domestic violence, and much more. There are also major issues of class, gender, and race that are likewise entwined. A brief review of the oppositional positions of the *social morality* and the *social hygiene* movements is important to an understanding of the social ethical engagement of early nursing with these issues.

The Social Morality Movement

The Social Morality Movement, also called the Social Purity Movement, was an Anglo-American, middle-class movement from the 1860s to about 1910 with some remnants persisting even today. The larger movement aligned disparate forces to the common end of the abolition of female prostitution. The movement is rooted in the work in England of the remarkable Josephine Butler (1828–1906). Butler, a middle-class woman married to an Anglican divine, campaigned for women's suffrage, for the right of women to better education; for the end of coverture in British (and American) law; for the abolition of female child prostitution, and for an end to "white slavery," that is, to trafficking of girls and young women from England into

Continental prostitution; and for an end to the prevailing sexual double standard. While this is a multi-pronged movement, its emphasis is on the end of prostitution and attendant venereal disease, and an end to the sexual double standard. A concern for justice for women generally, and prostitutes specifically, and a good bit of anger, propelled this movement, though for many there was also a religious commitment underneath. This was largely a woman and feminist, white, middle-class movement oddly joined by working-class men.

A socially unexpected tsunami of women and feminist efforts was precipitated by the surreptitious passage of the UK Contagious Disease Acts of 1864, 1866, and 1869, (contemporaneous with the founding of the Nightingale Training School for Nurses at St Thomas' Hospital, London (1860)). The initial act sought to reduce the incidence of venereal disease among military men by controlling prostitution that organized around military bases. The Acts required the forcible gynecological examination of any woman thought to be, or (falsely) reported to be, a prostitute. If she were found to be infected, she would be forcibly detained, for up to nine months, in a "lock hospital," until determined to be disease free.[43] There were plainclothes police, so called "morality police" who trolled for these women and had considerable independent discretion to bring charges.

In response to the Acts, Butler founded the Ladies National Association (LNA, 1869), a brilliantly organized, effective, grass-roots movement that brought in women who had never before been politically active. The ladies of the LNA published a "Women's Manifesto," which was signed by 2,000 women including Florence Nightingale.[44] Victorian society, both in the UK and the US, was unprepared for the force of this women's movement against the Acts and, more scandalously, for women to bring sex, sexual behavior, sexually transmitted diseases, reproductive anatomy, and the sexual double standard into open discussion in polite society. The women, and the confederate working-class men, held that these Acts were unconstitutional and morally wrong. The Acts simultaneously established the business of prostitution, *de jure*, and perpetuated both a sexual double standard and notions of male "sexual necessity." Butler maintained that her movement was an "abolitionist movement," not a "purity movement," as it sought to abolish the government sanctioning and regulation of prostitution.

The Social Hygiene Movement

The other side, the social hygiene movement, was furthered by the military and the medical profession. The military had a hardened general position that, "boys will be boys," and men could not be stopped from availing themselves of commercialized sex (prostitution) so that prostitution/prostitutes must be regulated. Eventually, medicine and the military came to see regulation as an ineffective means of control and called for its abolition.

Eventually, too, the social purity movement transitions into a social hygiene movement, the Acts are overturned; it is recognized that regulating prostitution is ineffective as a public health measure, that holding only women as the source and transmitter of venereal disease is absurd, and that the Acts did in fact violate the rights of women. This is an embarrassingly reductionistic version of the movements in their complexity and reach, but it is hoped sufficient to establish the context for the work of Albinia Broderick, Lavinia Dock, and Mary Burr in the early 1900s, who present successive, coordinated papers at the 1909 ICN Congress (the papers are transcribed in Appendix III, Chapter 4). While these are Congress papers that they presented, they had been backed up with political and social action. Though here limited to one large, exemplar issue, these papers represent and illuminate the scope and depth of social ethics in nursing in the early part of the 1900s.

Albinia Lucy Broderick—Be Uninfluenced by the Tyranny of Custom and Prejudice

Albinia Lucy Broderick, who later took the name Gobnait Ní Bhruadair, was a radical, Irish republican, firebrand nurse who sought the reform of nursing and entered into the abolitionist movement as a nursing leader. In 1909, she read the first paper, "Morality in Relation to Health," at the International Congress of Nurses."[45] Her paper began with a vividly detailed, gory, clinical picture of the three diseases, the discovery of the causative microorganisms, a bit of the global history of the diseases and their spread, and the wreckage the transmission of these diseases makes of lives from prostitutes to servicemen to husbands, to wives, to newborns, and to nurses in patient care. She makes note of the fact that physicians would hide the diagnosis from wives who were infected by their husbands, and from nurses who were caring for infected patients. She noted that "it was common practice to hide from the woman the nature of her disease. She only knew that 'she had never been well since her marriage'."[46] Broderick is knowledgeable of the spread of venereal diseases in Europe in the fifteenth century, during Charles VIII's (France) occupation of Naples, and even in Uganda of her day. The scope of her concern extended to global health. While she had first-hand nursing experience and knowledge of patients with venereal disease, she was knowledgeable beyond clinical practice and ably addressed the history, scientific knowledge, clinical treatment, and global reach of the disease. Her central concern, however, was for the abolition of the Acts regulating prostitution and the sexual double standard. Her speech notes that such regulation had failed in every European country that had attempted it; it only captured the older and regular prostitutes and not the younger freelancing prostitutes; and that (here she quotes a military report) "The isolation of a particular section of infected persons, namely of diseased prostitutes, cannot be considered an ideal method of arresting the disease, while large numbers of infected persons *of both sexes* remain free to spread the contagion."[47]

Broderick largely leaves the feminist issues for Dock to address but has several recommendations: (a) sex education for children, without deception; (b) teach children discipline and self-control; (c) notification, i.e., make venereal disease reportable as were other contagious diseases; (d) "open recognition. Bold acknowledgement of these diseases in our midst, and that they had to be met and treated"; (e) "free and easily accessible treatment to which no moral stigma is attached"; (f) punishment of infected persons who knowingly transmit the disease; and (g) the reduction of alcoholism. Much of her discussion is reminiscent of the early days of HIV/AIDS. She calls for nurses to be active in prevention, and that "scientific research should pursue its aims firmly and clearly, uninfluenced by the tyranny of custom and independent of prejudices."[48] She concludes her paper with a rhetorically effusive call to action:

> Form square and stand shoulder to shoulder, nation to nation, fighting for the human race, fighting for our national reputation, fighting for the good name of our century, fighting for the God-given right of health. For innocent women and children, fighting not against, but on behalf of, our poor sisters the prostitutes, who suffers from our culpable neglect and ignorance, fighting dear sister-women as which of us had not fought in our day, for the body and soul of the guilty, because his redemption is possible. So, let us stand steadfast, unfearing. We dare not fail. Nay, we cannot fail. For the weapons of our warfare are Knowledge, Unity, and Love unbounded; the legend on our banner is Light, and the aim of our strife is Peace. Hail comrades, and God speed to victory.[49]

Her paper is greeted with silence and "then the intense feeling it aroused found expression in a storm of applause which subsided only to be renewed again and again."[50]

Lavinia Dock—Rectifying the Social Causes of Disease

Lavinia Dock's paper "The Need of Education on Matters of Social Morality" followed. Dock applauds the growth of the "candid teaching of physiology and hygiene of sex and the newest developments of preventive medicine." But she has harsh words for society that "by reason of the deeply ingrained false shame, mock modesty, vulgar hypocrisy, and generally intensely pharisaic mental attitude that had been deeply ingrained in human society as the result of a double standard of morals, one for men and one for women."[51] This double standard meant that women were not taught about reproductive physiology. She was particularly concerned that nurses knew and witnessed the clinical aspects and tragedies of venereal diseases but that they were

> lamentably ignorant of the real extent of this so-called 'social' or venereal disease... no moral or historical, humanly truthful teaching was heard as to the *reason why* of these horrible diseases... though nurses might talk amongst themselves of tragedies witnessed, they usually seemed to regard them vaguely as fixed conditions of a mysterious universe.[52]

Dock discusses the inadequacies of nursing education and the need to improve teaching on the venereal diseases that took into account the social context of the diseases, the "*reason why*" they existed beyond the causative microorganism. Here, Dock moves into a discussion of prostitution,

> a subject so appalling and hideous that if one concentrated all one's thoughts upon it, especially on that branch called the white slave traffic, one could easily become deranged; yet in the efforts at the prevention of social diseases it could not be put aside.[53]

White slavery refers to the sex trafficking of British girls and young women over the age of consent (14+), though many were younger. Trafficking was essential to replacing the prostitutes who were disabled or died of venereal diseases, and to satisfy the men's appetite for younger prostitutes. Dock notes that in the US, there were an estimated 600,000 prostitutes whose "average life was 10 years, many dying after three to five years. Thus, to keep up the supply, about 60,000 fresh and once pure and healthy women were annually drafted into this death-dealing business."[54] She also notes that male prostitutes "were too often left out of consideration." Dock quotes Prince A. Morrow, a colleague and the founder of the Society of Sanitary and Moral Prophylaxis (US), and advocate for sex education: "Efforts should be directed not to making prostitution safe, but to prevent the making of prostitutes." Dock held that this was possible, but only if all women attained "the power such as could only be obtained through the possession of the franchise."[55]

In *Our Foreign Letter: The Nursing Profession and the Vote (British Journal of Nursing)*, Dock directly links nursing and women's power to eradicate untoward social conditions, to women's authority based on enfranchisement.

> Oh, how much there is to be done that will never get done until women have Power! Mrs. Kelley is convinced that child labor will not be ended in this country until women have the ballot. I am perfectly certain that the question of venereal disease, resting as it does, on the basis of prostitution, will never really be solved until that day, when women, realizing their sacred responsibility to the race, enact laws that will assist and encourage the educational propaganda which must, of course, go hand in hand with prevention. Education alone, in regard to disease alone, cannot accomplish everything... that has been made plain in the tuberculosis propaganda; but the glorious thing about education as to diseases is that it brings you straight and unerringly, and with no delay, down to the social causes which are contributory, and which need legislation for their removal. This strong light thrown on evil social conditions will show more urgent reasons for removing them than could be done in a century of argument.[56]

Dock, and all the leaders of early nursing, evidence an acute awareness of the social conditions that undermine health and give rise to disease, and the necessity for their amelioration. Here, in the case of prostitution and venereal disease, it was middle-class women advocating on behalf of outcast, lower-class women. Their position was not without flaws: they assume that all women in prostitution were forced or sold into the life. Some feminists (today) argue that the movement was patronizing and classist. It may well have been; however, there is an argument to be made that the close interaction nurses had with patients suffering from the devastating effects of venereal diseases engendered a measure of compassion as an impetus. Dock advocates for a fulsome agenda of teaching sex physiology and hygiene to the public, the abolition of the sexual double standard, and the educational preparation of nurses so that they might avoid becoming infected in the course of clinical practice. She also advocates for the improvement of education and wages for women, the ablation of social structures that reduce women to prostitution; for raising the age of consent; and for the criminal punishment of white slave traffickers. Research for her speech formed the basis for a book the following year.

Mary Burr—Be Outraged—Statistics on the Defilement of Girls Under 13

The third paper of the Congress was presented by nurse Mary Burr (Director of the National Council of Trained Nurses of Great Britain and Ireland) on "Some Statistics of Criminal Assault Upon Young Girls." She acknowledges the extraordinary difficulty in obtaining adequate statistics and that some organizations she approached "flatly refused to furnish information."[57] Burr investigates the number of cases of rape and sexual violence against girls, the number of subsequent prosecutions, the results of the prosecutions, and the ages of the victims. There were no comprehensive statistics to be had, so that she had to resort to the criminal statistics scrounged from various jurisdictions. The outcomes make for grim but not unexpected reading, even for today. For example, in one jurisdiction, in 15 years, there were reported 2302 "cases of defilement of girls under 13 [below the age of consent] and 2442 cases of girls under 16 reported to the police."[58] For this group, there were 145 convictions. Burr writes, "A curious fact in this grim document was the distinction between girls under and over 13. All the sentences of penal servitude were given in the former cases. Apparently, a girl over 13 and under 16 might be outraged [raped] and the sentence be anything from 14 days to 2 years."[59] Prosecutions were few, and convictions fewer still. "On inquiry why prosecutions in cases of assault were so few, the reply received from all quarters was that the culprit was so often the father, step-father, or brother of the victim." Often the children, as young as 10, were silenced, and if the girl were pregnant, she was "restrained by threats," and parents would not allow rescue workers to intervene. Burr was told that, in another jurisdiction, "convictions were very few, as relations were so often the culprits."[60]

Some of the defendants blamed "foreigners." But only one offender in all the reported cases for 1907 was an immigrant. "These men who defiled women and violated their own offspring were British."[61] She continues, in conclusion:

These men... had the power of helping to make the laws which women must obey, and of making them as easy as possible for the indulgence of their own lusts. Why must proceedings be taken within 6 months; why must a child, whose whole moral and physical nature had been so recently outraged, be subjected to cross-examination by a lawyer when there was corroborating evidence. Yet we are told that men could well be trusted to look after women's interests and welfare. If such a state of things were the result of their care, the sooner women took matters in hand the better it would be for the nation's moral and physical condition.[62]

Mary Burr persisted against odds to secure statistics for girl child sexual violence, rape, and trafficking needed to complete the full picture painted by Broderick, Dock, and Burr. The discussants following the paper were from Germany, New Zealand, and Finland. Their words corroborated similar conditions, from all three papers, in their own countries.

Dock would go on the following year to publish *Hygiene and Morality* (1910), written as a nursing textbook. It is a brilliant, incisive, social critique of British society that allows none of the police and political structures to escape unscathed. The jailers who abuse prostitutes; the disgruntled men who, in revenge, falsely accuse innocent women; the military that wants to assure safe semi-licit sex for its men; the judges who will not prosecute rapists and child molesters; the legislators and military who absurdly try to contain venereal disease by cooping up and treating women alone; the Parliament that establishes laws that severely punish the prostitutes but avoid actually abolishing prostitution; and the MPs who make it a misdemeanor to kidnap a girl under 16 for sexual purposes—all these and more are skewered by Dock's judgment. As a book for nurses, it was for all nursing to see and to take note, modeling both a vision for society, and for nursing activism.

Venereal disease is but one brief example that stands in for others that could also serve as exemplars, such as the need for uncontaminated milk for infants. What can be seen in these speeches is a concern for the individual person (prostitute), a concern for the individual within a subclass of disadvantaged persons (lower-class, prostitute, outcast), and the subclass within a larger class (women in society). But Broderick, Dock, Burr, Butler, and others undertake the critique of the entire ladder of social structures from the physicians and hospitals to the constabulary and their jails and lock hospitals, to judges, to legislators, to the laws and how they are enacted, and to the Parliament/Congress and the interpretation of their respective Constitutions. Along the way they critique legal, economic, political, military, medical, educational, and other social structures. And they act, as nurse-activists, to bring about social change.

These papers are important on multiple levels. First, they demonstrate a high level of social critique using different methods. Second, they display the extraordinary intellect of early nursing leaders. Third, their papers have bite, and are an implicit critique of contemporary nursing's tepid civic engagement. Fourth, they incorporate a thorough critique of society and medical practice and move from pathology-to-Parliament-to-practice in their recommendations. They are equipped with facts, statistics, prowess in social critique, a commitment to social change, and an activist and reformist commitment fueled by passion and values. In addition, they cross national borders in their critique, back and forth between the US and UK, and other nations as well, making common cause for shared nursing values and social ends. The health of society is at stake, and intimately entwined with the health of the individual. When the health of society is at stake, its remedies cannot and may not come at the expense of vulnerable persons.

Broderick's paper is a remarkable example of *epidictic discourse*, calling nurses to "stand square, shoulder to shoulder" in an affirmation of nursing values. As you read the papers in the Appendix, note especially how Broderick refuses to condemn prostitutes and instead embraces them. Dock's paper tackles the question of what nurses had not been, but should be, taught regarding venereal diseases. She then moves to a discussion of the social structures of prostitution (and thus the spread of venereal disease) where, take note, she does not pull her punches in condemning the sexual double-standard, the failings of male legislators, and the necessity of women's enfranchisement and political engagement. Burr's paper is armed with data collection, facts, and statistics, and unsparing condemnation of the failure of the judicial system to either protect these girls or to hold the men responsible to account. Broderick, Dock, and Burr are bold, courageous, and well-armed in their social analysis and critique. Their social and political engagement stands in stark contrast and as a reprimand to the drought in nursing's social ethics and social activism today.

Social Ethics

The work of Broderick, Dock, and Burr, as displayed in their Congress papers, are examples of nursing social ethics (see Chapter 10 for more extended discussion). Social ethics is that branch of ethics that engages in the critique of the social structures of a society with an emphasis on the sociopolitical conditions that foster social goods, the common good, and community, as well as social harms, including rigid social stratification, poverty, illness, exploitation, oppression, prejudice, and injustice. It engages in social criticism to the end of social change.[63,64,65] It is the broader framework under which concerns for social justice are explored, but also encompasses concerns for human dignity, well-being, and welfare; respect, fulfillment, community, harmony, peace, security, tranquility, unity, freedom, and equality; the common good, the one-and-many, virtue, and more. Social justice is but one among many concepts within social ethics, and it does not stand on its own and is not, itself, an ethics framework. Social ethics is intrinsically political in nature and directed toward social policy. As Winter notes, social ethics is concerned with "issues of social order—the good, right, and ought in the organization of human communities and the shaping of social policies. Hence the subject matter of social ethics is moral rightness and goodness in the shaping of human society."[66] Social ethics contains a vision for a good society, which forces us to ask, "What is nursing's vision for a healthy society, and how is nursing socially and politically engaged to realize that vision?"

Conclusion

Dock, Broderick, and Burr came up through the ranks of practicing nurses. They had in-the-trenches, ground-up, first-hand, experience of seeing persons suffer from diseases or conditions that were preventable, diseases that were the consequence of "evil social conditions." This is a strength of those who are nurses. Their vision for nursing was not limited to the medical situation of the individual patient. Instead, it extends to the context of the patient's illness and the social structures that affect health, illness, and treatment.

Again, contemporary nursing, by limiting its social concerns to those identified by bioethics, with its focus on *distributive justice*, betrays our brilliant and hard-fought heritage of social ethics. The justice literature in bioethics has broadened in recent years, to include environmental concerns, with some attention to poverty, and has generally been re-termed *social justice*, but it largely remains focused on access to care and the cost of care and rationing. In addition, in recent years, nursing education has developed a blinkered focus on evidence-based practice, science at the expense of humanities, and other constraining influences that diminish attention to philosophical, ethical, and social-ethical thinking. Today's nursing articles on sex trafficking (in CINAHL and PubMed databases), for example, are virtually entirely limited to the clinical recognition of persons who have been trafficked, particularly by nurses in the Emergency Department, and do not address social or justice issues. We are not shaking a fist at Parliament, or Congress, the judiciary, and the constabulary. Today's inattention stands in stark contrast to the vision and social compass of Broderick, Dock, Burr, Fenwick, Robb, and others. Any contemporary social critique of trafficking to be found resides within the social work articles, not in the bioethics or nursing bioethics articles. Social structures can and do wound large segments of society, further harming those already disadvantaged. A sticking plaster on the patient does not ameliorate the social forces that damage individuals, families, and communities; forces that nursing is equipped to address. As Hurlston notes in the *British Journal of Nursing* in 1911:

> To all thoughtful people who work among the poor in any of our large towns, the questions must often present themselves: What is the cause of all the disease we meet with among the children? Why, in the 20th century, in this so-called civilised country, is it allowed to exist? What are we all doing to improve this deplorable state of affairs?[67]

Indeed. Why are these conditions allowed to exist? What is nursing doing to improve this deplorable state of affairs? Perhaps remembering and reclaiming our social ethics could provide nursing a vision for its future.

Appendix III: Author's Note and 1909 ICN Speeches by Albinia Broderick, Lavinia Dock, and Mary Burr

Author's Note

The following three speeches are transcribed directly from the 1909 *British Journal of Nursing* (formerly the *Nursing Record*).[68] The speeches were recorded by an unnamed stenographer on-site and are a mix of the recorder's summative remarks and direct quotes from the speakers. The three speakers were Albinia Broderick, Lavinia Dock, and Mary Burr, in that order. Their papers were coordinated and sequential presentations. While there is a synopsis of the content of these papers in my comments above that duplicates some of the material in the speeches below, the full speeches are included here so that the reader might more directly access the voices of Broderick, Dock, and Burr in the entirety of their speeches. In addition, the full text of the speeches gives contemporary readers insight into the depth of social analysis and data collection these speeches reflect, and the ability to draw their own conclusions.

ICN International Congress of Nurses, July 23, 1909

Session: Morality in Relation to Health

Sister Agnes Karll, RN, President of the International Council of Nurses, presided at the session at the Caton Hall, on "Morality in Relation to Health" to which women only were admitted. She opened the proceedings by reading to the congress the letter from Mr. L.H. Shore Nightingale, cousin of Miss Florence Nightingale, O.M., already reported in these columns, and then said that today the Congress was to consider the darkest side of life, the most sorrowful side of nursing. It was hard to say how much illness, how many deaths, how many suicides, how much blindness among infants, had been caused by diseases resulting from immorality. What was the nurse's duty in regard to this question? Was it right that people should be kept in ignorance?

[Albinia Broderick's Speech] Morality in Relation to Health

The Honorable Albinia Broderick presented the first paper, and said that its title was "Morality in Relation to Health." More accurately, it should be "Immorality in Relation to Disease." The subject with which she had to deal was no matter of decency or indecency; she treated it neither from the point of view of sentiment, nor from the side of ethics or religion. She desired to bring forward from the scientific point of view a necessarily short and incomplete summary of the facts, which were strongly influencing the health of nations, facts of ordinary medical and nursing knowledge concerning three highly infectious diseases—soft chancre, gonorrhœa, and syphilis, which formed a group in medicine under the misnomer of venereal[69] diseases. Their causes are well defined; their manifestations and sequelae might well appall the most courageous. Ameliorative, and in some instances curative, treatment was an established possibility. They came under the head of preventable diseases. "If preventable, why not prevented?"

The speaker then described briefly the special characteristics of these three diseases: (1) soft chancre, exceedingly infectious, but amenable to treatment; (2) gonorrhœa, one of the genito-urinary diseases, attacking in its primary manifestations the mucus membranes, especially that of the urethra and the adult, and causing in the infant the so-called ophthalmia neonatorum, or gonorrhœal ophthalmia. It was familiar to the ancient world, but in 1879 Professor Neisser, of Breslau, revolutionised our knowledge by establishing the existence of a definite microorganism—the gonococcus—as the cause of gonorrhea. This disease was the chief cause of impotence and sterility both in male and female. Up to the date of Neisser's discovery and attack of this disease, it was regarded as a harmless urethral catarrh, a natural if not inevitable result of "sowing wild oats." Now we know that it was one of the most infectious diseases we had to meet, and that its consequences were far-reaching. We did not know yet when a case could be declared to have ceased to be infectious. Zweifel had noted a case in which a man infected a woman thirteen years after contracting the disease. After detailing the many serious sequelae with this disease, the speaker said, "At present, it is probable that we have not fathomed the depths of gonorrhœal complications. This we know, that they are far-reaching and capable of destroying health." If this were the case in the male, in the female the results were 10 times worse. Iwan Block, one of Germany's great authorities on this matter, said "the infection of a women with gonorrhœa is a disaster"; and Zweifel said, "This disease has, upon women, a miserably depressing effect, in contradistinction from men they are more likely to suffer for many years from intense pains. Whenever they execute certain bodily movements, it may be during ten years in succession, they experience pains, often horribly severe, and in most cases, they are condemned to a life of deprivation and misery, not usually from any faulty of their own, since most women are infected by their husbands." Still less than a man could a woman be declared "cured" of gonorrhœa with any certainty. It was the common practice to hide from the woman the nature of her disease. She only knew that "she had never been well since her marriage." Little girls might become infected through sharing the parent's bed, or using their towels. Infants were commonly infected, if at all, at birth. The resultant ophthalmia was too sadly well known to need description. By English and foreign writers, it was credited with from 30 to 79 percent of the cases of blindness in their respective countries.

Impotence, sterility, blindness—a goodly trio. Syphilis, the third disease of the group, was a chronic constitutional and infectious disease, described by Dr. F.W. Andrewes as having "the characteristics of a specific fever, running a chronic course, combined with those of an infective granuloma." In plain terms, syphilis was to be classified amongst the infectious fevers. It first made its appearance in Europe at the end of the fifteenth century, and first attracted notice when Charles VIII of France occupied Naples with his troops, when it spread with appalling rapidity, involving all countries of Europe, including our own. The infection was virulent to a degree now unknown amongst us, but, unhappily, repeated only too recently in the history of Uganda. The disease proved for a time as great a scourge as the plague itself; it obscured the less obvious gonorrhœa, and has since remained amongst us in a modified, but not for that reason a less dangerous form, common to all excepting a few of the uncivilised nations of the world. Like gonorrhœa, it was caused by a specific micro-organism, the *spirochete pallida*, a protozoan discovered by Fitz Schaudinn on March 3rd, 1905. Syphilis might be considered under two heads: (1) Syphilis acquired by fornication and other willful acts of unchastity, and (2) *syphilis insontium*, where wholly innocent persons were attacked. For this reason, it could not be classed as a purely venereal disease. Infection might occur from any syphilitic discharges. It could be spread by kissing, by the use of infected vessels or towels, or by anything which had been in contact with the infected mouth, even by licking an infected pencil. It could be contracted by a nurse or doctor in dressing, or operation, by a midwife during delivery; it could be transmitted through the placenta of the fetus, or acquired by the infant in suckling. The speaker described the three stages of development of the infectious disease, the primary, the secondary, and tertiary, the last of which, she said, might arise from one to three years after infection, or might even not occur for 50 years or more, so long drawn out was the possibility of the virus in this, the worst of the venereal group. The syphilitic gummata and hard nodules distinguishing this stage ultimately ulcerated, and in their ulcerative process caused loathsome disfigurement and often destroyed life. No part of the tissues of the body were immune from the disease.

Nor did the innocent escape. The disease contracted from prostitutes in the first instance might be communicated to the innocent wife and unborn child, the unfaithful and infected wife might infect her husband. *Syphilis infantium* crowned the mystery of pain. Shillitoe wrote, "Very many women are absolutely innocent, and altogether ignorant, of the serious nature of the complaint. Not infrequently we're asked to treat a woman for the whole course of the disease without once mentioning the word syphilis, or giving her any inkling as to the true nature of the ailment from which she is suffering…it is impossible to discuss the condition in the same open way as with men."

The wife seldom escaped; the mother might be infected by her syphilitic offspring. As to children, Fournier followed the cases of 90 married women infected by their husbands and pregnant in the first year. There were 50 abortions or stillbirths, 38 died in infancy, 2 only survived. It was estimated that syphilis of the father gave a mortality of 28 percent in the offspring, of the mother a mortality of

60 percent, of both parents of 68 percent. If the fetus survived, the syphilitic infant developed the secondary stage of the disease, the first being absent. It might be recognized by the wrinkled skin, the yellow old man's face, the excoriated buttocks, the syphilitic snuffle. Later, the child showed signs of degeneration, arrested development, malformation, epilepsy, mental weakness. Symptoms might not manifest themselves till later life. Even the second generation was not exempt.

Lunacy, mutilation, child murder, another and yet more likely goodly trio.

The speaker then gave some appalling statistics showing the widespread presence of venereal diseases, and their disastrous effects. Thus, Noeggerath had stated that of every 1,000 men married in New York, 800 had had gonorrhœa and 90 percent were uncured at the time of their marriage.

Dealing with the prevention of venereal diseases, the speaker repudiated the idea of regulation as effective. First, it had been tried in every European country but England and Norway, and the condition of affairs spoke for itself. Secondly, regulation touched only the older and regular prostitutes, leaving the younger and recently infected women, who were the great danger to the community, aside. Thirdly, a committee reported to the Advisory Board of our own Army Medical Service: "The isolation of a particular section of infected persons, namely, of disease prostitutes, cannot be considered an ideal method of arresting the disease, while large numbers of infected persons *of both sexes* remain free to spread the contagion." Her rhetoric would have been galvanizing in its day and not, as today, heard as over-the-top.

The speaker advocated:

1. Education, as the first plank. Children should be taught from their infancy to avoid masturbation, to regard the genital organs as sacred. They should each learn the simple physiology of sexual life, which could easily be taught from animals and plants. Lies should not be told them in regard to the birth of the little brother or sister. Habits of modesty, decency, and regularity in the accomplishment of the natural act should be inculcated.
2. Discipline the children. Self-control and self-discipline were more easily acquired in childhood than in later life.
3. Notification. Other preventable fall diseases were notifiable, why not this one, by far the most important of all? Take the seal of secrecy from the physician's lips and compel him to notify.
4. Open recognition. Bold acknowledgement of these diseases in our midst, and that they had to be met and treated.
5. Free and easily accessible treatment to which no moral stigma was attached.
6. The punishment of any infected person who knowingly exposed another to the risk of infection.
7. The diminution of alcoholism.

These diseases were eradicable from the human race; innocent and guilty alike desired to see them eradicated. Therein lay the chief strength of our cause.

The speaker concluded:

"I take it that we are at one upon the main point. As nurses, as patriots, we desire to limit as far as lies in our power, the physical, mental, and moral ills of humanity. We desire not merely to cure but to prevent. These of which we have treated are preventable diseases, remembering that fornication is no more a necessity of the body than our drunkenness or gluttony. And shall we not prevent them? Are we going to sit still, as we have sat still so long, and see the race to generate before our eyes? Are we going to watch the long, drawn-out sacrifice of life and health that is daily going on around us? Listen to Karl Marx: 'Society has hitherto failed to find a remedy, perhaps because only man has sought for one,' and 'all that is requisite for the attainment of this end is that those engaged in the study and practice of general hygiene, and those concerned in the safeguarding of public morality, should not weary in their efforts, and that scientific research should pursue its aims firmly and clearly uninfluenced by the tyranny of custom, and independent of prejudice.'

"The trumpet call to arms had sounded already. America has risen to rally round the white banner. Let us follow her lead. We are awakening. We, too, will get us from our sloth. We are ready to answer to the battle cry. Bitter opposition, a paralyzing indifference, will be encountered. We shall be evil spoken of. We shall be misunderstood, for we stand here, nurses and fellow citizens of this vast city called Life, face to face with a fight unparalleled in the history of nations.

"In serried battalions over against us are set the hosts of the ignorant, the prudish, the timid, the vicious, the alcoholic, the feeble-minded. We stand, the leaders of a forlorn hope, in the eyes of our fellow men, doubly disgraced if we fail, for by success alone can we be justified. We *must* succeed. What though each one of us be beaten to her knees in the struggle? we will fight on. What though we faint from this stress of conflict and weary for the loneliness of our toil? We will fight on. What though we fail? We will fight on.

"Form square and stand shoulder to shoulder, nation to nation, fighting for the human race, fighting for our national reputations, fighting for the good name of our century, fighting for the God-given right of health for innocent women and children, fighting not against, but on behalf of, our poor sisters the prostitutes, the sufferers from our culpable neglect and ignorance, fighting dear sister-women as which of us has not fought in our day, for the body and soul of the guilty, because his redemption is possible.

"So let us stand steadfast, unfearing. We dare not fail. Nay, we cannot fail. For the weapons of our warfare are Knowledge, Unity, and Love unbounded; the legend on our banner is Light, and the aim of our strife is Peace. Hail comrades, and God speed to victory."

For a few moments after the speaker ceased, the silence noticeable during the reading of the paper continued, and then, the intense feeling it aroused found expression in a storm of applause, which subsided only to be renewed again and again. It was the tribute of admiration of the nurses of the world to their comrade who so brilliantly, delicately, and courageously had drawn aside the veil with which mock modesty conceals the evil thing in our midst, and revealed it in its putrid enormity.

As lengthy applause subsided, Mrs. Bedford Fenwick reminded the Congress that a few days ago they had been asked to believe that the reader of that brilliant paper was not a trained nurse. This Congress was proud to claim her as a colleague and leader it was determined to follow.

The president of the session then called upon Miss L.L. Dock, RN.

[Lavinia Dock's Speech] The Need of Education on Matters of Social Morality

Miss Dock said that the crusade against venereal disease now being definitely waged by a campaign of public education, and the definite systematic, candid teaching of the physiology and hygiene of sex was the newest development of preventive medicine and the most helpful of all its promises—most hopeful because the evils it was attacking were the most horrible known to humanity.

As its promise was full of hope, its course was full of difficulties beyond the ordinary, by reason of the deeply ingrained false shame, mock modesty, vulgar hypocrisy, and generally intensely pharisaic mental attitude that had been deeply ingrained in human society as the result of many centuries of servile acceptance of a double standard of morals, one for men and one for women. From this false shame and hypocrisy had resulted in the dense ignorance prevalent as to the physiology of the reproductive organs and their functions, and, in addressing an audience of nurses on this topic, she might assume that even they were lamentably ignorant of the real extent of this so-called "social" venereal disease. She was made certain of this by recalling her own training, and by noting the result of inquiries made at the present time. She remembered very well the entire adequacy of her own instruction on this subject. Though in the immense hospital of city poor, syphilis and gonorrhœa were familiar terms, and though the pupils learned much about symptomatology, and something of precaution and the avoidance of infection, yet no moral or historical, humanly truthful teaching was heard as to the *reason why* of these horrible diseases, and she regretted to remember that in her own experience as a teacher in training schools, she did not realise the importance of doing more than skim the surface of this subject. Outside the hospital social conventions were in full control and inside a sort of professional fatalism dominated, so that, though nurses might talk amongst themselves of tragedies witnessed, they usually seem to regard them vaguely as fixed conditions of a mysterious universe. But today this fatalistic attitude was changing, and the deadly silence was breaking. Lagging last year in the rear of all other communicable diseases, venereal diseases had now been dragged out into the open light of publicity. There were evidences that the stir of propaganda was reaching into our training schools, and it was high time it should be so, for against the urgent call for the thousands of intelligent women in the nursing field to become missioners of prevention on these lines stands the fact that the great majority of nurses are, as yet, little more informed upon the great social facts of these diseases than are the laity.

Inquiries made of the training schools led to the conclusion that, while routine procedures of disinfection were generally taught, information was generally lacking as to the extent, prevalence, relation to conditions of society, and, above all, prevention of venereal disease.

A growing feeling of the need for more thorough teaching was, however, shown in the number of replies. One Superintendent of nurses wrote: "Personally, I think it a crime not to teach this subject to nurses." Women physicians seemed to have a special mission to carry this propaganda, and the first pioneer women in medicine did sound this note at the outset of their career, and if search were made, it would probably be found that their brave words set flowing the current of ideas now moving the leaders of the medical section of the societies of prophylaxis.

One Superintendent wrote that she determined that a system of very plain teaching should be substituted for the extremely fragmentary method that formerly prevailed. The lecturer on skin diseases had previously given some instruction on the subject of syphilis, but he had handled the subject so gingerly that most of the facts she desired emphasised were not touched upon. This year, a woman physician was asked to give the left pictures and demonstrations, describing the way the infection was carried, its effect on the organs and offspring, the causes of sterility, and finally the social aspect. Her manner of handling the subject was particularly fine, and her manner of gentle dignity quickly brought the class from a tense strained attitude to one of interest and attention.

In general, however, it seemed that the training school for nurses had a far more reserved mode of teaching venereal disease than other infectious diseases. Details regarding tuberculosis, its cause, transmission, and, above all, its prevention, were now published everywhere with copious fullness, and almost shouted from the house-tops, and in the case of nearly every other infectious disease, the mode of propagation of the germ, and prevention, are held to be of the most absorbing interest. Pupils in nurse training schools needed also to be taught that venereal diseases had causes that were perfectly understood, that they were propagated by the base use of the generative organs, and spread broadcast by our social institution of prostitution. Also, that the cause and dangers being perfectly well known to medical science, so, too, is prevention perfectly well understood, and that this whole class of hideous menaces to health and happiness *could* be made to disappear from the face of the earth; above all, they needed to be taught the unmitigated falsity and immorality of the double standard of morals in matters of sex.

Miss Dock said that many nurses did not even know enough to protect themselves from infection. She recalled two distressing cases where nurses caring for private patients were virulently infected, one losing an eye by gonorrhœal ophthalmia and the other's usefulness being destroyed by loathsome symptoms of syphilis. In these cases, the physicians had not given the nurses the smallest hint as to the nature of the cases they were exposed to, yet nurses were not expected to diagnose, and these unfortunates evidently did not.

Miss Dock said some might demur and suggest that precaution against infection was all nurses need to be taught. She earnestly insisted that they should be taught everything there is to know. They were women, and it was most urgent that all women should know the whole truth in regard to venereal diseases at the earliest possible time and to the fullest possible extent. Only when all women and men knew the truth in its fullness could we hope for a reduction of prostitution to its lowest possible limits, and only so could prevention be attained.

Prostitution was a subject so appalling and hideous that if one concentrated all one's thoughts upon it, especially on that branch called the white slave traffic, one could easily become deranged. Yet in the efforts toward the prevention of sexual diseases, it could not be put aside.

It was estimated that there were in the United States about 600,000 prostitutes. Their average life was ten years, many dying after three to five years. Thus, to keep up the supply, about 60,000 fresh and once pure and healthy women were annually drafted into this death-dealing business. Such a toll by an infectious and avoidable malady was heavy enough, but the true menace to the innocent women and children outside that number came from the male prostitutes, who were too often left entirely out of consideration. It was said that it took on average five men to support one prostitute, and they had horrible evidence in the social settlement where she lived that some of those poor creatures were visited by many more. In some houses of ill-fame there was a system by which women were paid by brass checks, which they afterwards exchanged, and one woman received 18 of such checks in one night. It was the men who visited these women who carried venereal infection into their own homes and distributed it amongst their wives and children.

The control and prevention of venereal disease lay in the control and prevention of prostitution, and Dr. Morrow, president of the American Society of Moral and Sanitary Prophylaxis, said: "efforts should be directed not to making prostitution safe, but to prevent the making of prostitutes."

Miss Dock said that her conviction, and that of many others wiser than herself, was that this was only possible through the attainment by all women of power and authority such as only could be obtained through the possession of the franchise. Women must have the power to make laws and enforce them; it was not enough to help to administer those made by a masculine, law-making body. Women must attain the capacity to legislate for the making and remaking of social conditions of work and labor, wages and salaries, education, home, business, and public life. Only by far-reaching changes in these basic things could prostitution be undermined and minimised, just as it was chiefly by the preparation of the soil that the farmer controlled his crops. Direct legislation against prostitution—*i.e.*, the various systems of policing and licensing—had been shown to be futile, and to those who argued that men cannot be made moral by law, we must reply that conditions which made women immoral by necessity must be altered by law.

First, society should be so organised that no woman need be unwillingly forced into prostitution. The President of the National Vigilance League in America, a physician of high standing, stated in a moderate, carefully weighed speech that of all the prostitutes in the country only 20 percent were willingly such. The other 80 percent had been tricked, betrayed, forced, kidnapped, or actually bought and sold for money into this slavery. Leaving moral and humane conditions aside, if this 80 percent were not forced into this life, the problem of eradicating venereal disease would be vastly simpler. What an outcry there would be if 80 percent out of 600,000 persons annually were compelled by inexorable destiny, the logical result of man-made social conditions, to be exposed to small-pox.

In combating venereal disease, there must be first the fundamental restriction of the traffic in alcoholic poison, for this was the main reliance and indispensable instrument of all corrupting agencies.

Next, better school laws, largely made and enforced by women. The last report of the Chicago Law and Order League stated that in the man-ruled schools of that city, conditions of sanitation were responsible for much of the infection that had sent 600 children into the venereal wards of the county hospital. Again, in New York City, when Miss Rogers, head of the school nurses there, tried in cooperation with earnest women principals to trace to its sources a series of cases of vaginitis which ran through the schools, their inquiries were stifled by the medical officers of health, who said that the nurses were going beyond their province.

Next, better labor laws. Miss Minor, Probation Officer in New York City, in the last report of the consumers league, said: "Hundreds are victims to our industrial conditions—low wages, irregularity, and lack of work." Child labor, to which male employers clung so tenaciously, was one of the first predispositions to immoral life, and to black as well as white plague, and vainly had the disenfranchised women appealed to the much-vaunted chivalry of man for the protection of the young.

The most painful evidence afforded in the United States of the vaunted chivalry of man had been the recent decision of the Supreme Court setting free a number of men who had been convicted of carrying on the white slave traffic as a business, on the grounds that the constitution of the United States did not enable the Federal Court to deal with them. The system of dealing with prostitution in the lower city Courts was, as everyone knew, nothing more or less than an organised system of blackmail of these defenceless women.

It was, therefore, impossible at the present time to punish dealers in the white slave traffic. This added satire to the brutality of the lynch laws for black men. The agents of the white slave traffic were all white citizens. The social order, with child labor abolished, young girls paid living wages, widowed mothers pensioned by the state, so as to enable them to stay at home and care for their children, etc., must go far towards reducing the *unwilling* numbers now forced into the ranks of those who propagate venereal diseases. Then only, when there were simply the prostitutes by preference to consider, could legislation be so directed as to be something more than a farce. Education must be estimated at its full value, but could not be relied on alone; it must go hand in hand with enlightened legislation.

As to the part nurses should take in this movement, Miss Dock said she was not one of those who insisted that the nurse's submissiveness must never lose its classic form; her professional subordination, right and indispensable in the sick room or hospital where she freely contracted to be under the absolute orders of those physicians who undertook and carried the responsibility of the patients, must not be carried unquestioningly into her social and human relations, but might there be modified by her opportunities and duties as a human being. The older and narrower idea of a nurse reduced her to a kindly and animated machine. Logically carried out, it made her capable of palliative labors only, whereas the only hope of humanity was in preventive work.

Preventive medicine was only in its early stages, and the nurse must not be shackled at the outset of her career with obsolete notions of self-effacement, but must be alert to follow and assist the advanced guard of medical progress.

Miss Dock urged that nurses should (1) Study and inform themselves on the moral prophylaxis question, so as to be capable of intelligent action when opportunity showed itself. (2) Join the national or international societies as working members. (3) Take every opportunity of giving simple talks and frank, plain instruction on sex physiology and sex hygiene, sex morality, and the dangers of ignorance in schools, social settlements, Young Women's Christian Associations, before groups of girls, mother's clubs, and young teachers; explain that the highest medical authority upholds the single standard of morality, and declare the old ideas of the physiological necessity of sex impurity for young men to be false. (4) Do all possible to promote fuller and broader instruction and training schools on the causes and prevention of venereal diseases, so that the oncoming generations of nurses might be better equipped than those of the past ages to enlighten, warn, teach, and, we might hope, legislate. Naturally, in the case of individual patients, the nurse's lips were sealed. Knowledge came too late, and truth would be a useless torment. But young mothers could be encouraged to teach their children. We must try to help to bring up a more intelligent race of women, who would in turn produce a more man-like race of men.

[Mary Burr's Speech] Some Statistics of Criminal Assault upon Young Girls

Miss Mary Burr, who presented the next paper, dealing with statistics of criminal assault upon young girls, said that statistics were usually considered very dry, but when they meant ruined lives, they demanded the closest attention. It was originally intended to draw as far as possible upon private sources, but those proved inadequate, and a dozen societies dealing with wronged women and children were approached for information on the following points:

1. The number of cases of criminal assault upon young girls and children met within their work.

2. The number in which prosecution followed.
3. The result of the prosecution.
4. The ages of the victims.

Only two associations—the National Society for the Prevention of Cruelty to Children and the Church Penitentiary Association—gave any definite information; even the National Vigilance Society referred her to the director of public prosecutions, and one lady flatly refused to furnish information which she considered private to a Congress of which she knew nothing. Was this work, which so closely affected the national well-being, a private preserve for those engaged in it?

One secretary, however, advised the speaker to buy the book of criminal statistics, which gave comparative statistics for 15 years, 1893–1907. In those 15 years there were 2,302 cases of defilement of girls under 13, and 2,442 of girls under 16, reported to the police.

Of these, 1,600 were tried for assault on girls under 13, and 1,765 for girls under 16. In 1907, the last year of which details were given, there were reported to the police 149 cases concerning girls under 13 and 178 of girls under 16. Two hundred and thirty-two cases were taken into the court of law. Of these, 4 were thrown out, 82 acquitted, 145 convicted. The punishment of those convicted was penal servitude in 23 cases, from 4 to 20 years, the usual term being from 5 to 7 years. One man was flogged. The remainder were imprisoned for terms varying from 14 days to 2 years.

A curious fact in this grim document was the distinction between girls under and over 13. All the sentences of penal servitude were given in the former cases. Apparently, a girl over 13 and under 16 might be outraged and the sentence be anything from 14 days to 2 years.

In addition, during the years 1893–1907, there were 3,407 cases of rape, and 12,280 of indecent assault upon women over 16, reported to the police, making an annual average for the 15 years of 1,362 lives wrecked. Those were statistics from the Blue Book.

In the pamphlet "Juvenile Delinquency," the Rev. T.G. Cree, Hon. Secretary of the Church Penitentiary Association, stated that 33 penitentiaries and refuges returned the number of cases of children under 16 dealt with by them as 347 and 745 respectively for a period of three years. Of these, 8 cases were between 6 and 8 years old, 18 between 9 and 11, 11 were 12 years old, 14 were 13 years old, and 301 were 15 years old.

In one town, the chief constable reported that there was hardly a child over 14 who had not fallen. In another, that children under 14 absolutely solicited in considerable numbers.

On inquiry of why prosecutions in cases of assault were so low, the reply was received from all quarters that the culprit was so often the father, step-father, or brother of the victim. In the covering letter, Mr. Cree further stated that fully 1,000 more cases were known, but parents would not allow the rescue workers to deal with them. He stated that convictions were very few, as relations were so often the culprit, also when there was danger of an infant being born the child was restrained by threats from saying anything until her condition was manifest. Again, young children were subjected to cross-examination by lawyers, and in one case a child of 10 was subjected to cross-examination for a full hour, but her evidence could not be shaken, and the case was sent to the Assizes [county court].

The National Society for the Prevention of Cruelty to Children reported 838 cases last year; 146 were prosecuted and 46 dismissed. In 20 collected cases, 18 were under 16, one child being 3 and another 5 years of age. In two cases, the fathers were the culprits, and in one, the brother was suspected.

Two of these cases were very bad, one of a girl who went to a gardener's for fruit midday Sunday, not returning until 6:30 p.m., when she went out again, it was supposed, to chapel. No more was seen of her till her body was taken from the river on Tuesday morning, when the child was found to have been violated. At the inquest the gardener was severely censured, and an open verdict returned.

The other case was one of a child of 10 outraged while her mother was lying dead. The father was supposed to be the delinquent, but as proof could not be brought forward, he was let off.

Out of 11 cases, 3 were discharged because there was, the judge said, "no corroboration," and one was "not proven." One was let off with a fine; the rest received sentences from 6 months to 10 years.

Of the two cases over 16, one was a girl mentally deficient, and the culprits, several youths, one of whom confessed to the wrongdoing, were all discharged by the magistrates.

The other was the case of a girl of 17, who was seized from behind, a drugged handkerchief stuffed into her mouth, and she was dragged into the bracken on a Surrey heath and violated. When she recognized her assailant, he tried to poison her, happily without much success. Chiefly for the attempt to poison, he was sentenced to seven years penal servitude.

If this number of cases were known, what about those unknown? If 327 cases were reported in a year, how many hundreds were unreported? Governments came and went, and yet this evil went unchecked. Did our lawmakers think it worse to kill the body than to outrage its honour and sully its soul?

Again, it was useless, as some were inclined to do, to blame foreigners. Only one offender in all the reported cases for 1907 was an alien.

These men who defiled women and violated their own offspring were British. They had the power of helping to make the laws which women must obey, and of making them as easy as possible for the indulgence of their own lusts. Why must proceedings be taken within six months; why must a child, whose whole moral and physical nature had been so recently outraged, be subjected to cross-examination by a lawyer on so delicate a matter; and was it likely in such cases that corroborative evidence could be obtained? Yet we were told that men could well be trusted to look after women's interests and welfare. If such a state of things were the result of their care, the sooner women took matters in hand, the better it would be for the nation's moral and physical condition.

International Congress of Nurses. "Morality in Relation to Health," *British Journal of Nursing*, August 28, 1909, XLIII (1117), 173–178.

Notes

1 Portions of this chapter also published in Marsha Fowler, "Remembering the Future," in Martin Lipscomb (ed.), *Routledge Handbook of Philosophy and Nursing* (London: Routledge, 2023).

2 Elizabeth Cady Stanton (1815–1902), "Declaration of Sentiments," Report of the Woman's Rights Convention, held at Seneca Falls, New York, July 19 and 20, 1848 (Rochester, NY: John Dick, 1948), The North Star office of Frederick Douglass, 1848. Elizabeth Cady Stanton Papers, Manuscript Division, Library of Congress (007.00.00). https://www.loc.gov/exhibitions/women-fight-for-the-vote/about-this-exhibition/seneca-falls-and-building-a-movement-1776–1890/seneca-falls-and-the-start-of-annual-conventions/declaration-of-sentiments/

3 Lavinia Dock, "The Need of Education on Matters of Social Morality," International Congress of Nurses. "Morality in Relation to Health," *British Journal of Nursing* XLIII, no. 1117 (August 28, 1909): 174.

4 Drawing of the Suffrage March Line order from the *New York Evening Journal* New York, Star Co., March 4, 1913, p. 2, col. 4, can be retrieved from: http://loc.gov/pictures/resource/ppmsca.02946/

5 Sheridan Harvey, "Marching for the Vote: Remembering the Woman Suffrage Parade of 1913" (Library of Congress, American Memory, American Women. 2001). Retrieved from https://memory.loc.gov/ammem/awhhtml/aw01e/aw01e.html

6 Barbara Welter, "The Cult of True Womanhood: 1820–1860," *American Quarterly* 18, no. 2, Part 1 (Summer 1966): 151–174.

7 Technological innovation will be addressed in Chapter 5.

8 Anne-Katrin Ebert, "Liberating Technologies? Of Bicycles, Balance and the 'New Woman' in the 1890s," *Icon* 16, Special Issue: Technology in Everyday Life (2010): 25–52.

9 Patricia Marks, "Women's Athletics: A Bicycle Built for One," in Patricia Marks (ed.), *Bicycles, Bangs, and Bloomers* (Lexington, KY: University Press of Kentucky, 1990).

10 Ebert, "Bicycles," 43.

11 Miliann Kang, Donovan Lessard, Laura Heston, and Sonny Nordmarken, *Introduction to Women, Gender, Sexuality Studies* (Amherst, MA: University of Massachusetts Amherst Libraries, 2017). https://openbooks.library.umass.edu/introwgss/front-matter/287-2/

12 Ibid.

13 Lucinda Canty, Christina Nyirati, Valorie Taylor, and Peggy L. Chinn, "An Overdue Reckoning on Racism in Nursing," *American Journal of Nursing* 122, no. 2 (Feb 1, 2022): 26–34. DOI: 10.1097/01.NAJ.0000819768.01156.d6. PMID: 35027524.

14 National Commission to Address Racism in Nursing. https://www.nursingworld.org/practice-policy/workforce/racism-in-nursing/national-commission-to-address-racism-in-nursing/

15 Vern Bullough, Lilli Sentz, and Alice Stein, *American Nursing: A Biographical Dictionary, Vol. 2* (New York: Garland Publishing, 1992), xiv.

16 Anon. "National Woman's Trade Union League of America Offers the Services of Miss Rose Schneiderman as a Lecturer on the Subject of The Working Woman in America," (announcement), *Life and Labor*, 20, 2, no. 8 (August 1912): 258.

17 Minerva K. Brooks, "Rose Schneiderman in Ohio," *Life and Labor*, 21, 2, no. 9 (September 1912): 288.

18 Diane Reay, "Sociology, Social Class, and Education," in Michael W. Apple, Stephen J. Ball, and Luis Armando Gandin (eds.), *The Routledge International Handbook of the Sociology of Education* (Abingdon: Routledge, 2010), 396–404.

19 Kupiri Ackerman-Barger and Faye Hummel, "Critical Race Theory as a Lens for Exploring Inclusion and Equity in Nursing Education," *The Journal of Theory Construction & Testing* 19, no. 2 (Fall/Winter 2015): 39–46.

20 Blythe Bell, "White Dominance in Nursing Education: A Target for Anti-Racist Efforts," *Nursing Inquiry* 28 (2021): e12379. DOI: 10.1111/nin.12379

21 Kechinyere C. Iheduru-Anderson, and Monika M. Wahi, "Rejecting the Myth of Equal Opportunity: An Agenda to Eliminate Racism in Nursing Education in the United States," *BMC Nursing* 20 (2021): 30. DOI: 10.1186/s12912-021-00548-9

22 Sharissa Hantke, Verna St. Denis, and Holly Graham, "Racism and Antiracism in Nursing Education: Confronting the Problem of Whiteness," *BMC Nursing* 21 (2022): 146. DOI: 10.1186/s12912-022-00929-8

23 Accessioned at the Huntington Library, San Marino, California.

24 Marsha Fowler, unpublished personal research accessed at the Huntington Library, rare documents archives, 1984.

25 Bureau of Registration of Nurses, California State Board of Health, *Schools of Nursing Requirements and Curriculum* (Sacramento, CA: State Printing Office, 1916).

26 Marsha D. Fowler, "The Influence of the Social Location of Nurses-as-Women on the Development of Nursing Ethics," in Helen Kohlen and Joan McCarthy (eds.), *Nursing Ethics: Feminist Perspectives* (New York: Springer, 2020). DOI: 10.1007/978-3-030-49104-8_1

27 National League for Nursing Education, *Standard Curriculum for Schools of Nursing* (New York: NLNE, 1917).

28 Marsha D. Fowler, "The Influence of the Social Location of Nurses-as-Women on the Development of Nursing Ethics," in Helen Kohlen and Joan McCarthy (eds.), *Nursing Ethics: Feminist Perspectives* (New York: Springer, 2020). DOI: 10.1007/978-3-030-49104-8_1

29 Harriet C. Camp, "The Ethics of Nursing: Talks of a Superintendent with Her Graduating Class," *The Trained Nurse and Hospital Review* 2, no. 5 (1889): 179.

30 American Nurses Association. *Code of Ethics for Nurses with Interpretive Statements* (Silver Spring, MD: ANA, 2015).

31 Editor, "Votes for British Nurses," *The Nursing Times* XIV, no. 664 (January 19, 1918): 61–62.

32 Anon. "Nurses and the Vote," *The Nursing Times* XVI, no. 781 (April 17, 1920): 475.

33 Anon. "Nurses and the Vote," *The Nursing Times,* 1920, 475.

34 Anon. "Nurses and the Vote," *The Nursing Times* XV, no. 749 (September 6, 1919): 893.

35 Lavinia L. Dock, "The Nursing Profession and the Vote," *British Journal of Nursing* XLII, no. 1089 (February 13, 1909): 135.

36 Ibid.

37 Editor. "How Shall I Vote? *The Nursing Times* XIV, no. 708 (November 23, 1918): 1171.

38 Ibid.

39 Lavinia Dock, "The Duty of This Society in Public Work," *The American Journal of Nursing* 4, no. 2 (Nov. 1903): 99.

40 Ibid., 99–100.

41 Broderick was a nurse but not a trained nurse per se.

42 Anon. *Address to Women on the Prevention of Venereal Disease,* (book review). *The Nursing Times,* Some New Books section, XIX, no. 955 (August 18, 1923): 782.

43 Judith Walkowitz, *Prostitution and Victorian Society: Women, Class, and the State* (Cambridge: Cambridge University Press, 1980); 1–9.

44 Josephine Elizabeth Grey Butler, *Personal Reminiscences of a Great Crusade* (London: Horace Marshall & Son, 1896).

45 BJN International Congress of Nurses, Friday Morning July 23, 10 a.m. to 12:30 p.m. *British Journal of Nursing* XLIII, no. 1117 (August 28, 1909): 171–173.

46 Albinia Broderick, "Morality in Relation to Health," ICN Congress, *British Journal of Nursing* XLIII, no. 1117 (August 28, 1909), 171.

47 Ibid., 172.

48 Ibid., 173.

49 Ibid.

50 Ibid.

51 Dock, Lavinia, "The need of Education on Mattters of Social Morality," *British Journal of Nursing*, vol. XLIII no. 1,117 (August 28, 1909): 173.

52 Ibid.; italics as in original.

53 Ibid., 174.

54 Ibid.

55 Ibid.

56 Lavinia L. Dock, "Our Foreign Letter: The Nursing Profession and the Vote," *British Journal of Nursing* XLII, no. 1089 (Feb. 1909): 135.

57 Burr, Mary, "Some Statistics of Criminal Assault Upon Young Girls," *British Journal of Nursing*, vol. XLIII no, 1,117 (August 28, 1909): 175.

58 Ibid., 176.

59 Ibid.

60 Ibid.

61 Ibid.

62 Ibid.

63 Marsha D.M. Fowler, "Nursing and Social Ethics," in N.A. Chaska (ed.), *The Nursing Profession: Turning Points* (St. Louis, MO: C.V. Mosby, 1989), 24–30.

64 Marsha D.M. Fowler, "Professional Associations, Ethics and Society," *Oncology Nursing Forum* 20, no. 10 (Supplement to Nov./Dec. 1993 issue): 13–19. PMID: 8278287

65 Marsha D.M. Fowler, "Social Advocacy," *Heart & Lung* 18 (Jan. 1989): 1, 97–99. Also in M. Snyder and R. Lindquist (eds.), *Alternative/Alternative Therapies in Nursing* (New York: Springer Publishing, 1998). PMID: 2912930

66 Gibson Winter, *Social Ethics: Issues in Ethics and Society* (London: SCM Press, 1968), 6.

67 Julia Hurlston, "Stray Thought for Nurses," *British Journal of Nursing* 1, no. 188 (Jan. 7, 1911): 6–7.

68 International Congress of Nurses. "Morality in Relation to Health," *British Journal of Nursing*, August 28, 1909, XLIII (1117), 173–178.

69 From the Latin for Venus, the goddess associated with love and beauty

5

AN UNAUTHORIZED BIOGRAPHY OF BIOETHICS

Its Social Context

Most of the histories of bioethics focus on organizational developments, "great men," clinical-technologically driven issues, and federal legal developments. Social movements are mentioned only in passing, and even then, as having influence upon medicine, not bioethics. There is no need to duplicate historical ground here that is already ably addressed elsewhere in various histories of bioethics. Instead, we will walk through some of the social movements that formed the context of the emergent bioethics. These movements have, in varying ways, influenced the shape of its development and content, more specifically the issues and questions bioethics chooses to address. Some of these movements have roots in the 1800s but reach an apex at the time that bioethics is born. Others are located within the period of the development of bioethics. To the extent that it can be, their arrangement is as contiguous and linear as possible. Yet, as a friend has recently reminded me, in this book there are "so many interrelated threads it is almost impossible to write linearly; history is chronological but it is not linear."[1] The movements discussed below do interact, some intertwine, some stand alone; however, all affect various aspects of the field of bioethics.

A problem with bioethics in general (and bioethics in nursing) is its ostensible reliance upon *reason*, i.e., the use of abstract, decontextual, Continental philosophy, a philosophy "divorced" from the sociopolitical setting in life that shaped it, as if, in reality, reason were untouched by its own *sitz im leben* (setting in life). *Sitz im leben* is a term originating with German theologian Hermann Gunkel in the early 1900s. It refers to an aspect of literary form-criticism; that is, the analysis of the meaning, function, and purpose of a text, written or orally transmitted in a previous era. Texts have meaning in the period in which they were written. This means it was shaped by the sociopolitical and cultural circumstances of the day, including the author's own situatedness and the community for which it was

DOI: 10.4324/9781003262107-6

written; circumstances that may be obscure to a reader chronologically removed from the text. *Sitz im leben* must be considered in order to promulgate a contextual interpretation of a text.

A consideration of the history and development of nursing ethics and bioethics is necessarily bound to written texts, many written in a prior era. Though hardly ancient texts, Beauchamp and Childress' textbook *The Principles of Biomedical Ethics*[2] and *The Belmont Report*[3] are foundational texts for bioethics that come from a different cultural and sociopolitical period than our own, one in which bioethics had not yet been established as a discipline. Additionally, these texts draw from predecessor texts, some ancient, but principally from the 1600s to the 1800s. Borrowing and elasticizing the concept of *sitz im leben*, we will look at a few of the contextual influences upon these "founding" written bioethics texts and, thus, the development of the field. Today, some of these influences have largely receded from the memory of nurses in ethics. In succession, we will look at inhumane experimentation, medical power and sovereignty, the role of ethics in professions; power, paternalism, and patriarchy; the corporate betrayal of social trust, whistle-blowing, medical misogyny, the social critique of medicine, and technology. This is a full plate, so perhaps it would be good to eat dessert first by beginning with a bit of philosophical gossip and a not-so-rational influence upon the adoption of reason as the basis of ethics (and its importation into bioethics). Then we will take a more leisurely gaze at the confluence of sociopolitical and economic forces that affected the content, development, and scope of bioethics.

Unseemly Academic Gossip to Make a Quick Point

Occasionally, buried deep within yellowed books, often in the footnotes, one may encounter a delicious and extremely artfully, if abstrusely written, bit of academic gossip. Johann Gottfried Herder was the greatest eighteenth-century philosopher whom no one has read. He was Immanuel Kant's best student, then became an exceptionally capable rival and opponent. It is in a book on the Herder–Kant rivalry that we find the story of Kant's turbulent years and the redirection of his life and philosophy. It is more than possible that it was Kant's personal experience, and not an illuminative rational moment, that accelerated his philosophical redirection.[4]

Kant turned 40 in 1764, and his work took what is commonly referred to as "a critical turn" in that decade. These are years in which he sought to marry, but was too poor to make a "good" marriage; that is, one of a higher social standing. While the meaning of the evidence is subject to academic debate, Kant is known to have had an intimate (possibly amorous—this is the debate) relationship with three women, two married and one unmarried.

There are two women for whom *marriage* is not an issue, but personal intimacy quite definitely is. Kant eagerly spent time with each of these women, and their fondness for him is documented. The first is Countess Karoline Charlotte

Amalie von Keyserling. The other is the woman whose scandalous personal life and one flirtatious letter to Kant have always occasioned the most speculation, Frau Maria Charlotte Jacobi. Both of them were married women when Kant came to know them, but women married very young to men much older.... The question of an erotic dimension to this important relationship [with von Keyserling] is one that has been for the most part unwelcome among Kant scholars.[5,6]

Frau Maria Charlotte Jacobi was married to Kant's good friend Conrad Jacobi, though in the mid-1760s she became interested in two men: Kant and his friend Göschen. Kant spent considerable time with her, going to the theater with her and sitting in her box, attending her social gatherings, and more. In 1768, she divorced Jacobi and married... not Kant, but Göschen. Kant became conspicuous about maintaining a relationship with Jacobi thereafter.

Kant is known to have had a third relationship, with Fraülein Charlotte Amalie von Knobloch though there is less documentation, so the relationship remains a matter of speculation and debate. Note that in these instances that *von* preceding the surname is a nobiliary particle that signals the nobility of the family. As the son of a harness maker, from a Lutheran Pietist family, Kant was reaching upward in his relationships, in a class-stratified German society. Vorlander notes that Kant had said, "When I needed a woman, I couldn't feed one; when I could feed one, I didn't need one."[7]

After at least three sustained relationships of some intimacy, Kant loses out in the marriage lottery and his judgment of women becomes "sour."[8] Kant, however, is a philosopher, so his sourness seeps out of the pages of his *Observations on the Feeling of the Beautiful and Sublime.*[9,10] Among other brutal declarations, he writes:

> Women will avoid evil not because it is unjust but because it is ugly, and for them virtuous actions mean those that are ethically beautiful. Nothing of ought, nothing of must, nothing of obligation.... They do something only because they love to, and the art lies in making sure that they love only what is good. It is difficult for me to believe that the fair sex is capable of principles, and I hope not to give offense by this, for these are also extremely rare among the male sex.[11]

Woman, then, is not capable of deciding the moral *ought* based on principles, that is, by reason. To be fair, Kant says that men are capable but do not. Zammito, citing others, gives a train of Kant's comments on women:

> In matters of understanding women are pretty much children. Brutally, Kant observes: "women... have little character at all. When one knows one, one knows them all." He restates the point elsewhere: "the feminine sex has more good humor and heart than character." In women, "even if they have understanding, sense dominates."[12]

Kant embraces the gender norms of his period, but here we apparently see his personal experience seeping through as well. In summarizing this period of Kant's life, Zammito writes:

> This is what Kant came to believe and then set about to achieve in the second half of the 1760s, after his own fortieth year and in the context of disappointments that induced "disgust at the unsteady condition of [sexual] instinct." What exactly might these disappointments occasioning disgust have been? We can formulate them in three echelons of increasing intimacy. First, he was disgusted at the decadence of society. Second, he was disgusted at the decadence of scholarship... finally, and perhaps most pointedly, he was disgusted at his own susceptibility to the sexual allure of women. His resolve was to have none of the last, little of the first, and to purify the second into the most "rigorous" and impersonal inquiry possible.[13]

Kant thereafter withdraws to a life of ascetic renunciation of happiness and pleasure, an extreme regimentation of daily life, an intense application to the work of philosophy, in which, ultimately, a resolute defense of reason as the basis of ethics would evolve. This is his "silent decade" of 1770–1781 in which his ethics takes its critical turn. In his early, called *pre-critical*, years, Kant was influenced by British philosopher Francis Hutcheson, the core of whose moral philosophy was that we possess a *moral sense*, a perceptive faculty. This moral sense enables us to *feel* "a kind of pleasure upon perceiving benevolence, and to appraise such benevolence as morally good on the basis of this *feeling*."[14] In *Observations on the Feeling of the Beautiful and Sublime*, Kant's ethics is not yet *a priori*; feeling, inclination, and moral sense, the empirical, have a role in morality; freedom and autonomy are not central concerns as they will become in his critical period. In his 1785 *Groundwork of the Metaphysics of Morals*,[15] however, Kant rejects feeling, inclination, moral sense, anything empirical, as having a role in ethics. His ethics now has an *a priori* foundation where freedom and autonomy are central, and the *categorical imperative* becomes his supreme principle of morality.

Philosophers reasonably tend not to draw a straight line of causation here, and simply toy with correlation. Though Kant had been moving toward a rationalist ethics, it is not unreasonable to suggest that the later strict Kantian rationality (that is often presented in bioethics in nursing) is colored by Kant's failure to secure a wife, his failure in a series of intimate relationships, his broader unhappiness, and his rejection of a normal life. The point here is that the setting in life of a text influences its content and interpretation, often outside the author's own awareness, and here part of that context is the "sourness" of Kant's personal life. Kant and Mill predominate in bioethics in nursing, with a dash of Rawls, customarily through secondary and partial sources. Nursing did not choose Kant and Mill; nursing chose Beauchamp and Childress. Though an excellent work in its own perspective, as mentioned above, it had roots in Kant, Mill, and Rawls. By nursing's uncritical adoption and utilization of *The Principles of Biomedical Ethics*, in a sense Kant and Mill were chosen *for* nursing without nursing's critical reflection—suppose nursing bioethics had chosen to follow a different philosophical stream, perhaps the early Kant, or Hutcheson, or Herder or another?

Context Makes a Difference: A Confluence of Social Forces That Affected the Emergent Bioethics

Bioethics arises as a modern discipline in the 1960s, solidifies over the next 20 years or so, and in the 1990s and thereafter cements its position in academics, health care, and the public arena It is not untouched by the sociopolitical and economic movements swirling around it. These movements vary in kind; some are social and political, some international, and some are medical in and of themselves. These social forces are contemporaneous with one another, and influence the field of bioethics, though they are not necessarily directly interactive with one another.

Inhumane Experimentation on Human Subjects

When they came to light, the infamous hellscape of Nazi experiments on involuntary human subjects (prisoners) during World War II subsequently precipitated the creation of international regulations governing the use of human subjects in research. The *Nuremberg Code of 1947*[16] and the World Medical Association *Declaration of Helsinki*[17] (1964) require a number of safeguards for the protection of human subjects in research. While the *Nuremberg Code* predates the emergence of bioethics, the *Declaration of Helsinki* falls within bioethics' neonatal period. Though, Albert Jonsen notes, surprisingly, that the concerns that emerged from Nuremberg did not galvanize a response within American medicine.[18] It would take the exposure of unethical experimentation closer to home to move medicine.

Four studies conducted in the US are held up as morally unacceptable: the medical Tuskegee USPHS Syphilis Experiment,[19] 1932–1972; the Willowbrook Hepatitis Studies, 1956–1970; the Laud Humphreys ethnographic Tearoom Trade Experiment, 1970; and the social-psychologist Stanley Milgram's Obedience Experiment, 1961–1964. However, in 1966, Henry Beecher published his article "Ethics and Clinical Research" in the *New England Journal of Medicine*.[20] Beecher's article identifies 22, deeply disturbing, medical research projects, conducted from prestigious universities, all of which were ethically questionable or worse, and published in respected medical journals.[21] In 1962, British physician Maurice Pappworth published "Human Guinea Pigs: A Warning" in the lay magazine *Twentieth Century Magazine*, followed by a book *Human Guinea Pigs: Experimentation on Man*, and a subsequent reflection (1990).[22,23,24] In his initial article for a public readership, Pappworth identifies 14 morally objectionable medical research experiments. He later expanded this article into a book in which he details 78 medical experiments that violated provisions of the *Nuremberg Code*. In his 1990 reflection, he notes that "whenever I read an account of an unethical experiment, I wrote a letter to the journal protesting, often as not to have it rejected. Medical research had become sacrosanct, based on the dubious dogma that its continuation must be the prime concern of teaching hospitals."[25] While research review committees had yet to come into being, the obscenity of these experiments should nonetheless have met with alarm and action; the guild had essentially stonewalled Pappworth. One hopes that the safeguards in place today will be sufficient to prevent unethical research, including research conducted by American companies outside the United States.

Medicine Agglutinates, Associates, and Promulgates a Code of Ethics for Medicine

In the late 1800s, at the time that modern nursing education is becoming more rigorous, scientized, and standardized, medical education is a snake pit, filled with snake oil salesmen, quacks, and some legitimate university medical programs. There were many competing theories of medicine including allopathy, homeopathy, mesmerism, phrenology, naturopathy, Grahamism, and a delightful variety of others. To the consternation of university physicians, proprietary schools and apprenticeships recruited men from the working and lower middle classes—as well as from some the rigorous university medical schools that had not, as yet, become sovereign. Though there were 17 medical schools for women that were founded in the latter half of the nineteenth century, women were not admitted to the elite university schools, until 1890 when, strapped for money, Johns Hopkins University Medical School agreed to admit women in exchange for a half million dollars to be contributed by wealthy philanthropic women.[26] The women's medical colleges and admission of women to co-educational medical schools would decline in the early 1900s, when the American Medical Association worked to entrench allopathic medical education, to extinguish rival theories of medicine, and to solidify the profession. Medicine had embarked upon a plan to consolidate its power, prestige, and authority. Paul Starr's excellent popular and Pulitzer Prize winning work *The Social Transformation of American Medicine: The Rise of a Sovereign Profession and the Making of a Vast Industry* chronicles the development of medicine as a formidable social institution and power.[27]

The American Medical Association Code of Ethics for Medicine

The American Medical Association formulated its first code of ethics in 1847, the year of its founding. While medicine, clergy, and law had long been well-regarded professions, medicine at this point in American history was only nascently organized and not standardized in education or practice. The first *Code of Medical Ethics*[28] reflects this. It does detail the responsibilities of the physician to patients, to other professionals, and to society, as well as the duties of patients, other professionals, and society to individual physicians. The specification of reciprocal duties is based on "a few considerations on the legitimate range of medical ethics... Every duty or obligation implies, both in equity and for its successful discharge, a corresponding right."[29] The *Code* does, however, attempt to situate medicine among the classical professions, and set an impermeable membrane around who is in and who is out. There is a somewhat defensive assertion that

> His position, purposes and proper efforts eminently entitle him to, at least, the same respectful and considerate attentions that are paid, as a matter of course and apparently without constraint, to the clergyman, who is admitted to administer spiritual consolation, and to the lawyer, who comes to make the last will and testament.[30]

The social eminence of the physician and medicine is one consideration, but the *Code* is also concerned to limit who may be regarded legitimately as "regularly initiated members of the medical profession, also known as *regular physicians*, over against 'the host of quacks who infest the land.'"[31] Under obligations of the public to physician, the *Code* states:

> The benefits accruing to the public directly and indirectly from the active and unwearied beneficence of the profession, are so numerous and important, that physicians are justly entitled to the utmost consideration and respect from the community. The public ought likewise to entertain a just appreciation of medical qualifications;—to make a proper discrimination between true science and the assumptions of ignorance and empiricism...[32]

Terence Johnson, a sociologist of professions, writes that

> In periods in which it is claimed that charlatanism is rife and needs to be stamped out are just those periods when an occupation is attempting to establish or struggling to maintain a monopolistic position. Practice can be unqualified only where a monopoly skill by one group exists.[33]

The *Code* identifies proper medical qualifications:

> A regular medical education furnishes the only presumptive evidence of professional abilities and acquirements, and ought to be the only acknowledged right of an individual to the exercise and honours of his profession... who has license to practice from some medical board of known and acknowledged respectability, recognized by this association, and who is in, good moral and professional standing in the place in which he resides, should be fastidiously excluded from fellowship, or his aid refused in consultation when it is requested by the patient. But no one can be considered as a regular practitioner, or a fit associate in

consultation, whose practice is based on an exclusive dogma, to the rejection of
the accumulated experience of the profession, and of the aids actually furnished
by anatomy, physiology, pathology, and organic chemistry...[34]

This is a period of patent medicines, and regular physicians had an obligation to
protect the public from quackery—which simultaneously drew a boundary between *regular medicine* and all others as quacks.

It is the duty of physicians, who are frequent witnesses of the enormities committed by quackery, and the injury to health and even destruction of life caused
by the use of quack medicines, to enlighten the public on these subjects, to
expose the injuries sustained by the unwary from the devices and pretensions of
artful empirics and impostors.[35]

For their part, "the first duty of a patient is, to select as his medical adviser one who
has received a regular professional education"[36] and "the obedience of a patient to
the prescriptions of his physician should be prompt and implicit."[37]

The intent here is not to analyze this 1847 *Code of Ethics for Medicine*, but rather
to situate the *Code*'s self-aggrandizement and protectionism within considerations
of the sociology of professions. These considerations affect nursing as well, and,
for our purposes here, are relevant to the role of ethics within professions.

How Ethics Functions in Professions

The zenith of the sociology of professions coincides with the rise of the discipline
of bioethics, and while it is more concerned with the attributes of professions per
se, it raises questions of the function of ethics for professions.[38] Defining what constitutes a profession has been addressed by two main approaches: *trait definitions*
and *functionalist definitions*. Trait definitions of professions generally represent the
approach that nursing takes: identify a set of attributes that, together, are hallmarks
of a profession. They include the familiar assortment: (a) a well-defined body of
specialized knowledge, (b) specialized higher education and expertise, (c) provision of a practical service, (d) a discipline-specific professional association, (e)
autonomy of practice, (f) profession-determined standards of education and practice, (g) adumbration[39] of a code of ethics,[40] and (h) altruistic motivation.[41,42,43,44,45,46]
The second approach to defining a profession relies upon functionalist models that
stress "the functional value of professional activity for all groups and classes in society."[47] In functionalist models, "there is no attempt to present an exhaustive list of
'traits': rather the components of the model are limited to those elements which are
said to have functional relevance for society as a whole or to the professional–client
relationship."[48] In the trait models, ethics, or more specifically a code of ethics (not
necessarily written), is a defining attribute. In functionalist models, "professional
ethics has a social utility because it assures that the values of the profession are

reinforced and displayed by individual practitioners, and it constrains the negative effects that monopolization of practice may have for the consumer."[49] In both functionalist and trait models of profession, ethics serves as a defining attribute.

And yet, there are differing views on the relationship of professions to society that produce different views of the role of ethics in professions. In Emil Durkheim's view, as a consequence of the societal division of labor, there is a general disintegration of social ties, and morality becomes less binding. Professions are altruistic moral communities that are self-policing, that replace (or at least augment) the moral ties that have loosened in society. Professional ethics is enforced through various forms of moral pressure—*moral suasion*, disapproval, censure or ostracism—which serve to restrain individual professionals from tarnishing the guild, or from engaging in rampant self-interest at the expense of clients, the profession, or society. This is an idealized view of professions, partly undermined by evidence of lobbying and power-brokering at the macro level, as well as evidence of misconduct, the failure of self-policing, and a lack of altruism. A second view of professions is substantially more cynical but perhaps more consistent with evidence. In this perspective, professions are occupationally narrowly specialized, monopolistic, power elites that serve their own purposes and ends. Ethics is so structured as to further the power and dominance of the group, grant it exclusive authority, suppress competition, secure its social stature and authority—through the exploitation of a social need. Stamey writes that

> Every concretely specified ethic of the past has tended to function as an ideology rather than as an instrument of critical ethical reflection. Ethical reasoning has functioned not only to translate universal ethical principles into concretely specified situational duties; it has served to validate and perpetuate (unjustifiable) privileges of a limited segment of the human community.[50]

Deats notes that Stamey is only partially correct "for there have been challenges to privilege, and there has been a stream of more universal, more prophetic, more critical ethical thought."[51] Codes of ethics and professional ethical literature, then, should be read against these views of the role of ethics in professions and analyzed for their perpetuation or challenge to unjust guild privilege.

Johnson, a sociologist of professions, adds a further dimension to the discussion of ethics in professions. Johnson sees a profession not as an occupation, but as a social division of labor with a specific form of occupational control. His theory of professions begins with the social division of labor. More specifically, his emphasis is on the social division of labor and its consequences for the professional–client relationship. While he details a fascinating range of effects, his discussion of three forms of occupational control has direct implications for the role of professional ethics.

In brief, Johnson posits three forms of occupational control: *collegiate, patronage*, and *mediative. Collegiate* occupational control is what is considered the classical professions, such as law, medicine, and ministry. Under collegiate control there is a significant power differential between professional and client. The professional determines the nature of the relationship, when it begins, when it ends, the needs that are to be served, and what transpires. The professional is highly specialized and the client highly unspecialized, and thus dependent and vulnerable to exploitation. In collegiate occupational control, the profession autonomously establishes its ethics; its ethics might look like either of the two views of professions—as a reinforcement of a moral community, or as a self-protective offensive. In the second form of occupational control, *patronage*, the professional uses her or his specialized knowledge in the service of the goals of the patron. It is the patron, not a client, who determines the need to be met, when the relationship starts, when it ends, and the quality of the performance. Artists and architects customarily serve under patronage control. Ethics in this form of occupational control consists in the proficiency and excellence in performance of a specific task. *Mediative* occupational control exists where the state exercises control over both the professional and the client. The state controls the needs that can be met, how they will be met, when the relationship begins and ends; that is, the state controls the content of practice and professional and consumer choices are circumscribed.[52] With mediative control, Johnson writes that, "the clear-cut ethical prescriptions of professionalism which specify 'client' and colleague relationships are no longer entirely applicable"[53]

Medicine has moved into a hybrid position of maintaining the social stature of a profession, i.e., of collegiate occupational control while, in practice, having moved into a mediative control, mediated by insurance companies, state and government programs of medical coverage, and a range of political and economic forces. Still, Johnson notes a number of factors in collegiate occupational control, *professions*, that reinforce the authority and privilege of the physician within the physician–patient relationship, and the stature and privilege of medicine in society.

Medical Malefactions: Power, Paternalism, Patriarchy

Consolidating Professional Sovereignty

Star's historical study of American medicine addresses "first, the rise of professional sovereignty; and second, the transformation of medicine into an industry and the growing... role of corporations and the state."[54] Starr details medicine's consolidation of practice authority. The next step was to secure economic, social, and political power.

> The conversion of authority into high income, autonomy, and other rewards of privilege required the medical profession to gain control over both the market for its services and the various organizational hierarchies that govern medical practice, financing, and policy. The achievement of economic power involved more than the creation of a monopoly in medical practice through the exclusion of alternative practitioners and limits on the supply of physicians. It entailed

shaping the structure of hospitals, insurance, and other private institutions that impinge on medical practice... these organizational and political arrangements have become more important as bases of economic power than the monopolization of medical practice.[55]

Starr's popular book, though not an academic book, is well researched, and winner of the Pulitzer and Bancroft Prizes. It pulls together a number of forces that allowed medicine to achieve sovereignty, authority, monopoly, and economic and political power. That sovereignty, of course, included physician dominance of the physician–patient relationship, manifest in paternalism, and reinforced by factors of dependence, distance, uncertainty, and indeterminacy.

Terence Johnson specifies that the effects of the social division of labor on the professional-producer/consumer-client relationship consists of interrelated factors of *social and economic dependence, social distance, uncertainty*, and *indeterminacy*.[56] Social and economic dependence arises when the occupational skill is highly specialized; the more the occupational group becomes *specialized* the more the consumer becomes *unspecialized* and dependent upon the profession for the provision of services that the consumers are unable to evaluate or to produce for themselves. *Social distance* results. Social distance creates a structure of *uncertainty* or what Jamous and Peloille term *indeterminacy*.[57] Indeterminacy has a proportionate relationship with *technicality*, the technical skills of doing medicine. Jamous and Peloille propose an Indetermination/Technicality, or I/T ratio.

> The I/T ratio expresses the possibility of transmitting, by means of apprenticeship, the mastery of intellectual or material instruments used to achieve a given result. This makes it possible to appreciate the limits of this transmissibility; i.e. the part played in the production process by "means" that can be mastered and communicated in the form of rules (T), in proportion to the "means" that escape rules and, at a given historical moment are attributed to virtualities of producers.[58]

Where indeterminacy is higher, on balance, than technicality, social distance is greater than where indeterminacy is low and technicality high. The higher the indeterminacy, the greater the social distance. Where social distance is great, there is greater potential for professional autonomy or sovereignty at the expense of the consumer. Indeterminacy can be enhanced by professionals through *mystification*. Mystification further distances in symbolification through such means as white coats, stethoscopes around the neck, medicalese, and more. Johnson writes that

> The power relationship existing between the practitioner and client may be such, then, as to enable the practitioner to increase the social distance and his own autonomy and control over practice by engaging in a process of "mystification". Uncertainty is not, therefore, entirely cognitive in origin but may be deliberately increased to serve manipulative or managerial ends.[59]

Jamous and Peloille note that "It is possible to say that the system includes dominant members and dominated members."[60] Patients in the medical system found themselves to be the dominated members. It did not sit well. Their discontent will give rise to the development of the patient's rights movement, and ultimately a *Patient Bill of Rights.*[61]

It was the 1970s, the later end of the US Civil Rights Movement with its concern for rights and the individual in the face of constituted authority. Bioethics was all fueled-up and on the launch pad. So was the consumer movement. Robert Mayer notes that "the term 'consumer movement' refers to... nonprofit advocacy groups and grassroots activism to promote consumer interest by reforming the practices of corporations or policies of the government."[62] For consumers, enough was enough: medical and physician sovereignty and paternalism had reigned over the health of society and its individual members for well over a century. Medicine, however, was not the only broken profession, and not the only provocation of public ire and loss of social trust. It was a period of banking failures, and the collapse of Enron that left 20,000 employees with a loss of $2 billion in pensions. There were many other betrayals of trust in the national awareness. Two such examples are those of the Challenger Shuttle O-rings failure and the Ford Pinto gas-tank explosions.

Betrayal of Social Trust: Morton Thiokol, Pintos, and Whistleblowing Traitors

Morton Thiokol

The space shuttle *Challenger* (1986) was fitted with an O-ring seal, a type of gasket, made by Morton Thiokol. The O-rings sealed the joints on the solid rocket booster preventing hot pressurized gas from leaking. Shortly after liftoff the O-rings in the right rocket booster had failed. This caused structural failure that caused aerodynamic forces to break the shuttle apart—as millions of Americans viewing the launch on television saw the Challenger explode, instantly killing the entire seven-person crew. The commission investigating the disaster found that the flaws in the O-ring seals were known, and had been reported, and that the disaster could have been avoided. The commission further found that the disaster was largely a consequence of NASA's organizational culture and decision-making processes where warnings were ignored, and NASA did not adequately communicate engineering-technical concerns.[63]

Ford Pinto

The regulatory requirements for cars in the 1970s were in flux. In the case of the Ford Pinto, the car had a design flaw in the placement of the gas tank in relation to rear bumper design and other engineering issues. There were also economizing production measures that were taken in the construction of the mounts that would also prove to increase risk. In rear collisions over 25 miles per hour (40 km/hour), a bolt could puncture the gas tank, causing the tank to leak and spark, further causing the gas tank to engulf the passenger compartment in flames. Passengers were at risk of severe burns and burn death. The flaw was discovered during testing; however, in Ford's risk–benefit analysis, it was decided that it would cost more to re-tool production and to correct the flaw, than to compensate victims for burn injuries or death.[64] In Ford's profit-based risk–benefit equation, human life was inadequately valued against corporate costs of recall and redesign. The Pinto story became the "textbook case" in business ethics and tort law circles as an instance of morally bankrupt corporate behavior that plagued American society. A Pulitzer Prize winning article by Mark Dowie, published as "Pinto Madness" in *Mother Jones* magazine (1977), established this as the prevailing narrative, which inflamed public ire and fueled the larger consumer movement. He referred to the Pinto as a "firetrap."[65] Subsequent analyses were made and the case became both more nuanced and its interpretation more contested.[66,67] Nonetheless, whatever the arguments over the merits of the case, public opinion remained firm and enlarged the social mistrust of corporations.

A Few Ethical Outcomes

Breaking faith with the public has consequences. In terms of the loss of faith in institutions such as medicine, and in mega-corporations such as Enron, Ford, and Morton Thiokol, a varied ethical literature arose. William Lawrence's 1976 book *Of Acceptable Risk: Science and the Determination of Safety*[68] became a foundational text for discussions of risk versus safety and was followed by a number of similar works.[69] In the government report, Baruch Fischoff et al. write that

> Acceptable-risk decisions are an essential step in the management of technological hazards. In many situations, they constitute the weak (or missing) link in the management process. The absence of an adequate decision-making, methodology often produces indecision, inconsistency, and dissatisfaction. The result is neither good for hazard management nor good for society.[70]

One of the conclusions of the report is that

> Values and uncertainties are an integral part of every acceptable-risk problem. As a result, there are no value-free processes for choosing between risky alternatives. The search for an "objective method" is doomed to failure and may blind the searchers to the value-laden assumptions they are making.[71]

Discussions of acceptable risk are meant to be applied at the macro, not the individual level. At the macro-level, competing values exist: social values, political values, economic values, corporate values, and more, and of course human values.

The way to reconcile the values resident in decisions on risk is to have the voices of those groups with a vested interest represented at the table, which is rarely the case.

Exit, Voice, and Loyalty

Another body of literature followed, including Albert Hirschman's influential book *Exit, Voice, and Loyalty: Responses to Decline in Firms, Organizations or States* (1970).[72] His book fundamentally deals with the response of human groups, such as consumers, to a decline in the quality whether of goods, services, function, or values. The book came to be applied in a wide range of issues such as membership organizations, employment situations, political situations, transnational migration, emigration, asylum seeking, and more. Hirschman's analytical framework maintains that there are two possible responses to decline in organizations, firms, or states: *exit* and *voice*. *Exit* refers to withdrawal from the group in question. *Voice* refers to expressing grievance, concern, or recommendations for change. As an economist and political theorist, in Hirschman's scheme, *exit* represents economic action (think strike or boycott), *voice* represents political action (think confrontation, dissent). *Loyalty* (or its degree thereof) affects whether one chooses to exit or to engage in voice (think patriotism, religious devotion, organizational allegiance or brand loyalty). All three concepts could be expressed collectively. The concepts of exit, voice, and loyalty had great bearing within the context of a disaffected public and the consumer movement. Exit, voice, and loyalty were means of applying pressure to effect change, especially with collective action (e.g., unions), though significant exit is a signal of the decline of a group, organization, or state. Within nursing, Hirschman's concepts came to be applied individually when the work environment was deemed less than satisfactory.

Whistleblowers

In work settings, exercising voice can risk reprisal, particularly where it is a single voice. Such was the case in the *Challenger* disaster and the Ford Pinto case, and perhaps the majority of whistleblowing cases. Whistleblowers are persons, often employees, who disclose information about a private or public sector firm, corporation, organization or agency.[73] The disclosure relates to organizational actions that the person believes to be ethically wrong-making, unsafe, potentially dangerous, illicit, illegal, fraudulent, out of compliance with standards, fraudulently misrepresented, violating human or worker rights, or any form of organizational or group (e.g., research group in drug trials) misconduct. The disclosures may be made to a superior (within the organizational ladder), to an outside party (regulatory body, the press), or to a third party (an external anonymous reporting mechanism). Whistleblowers are held in contempt and are commonly subject to reprisal of varying degrees, from being shunned by colleagues, to ostracism; being discredited; suffering defamation and character assassination; vilification; demotion, dismissal, blacklisting, and in the case of a state, charges of treason or sedition, incarceration, or execution. As there is a general ethical expectation that misconduct must be addressed, whistleblowing is a moral good. And yet, informers are regarded as traitors and snitches, or in the vernacular of the day, as rat finks,[74] a pejorative term associated with police informants. The whistleblowing literature largely discusses whistleblowing in the context of organizational misbehavior, or that of a group (such as a group of researchers that falsifies data), rather than instances of reporting an individual, for example a health-care professional practicing under the influence of alcohol or drugs.

Within the context of the developing field of bioethics, a pivotal document, *Whistleblowing in Biomedical Research*,[75] was published in 1981 by the President's Commission for the Study of Ethical Problems in Medicine and Biomedical and Behavioral Research. The report specifically targets whistleblowing in the various phases of biomedical research, from Institutional Review Board (IRB) proposal to publication. It does not address reporting, for example, of a pharmaceutical corporation, or a medical center. In the chapter "The Whistleblower as a Deviant Professional: Professional Norms and Responses to Fraud in Clinical Research,"[76] Judith Swazey and Stephen Scher address the core moral norms that conflict. They begin by citing Westin on the 1960s phase of whistleblowing. It was led

> Primarily by employees who were impelled to action during the consumer-protection, civil rights and [Vietnam] anti-war movements of the 1960s. There were the first people to break out of the "Organization Man" ethos of total company loyalty that corporate policy dictated and social mores accepted in the forties and fifties. Almost all of these first-stage protestors lost their jobs, and also any protests they took to the courts... the second stage of corporate whistleblowing, from the early 1970s down to the present, has been marked by two parallel trends: the enactment of dozens of... laws... and a steady rise in whistleblowing incidents.[77]

Despite the range of legal protections for employee and public protection, corporations managed to proceed, business as usual. Westin notes that "the result was that most whistleblowers of 1970–1979 fared only a little better than their predecessors."[78] As Swazey and Scher and many others note, whistleblowers rarely emerge unscathed.[79] By their reckoning, the moral crux of the issue is that

> The whistleblower may be—and within the group usually is—perceived and treated as [one] who has committed a disloyal, indeed treasonable act... both the negative responses to and sanctions against the whistleblower... seem to have two major sources. First, in terms of the group or organizational norms, the whistleblower is seen by those within the group as having violated a moral obligation of loyalty, particularly if he has gone public. Second, if whistleblowing occurs in the context of a professional group, such as scientists or physicians, it is seen from within the group as violating professional norms of [respecting professional] autonomy and self-regulation.[80]

It also calls into question the ability of the profession, not just the individual professional, to self-police its ethical behavior. Given that the document focuses on biomedical research, it does not explore the moral norms of reporting, for example, physician groups or hospitals. The persistence of reprisal for whistleblowing led to the creation of the National Whistleblower Center in 1988. Its "mission is to support whistleblowers in their efforts to expose and help prosecute corruption and other wrongdoing around the world."[81] Whistleblowing is an issue globally, not just in the US, and not simply in medical research. At least 50 countries now have a range of laws governing whistleblowing in private and public sectors.[82] And, still, whistleblowers do not fare well.

Whistleblowing on a Serial-Murdering Nurse

Amy Loughren, RN was a whistleblower. She was a single mom with two daughters, severe cardiomyopathy that she tried to hide while trying to make ends meet financially. She worked nights in the ICU with nurse Charles "Charlie" Cullen so that she could be available to her daughters in the daytime. She and Cullen became friends while working together. Cullen had worked in nine hospitals, in two states, over a period of 16 years. In that time, he skillfully used insulin, digoxin, and epinephrine to murder patients, leaving a trail of murders behind him as he moved from hospital to hospital and to one nursing home. When arrested, he was charged with 26 murders, but he thought that he had probably killed about 40. Police estimates are that there may have been as many as 300–400 murders. In 2003, he confessed to 29 murders and additional attempted murders by lethal injection. But this is about whistleblowing and not a nurse who serially murders patients.

At every turn, the police were stymied by the hospital, all of the hospitals, who stonewalled them. It is called risk management. The hospitals had suspicions, yet Cullen was passed along from hospital to hospital, with evidence left behind, admittedly expertly concealed, and dead patients. He was followed by neutral performance evaluations so that he could move from position to position. No one stopped him, until Amy Loughren who, under threat of dismissal, clandestinely cooperated with the police detectives.[83]

Why Can't a Woman Be More Like a Man? Protectionism, Paternalism, Sexism

In the 1800s, medicine's attitude toward women is one of protectionism. For her own benefit, girls and women, the weaker sex, had to be protected, lest their health suffer. Physicians of the period would argue that the demands of education, particularly higher education, with its intense mental application, would redirect blood flow to the brain, and cause withering of the female reproductive organs, thereby subverting a woman's "vital functions," that is childbearing.[84] Protectionism was simply one aspect of medical paternalism and sexism. Paternalism is somewhat less pervasive today, but sexism in health care persists. Rachel Gross' recent article "Please Don't Call My Cervix Incompetent: There's No End to the Weird Ways Medicine Describes Women's Bodies" is a more humorous example, though it is "kidding on the level."[85]

Sexism pervades society in many ways that affect the health and safety of women. For example, the safety regulations and mechanisms in the design of automobiles protect male bodies. Susan Molinari and Beth Brooke write that

> We live in a world designed for men. The top shelves in many supermarkets are too high for many women to reach. Many cellphones are too big for an average woman's hand. And because women's bodies have a lower metabolic resting rate than men's, the typical office is about five degrees too cold for women... But in some instances, unequal design costs lives. For example, more than 40,000 Americans are projected to die in automobile crashes this year... Importantly, those deaths are not suffered equally. While men are more likely to cause crashes, women are more likely to die in them.... a woman is 17 percent more likely to die... and 73 percent more likely to be seriously injured... Why? All the crash test dummies are male. Even the "female" dummies the government requires in tests are just smaller versions of male dummies... many cars are not primarily designed to keep women safe.[86]

In "a world designed for men," women's health, safety, and survival is plagued by regulatory and legislative blind spots worthy of nursing input.

Second-wave feminism (1960–1980s) would undertake the overturn of medical paternalism toward women, not simply for reproductive issues, but also general medical misogyny.[87] Sociologist Ruth Rosen writes that "generally treated as ignorant or hysterical patients, women had long suffered the medical establishment's arrogant attitude toward their ailments. The experience could be humiliating, enraging and... induces visceral understanding of women's secondary status."[88] The subordinate status of women is nowhere more in evidence than in the issue of drug testing.

The Thalidomide Scandal and the DES Tragedy

Thalidomide

Thalidomide, a tranquilizer that was used to quell morning sickness, was first given in the 1950s without having been tested on pregnant women. The US Food and Drug Administration had not approved the drug, but tablets were distributed to physicians to use in clinical trials. Thalidomide was teratogenic. Fetal exposure prior to day 42 of pregnancy resulted in children born with brain damage and phocomelia; severe eye, ear, and face damage; urinary tract and cardiac defects. Approximately 40 percent died shortly after delivery. Of the 2,000 infants born in the

UK with thalidomide damage, 466 survived. Because the drug had not yet been approved in the US, the incidence of surviving infants with severe defects was lower, numbering 17. However, Thalidomide raised another issue in the US, one that became quite public.

During the pregnancy with her fifth child, Sherri Finkbine, an Arizona resident, took sleeping pills that contained Thalidomide. She learned that the fetus had deformities and sought to obtain an abortion. She could not in Arizona, and because her case had become nationally known, hospitals in other states would not accommodate her for fear of adverse publicity. She flew to Sweden where the abortion was performed (1962). The fetus was severely deformed. Finkbine's situation stoked long-simmering discontent with the legal strictures surrounding abortion. This galvanized a movement that would ultimately end with according women the right to abortion, in the legal case *Roe v. Wade* (1973).[89] The drug companies had systematically suppressed evidence of Thalidomide's teratogenicity, and with the aid of various agencies managed to gag physicians regarding its damaging effects.[90] Though not all have been detailed here, Finkbine's case represents a convergence of a number of issues discussed above: bad faith and greed on the part of "Big Pharma"; inadequate oversight of and restraints upon corporate power, public loss of trust in medical structures, inadequate drug approval mechanisms internationally; paternalism and sexism in US medicine and the courts; and the denial of reproductive rights to women. However, Thalidomide was not the only drug at issue.

Diethylstilbestrol (DES)

Thalidomide was not the only tragedy in women's care. From about 1940 to 1971, diethylstilbestrol, known as DES, was a drug used to prevent complications of pregnancy (miscarriage, premature labor) and to stop lactation. It was widely prescribed in Europe and anglophone nations. It was shown to be ineffective in preventing miscarriage and premature labor, so ceased to be prescribed for that, but continued to be used to stop lactation, for emergency contraception, and to treat symptoms of menopause.[91] Millions of women received DES during pregnancy. While there was evidence of a modest increase in risk for breast cancer in women who took DES, the most profound effects are found in DES daughters exposed *in utero*, with epigenetic effects also found in DES granddaughters. DES sons exposed *in utero* were at higher risk of urogenital abnormalities and an increased risk of testicular cancer. DES grandsons were at increased risk of hypospadias. In a 2011 study, researchers found that daughters exposed to DES *in utero* had

> a twofold higher risk of infertility and a fivefold increased risk of having a preterm delivery... about 40 times the risk of developing CCA [clear cell adenocarcinoma] than unexposed women... The research now shows that the risk for DES-exposed daughters continues through at least age 40. In addition, these

women are more than twice as likely to develop... cervical intraepithelial neoplasia and have an 80 percent higher chance of developing breast cancer after age 40. According to the results of this study, by age 55, 1 in 25 DES-exposed daughters will develop abnormal cellular changes in the cervix or vagina, and 1 in 50 will develop breast cancer due to their DES exposure.[92]

DES has affected at least three generations: mother, child, grandchild, and possibly additional generations as well. Pilar Zamora-León makes note of an additional tragedy of this situation:

It has been known for decades that xenoestrogens are associated with the development of tumors. Since the late 1930s, studies in mice have shown that DES exposure could induce neoplasms in genital and breast tissues. Unfortunately, the experimental results were ignored, and the FDA approved the use of DES as a "safety drug." DES has the ability to cross the placenta, altering the development of the fetus, behaving as an endocrine disruptor, teratogen, and carcinogen. DES can induce severe alterations in the reproductive tract of the fetus that can lead to disease decades later.[93]

Every Cell Has a Sex

Women have not been equitably served by modern medicine. They have been, and remain, disadvantaged at every stage of development of research and science. The Brigham and Women's Health Report (2014) states:

The science that informs medicine—including the prevention, diagnosis, and treatment of disease—routinely fails to consider the crucial impact of sex and gender. This happens in the earliest stages of research, when females are excluded from animal and human studies or the sex of the animals isn't stated in the published results. Once clinical trials begin, researchers frequently do not enroll adequate numbers of women or, when they do, fail to analyze or report data separately by sex. This hampers our ability to identify important differences that could benefit the health of all.[94]

While this is seen in both the Thalidomide and DES tragedies, to the continuing disadvantage of women's health and lives, sexism persists in medical and pharmacological research, including disproportionate funding of research for male-dominant diseases, sexism in clinical medical practice, and even in medical schools where women physicians suffer hostility, humiliations, and indignities; that is, in every aspect of medicine.[95,96,97,98,99] Measures, in the form of policies and guidelines, have been taken to ameliorate gender differences in preclinical research and clinical care.[100,101,102] But those policies and guidelines are not necessarily surveilled or enforced and in clinical practice do not eradicate entrenched sexist (or racist) attitudes.

And Still It Persists

Paternalism and sexism in medicine and medical care have not gone away. To be clear, not all paternalistic physicians are sexist as well. In the 1960s, the full force of second-wave feminist, and even non-feminist, women's fury took aim at paternalism and sexism in medicine and became the *women's health movement*. Ruth Rosen's *The World Split Open: How the Women's Movement Changed America*[103] (2000, 2006) provides an excellent broader contextual work with a section on the movement. The definitive work on the movement is Sheryl Burt Ruzek's *The Women's Health Movement: Feminist Alternatives to Medical Control* (1979).[104] This was a complex movement that channeled women's ire in an attempt to change the medical system to improve both medical knowledge about women, and to end the mistreatment of women in the medical system. It would be remiss to fail to mention that this was a white, middle-class feminist and women's movement that largely did not address the issues of health care for women of color. The movement sought to improve women's health *en toto*, not solely reproductive health. Two classic works of the period are the Boston Women's Health Book Collective's *Our Bodies, Ourselves: A Book By and For Women* (1973),[105] and Barbara Ehrenreich and Dierdre English's *Witches, Midwives, and Nurses: A History of Women Healers* (1973).[106]

A deeper treatment of this movement is warranted, though not here. Like first-wave feminism, the second wave contained numbers of colorful, informed, brilliant, and vilified, uppity women. By addressing the politics, economics, and sexism of medical science, physician ignorance of female anatomy and physiology, and physician clinical behavior, these feminists managed to attenuate medical paternalism and sexism, though more successfully with paternalism than with the sexism that seems refractory to ablation. Heta Häyry's short 1991 book *The Limits of Medical Paternalism* brings together an extended discussion of physicians' justifications for paternalism in a case of egregious sexism.[107]

As social trust in medicine and physicians plummeted, women's voices coalesced into a roar. Helen Reddy's song "I Am Woman" became the feminist anthem: "I am woman, hear me roar, In numbers too big to ignore..."[108]

> Perhaps nowhere was the distrust of professional domination more apparent than in the women's movement. Feminists claimed that as patients, as nurses, and in other roles in health care, they were denied the right to participate in medical decisions by their paternalistic doctors who refused to share information or take their intelligence seriously. They objected that much of what passed for scientific knowledge was sexist prejudice and that male physicians had deliberately excluded women from competence by keeping them out of medical schools and suppressing alternative practitioners such as midwives.[109]

Paternalism has largely given way to norms of informed consent and respecting patient wishes, the obverse of paternalism, in large part because of the women's health movement. The women's health movement had a direct effect upon exposing paternalism and yet the pristinated version is that respect for patient choice and informed consent arose from Nuremberg. Certainly they are related but, as noted previously, American medicine was not particularly responsive to the concerns that emerged from Nuremberg.[110] As women, and as nurses, surrounded by feminism and physicians in the 1960s and 1970s, the dynamism, vitality, breadth, numbers too big to ignore, and clamorous roar of the women's movement against the sexism, paternalism, and abuses of women in medical science, clinical and academic medicine was an irresistible force for change, even as other social forces would also contribute to that change.

Medicine under the Macroscope

In this period, medicine comes under scrutiny, not by consumers alone, but also by sociologists, philosophers, theologians, social historians, social critics, political activists, and more. The birthing and infancy of bioethics is surrounded by a cloud of critics with rather pointed analyses of medicine. In some instances, those analyses compare the US with medicine in the UK. They critique various aspects of medicine and its social and political power; its clinical sovereignty, its hegemony over an ever widening and encompassing medicalization of life; its interaction with a medical-industrial complex; its complicity in iatrogenesis—in short, the critiques are generally scathing. Illich, for example, writes:

> Within the last decade, medical professional practice has become a major threat to health. Depression, infection, disability, dysfunction, and other specific iatrogenic diseases now cause more suffering than all accidents from traffic or industry. Beyond this, medical practice sponsors sickness by the reinforcement of a morbid society... the so-called health-professions have an indirect sickening power—a structurally health-denying effect.... By transforming pain, illness, and death from a personal challenge into a technical problem, medical practice expropriates the potential of people to deal with their human condition in an autonomous way and becomes the source of a new kind of un-health.[111]

These works did not simply sit on academic bookshelves; many, but not all, made their way to a public readership. They brought new schemata and concepts to the public, such as Illich's *iatrogenesis*. A few of the more widely known works of this period are (chronologically):

- Philip Rieff. *The Triumph of the Therapeutic*. New York: Harper & Row, 1966.
- Barbara Ehrenreich and John Ehrenreich. *The American Health Empire: Power, Profits and Politics*. A Report from the Health Policy Advisory Center. New York: Random House, 1970.
- Eliot Freidson. *Professional Dominance: The Social Structure of Medical Care*. New York: Atherton Press, 1970.

- David Mechanic. *Politics, Medicine and Social Science*. New York: John Wiley, 1973.
- Thomas Szasz. *The Myth of Mental Illness*. New York: Harper, 1974.
- Ivan Illich. *Medical Nemesis: The Expropriation of Health*. London: Calder & Boyars, 1974. https://archive.org/details/medicalnemesisex00illirich
- John Knowles. *Doing Better and Feeling Worse: Health in the United States*. New York: W.W. Norton, 1977.
- Susan Sontag. *Illness as Metaphor*. New York: Farrar, Straus & Giroux, 1978.

The nature and scope of bioethics is better and more fully understood where the contemporaneous critique of medicine as a social and political structure, and physicians as professionals, is accessed. All are thoughtful, some are polemic, and some are more narrowly focused, but all are worthy reads. Their focus varies from the social construction of illness, to medicine as empire, the high cost of American medical care without proportionate positive outcomes, the use of technology, and more.

Technological Society, Technological Imperative, and Medicine

The mid-1900s was a period of acceleration of technological development in science, engineering, and medicine. In medicine, the development of technology escalated, and, for this, poliomyelitis presents a good case study. The poliomyelitis epidemics of the 1940s and 1950s gave rise to the development of the Salk (1952) and Sabine (1957) vaccines, and a feud between the two men. The 1954 Salk vaccine field trial was the largest trial that had ever been conducted on a human population.[112] Unfortunately, in the Western states, 200,000 children received vaccines, in which the inactivated live virus had not been inactivated.[113,114] Public vaccine anxiety increased, causing a crisis, even though the defective vaccines were those produced solely by Cutter Laboratories.[115,116] Polio caused paralysis of the respiratory muscles requiring ventilatory assistance with the negative pressure ventilator, called the *iron lung*, first developed in 1928, but with origins as far back as the 1700s. In the 1950s, one could see rows of children in iron lungs in large wards of the hospital; iron lungs were cumbersome and psychologically problematic for the patient, and eventually led to the development of the cuirass ventilator, and ultimately to positive-pressure ventilators. Positive-pressure ventilators spurred the development of intensive care units (ICUs) in teaching hospitals and medical centers, later to enter community hospitals as well.[117,118,119]

As medical science and technology ramped up, ICUs became differentiated in terms of specialized care, with an increase in specialties in both medicine and nursing.[120,121,122] Technology developed explosively, not only in medicine, but across the whole of society and in every personal and public domain. By the mid-1950s, many families had television! With seven channels! Each technological or scientific development gave rise to additional developments, both technical and scientific, and not. The isolation of the polio virus allowed the development of a vaccine, which had to be undergirded by research facilities, funding, and federal support; drug approval structures; vaccine manufacturing facilities and supply lines; a public health system and personnel for distribution; the development of the iron lung and manufacturers; materials and distribution supply lines to manufacture them; transportation of goods by land or air; and other social structures. These structures further lent themselves to the development, distribution, and utilization of positive-pressure ventilators, and a cascade of other developments affecting every aspect of society.

The literature surrounding technology is initially promulgated by those in science or engineering, but later shifts to those in the humanities and social and political sciences who develop a *humanities philosophy of technology*. Their critiques of technology range from broad technology-and-society critiques, to more focused analyses of technological change in relation to politics, to critiques of technology itself, to narrower examinations of the effects of technological development on education, communications, medicine and more, and for our purposes the physician–patient relationship specifically.

In the period surrounding the emergence of bioethics, the most well-known social critique was also the most contested, yet pivotal to the emerging humanities philosophy of technology literature. In 1954, French sociologist, philosopher, and theologian Jacques Ellul presciently warned against *La Technique ou L'enjeu du Siècle*.[123] His warning entered the English language in 1964 as *The Technological Society*.[124] Ellul was concerned about *technique*, which is not to be confused with *technology*.

> The term *technique*, as I use it, does not mean machines, technology, or this or that procedure for attaining an end. In our technological society, *technique* is *the totality of methods rationally arrived at and having absolute efficiency* (for a given stage of development) and in *every* field of human activity.... Technique is not an isolated fact in society (as the term technology would lead us to believe) but is related to every factor in the life of modern man; it affects social facts as well as all others. Thus, technique itself is a sociological phenomenon.[125]

Technique does not refer to specific technologies, nor to the universe of technology, *the machine*. *Technique* is a sociological phenomenon in which the societal perspective is one of "the consciousness of the mechanized world." It is a societal attitude toward technology. As the *technological society* embraces technology, it becomes a *technological system* in which technology recreates the human world, essentially commanding the way in which humans will live, and becoming in itself, autonomous at the expense of human autonomy. Ellul writes

> Technique has penetrated the deepest recesses of the human being. The machine tends not only to create a new human environment, but also to modify man's very essence. The milieu in which he lives is no longer his. He must adapt

himself, as though the world were new, to a universe for which he was not created. He was made to go six kilometers an hour, and he goes a thousand. He was made to eat when he was hungry and go to sleep when he was sleepy, instead, he obeys a clock. He was made to have contact with living things, and he lives in a world of stone. He was created with a certain essential unity, and he is fragmented by all the forces of the modern world.[126]

Ellul's argument is that, in an assumption that technological progress is always beneficial, humankind has become obsessed with scientific and technological development, which has resulted in greater scientific and technological evolution and expansion, and expansion into every nook and cranny of our lives. His warning is that technology, that is, *the technological system*, would outpace our ability to control it, and that humanity would, instead, become recreated, reshaped, and controlled by its own technology. (Here, the current debate over the regulation of artificial intelligence comes to mind.) For Ellul, "the fixed end of *technique* [is]— *efficiency*"[127] with technology accomplishing its bidding. While technique aims at rational, abstract, mathematical *efficiency*; humans are anything but efficient. Ellul notes that "to obey a multiplicity of motives and not reason alone seems to be an important keynote of man."[128] That multiplicity of motives includes the aesthetic and the moral. He continues:

> When in the nineteenth century, society began to elaborate an exclusively rational technique which acknowledged only considerations of efficiency, it was felt that not only the traditions but the deepest instincts of humankind had been violated. Men sought to reintroduce indispensable factors of aesthetics and morals.[129]

The aesthetic, artistry, and ethics are the antithesis of efficiency. Hence, many of the antiques we see have "inefficient" artistic embellishments: the elaborately decorated sword hilt, engraved and embellished suits of armor, the decoratively flourished steam engine, the Art Deco motif on the sewing machine face plate, the decorative guides on the woodworker's plane, or the hearts in the cast iron of my grandmother's apple peeler. Unadorned and stamped out, in any realm. Is more efficient. In much the same way, ethics, too, is an impediment to efficiency.

> Abstract techniques and their relation to morals underwent the same evolution. Earlier economic or political inquiries were inextricably bound with ethical inquiry, and men attempted to maintain this union... Modern society is, in fact, conducted on the basis of purely technical considerations.[130]

The *technological society* adapts social conditions to accommodate *the machine*. One need only look at the movement from handwritten letters, with dipped pen and ink, perhaps in a beautiful Spencerian hand, to typed letters sent by "snail mail," to email, to text messages with their initialisms (LOL). The efficiency of email and text messages is undeniable and their use essentially required today. A postal letter might take a week to receive and turn around, giving time to reflect. Emails and text messages demand immediate response. Still, that which is important, such as wedding invitations (printed on special paper, often in computer-generated cursive font, but hand addressed), is sent via the (now struggling) postal service; it represents a resistive force and the "indispensable factors of aesthetics and morals" in our "multiplicity of motives." Digital technology has changed personal communication, teaching and learning, purchasing, travel, music, listening, viewing, reading, and much more. The changes wrought by digital communications are no less monumental than those wrought by humanity's shift from orality to literacy with the development of writing. As Ellul notes, technological innovation brings benefits, and yet those innovations change us and society. Social media is a case in point, as is the focus on science, technology, engineering, and mathematics (STEM) in education, with its efficiency-targeted focus on contributions to the technological system, at the expense of the liberal arts with their emphasis on understanding, aesthetics, ethics, and reflections upon human experience.

Despite his assertion that the technological society is the defining attribute of the twentieth century, that its technological development has benefitted humankind, and that it nonetheless undermines human autonomy and freedom, Ellul claims that he is neither deterministic nor technophobic. What he calls for is an embrace of the dialectic tension between technique and humanity's multiplicity of motives. He himself holds that *The Technological Society* is only one side of the dialectic. Matlock correctly notes that

> The closest Ellul ever came to proposing a solution was in later essays in which he calls for an "ethics of nonpower," whereby "man will agree not to do all he is capable of." This includes choosing not to maximize certain technical means in one's private life as well as in the public sphere. It is not until we are capable of this kind of relinquishment that we can be free, both from technical determinism and for rational control of technique, as neither type of freedom is a simple given.[131]

For Ellul, technique moves inexorably toward efficiency, enacted by the technological system that is itself efficient. The point of intervention is to break the link between efficiency as means and efficiency as end, or more specifically to challenge efficiency as means, end, and goal by holding them in dialectic tension with the multiplicity of motives—and goals—that affirm human autonomy, freedom, ethics, art, and progress.

Questions of not doing all that we are capable of continue in the related and subsequent discourse on *autonomous technology*, or the *technological imperative*. Technological development enables much that humans *can* do, but does not ask *may, should, ought* we to do it? This is, in part, Ellul's question and solution. In his book *Autonomous Technology: Technics-out-of-Control as a Theme in Political Thought* (1977),[132] Langdon Winner both shares and challenges Ellul's synthesis.

Autonomous Technology and the Technological Imperative

There are several ways in which the concept of *autonomy* is used in bioethics, though it is predominantly (and almost exclusively) understood to mean respect for patient choices. It is secondarily understood as the physician's (or nurse's) autonomy of practice, free of non-professional, external constraints. Another use of *autonomy* includes the freedom to develop research, science, and technology independent of political or commercial forces of influence, a particular concern in relation to corporate-sponsored university research. Ellul raises the issue of the technological society, operationalized by technology which has an expanding and autonomous life of its own in the whole of society, each development leading to another and another—and having its own ethical implications for human autonomy.

Autonomous technology does not refer to any one technology, but to the technological system as a whole. The notion of *autonomous technology* is variously associated with the dis-ease with rapidly advancing industrialization and its resultant social and technological change (e.g., Mary Shelley's *Frankenstein*),[133] with the dehumanizing effects of technology (e.g., Lewis Mumford, Herbert Marcuse, Martin Heidegger, and members of the Frankfurt School), and with the view that technological systems define and shape aspects of human culture and activity (e.g., Jacques Ellul, Langdon Winner).

Langdon Winner both agrees and disagrees with Ellul, particularly on the issue of *autonomous technology*. Winner maintains that autonomous technology is most clearly in evidence in politics, specifically in the political mandate for the advance of technology. He notes that technology can be ill-used and can lead to "an ever-increasing array of rules,... regulations... to maximize the benefits of technological practice while limiting its unwanted maladies."[134,135] Winner's approach to technology

> begins with the crucial awareness that technology in a true sense *is legislation*. It recognizes that technical forms do, to a large extent, shape the basic pattern and content of human activity in our time. Thus, politics becomes (among other things) an active encounter with the specific forms and processes contained in technology... *technology is itself a political phenomenon*.[136]

Winner generally agrees with Ellul; however, he diverges from Ellul's perspective in his emphasis on the political dimensions of technology, and in according human agency greater strength of force through the political process. He does, like Ellul, argue that technology is out of control and pervasive in its influence upon society and individuals, but differs in that he regards technology as only semi-autonomous, capable of being redirected through human agency, that is, through human autonomy.

The *technological imperative* refers to existing technology that necessitates decisions on additional technology. For example, rockets and shuttles for manned space flights required the development of space suits for space walks; the Hubble telescope needed a new lens ground as "glasses" for the aging telescope; or digital communications and data storage, necessitating malware, virus, and identity theft protections. John Weckert states this clearly:

> the level of technological optimism in society leads to the technological fix being the first option considered for many problems and that this in turn generates a technological treadmill. Many, if not most, technological fixes cause new problems to which technological fixes are again applied. Fixing or alleviating problems caused by this human propensity for technological fixes creates a new technological imperative.[137]

Autonomous technology and the technological imperative should not be mistaken for *technological determinism*; i.e., that "because a particular technology means that we *can* do something (it is technically possible) then this action either *ought* to (as a moral imperative), *must* (as an operational requirement) or inevitably *will* (in time) be taken."[138] Redefining the technological imperative in this way is infelicitous to the literature, emphasizes individual technologies, denies the political means of restraining the ill effects of technology, and in the end denies any human autonomy in relation to technology.[139]

This is not simply a period discussion; it has resurfaced more recently in discussions of various computer and software applications ransomware, digital fraud, the dark web, AI cloning, identity theft, data collection and spying, drones, facial recognition, motes and smart dust, disinformation bots, widespread use of artificial intelligence, and more. The discourse surrounding the development, use, misuse, untoward consequences, and restraint of technology is, and will remain, relevant.[140]

Bioethics only gave passing, if any, notice of this literature. Tina Stevens writes:

> There is evidence that some early bioethicists had been influenced by intellectuals concerned with the philosophy of technology, the likes of Lewis Mumford, Jacques Ellul, or Herbert Marcuse. In their attachment to the tools of moral philosophy, however, bioethicists let slip away the early influence of this other philosophical area. The inquiry begun by these social critics in the nineteen fifties and sixties and continued more recently by those few who, like Langdon Winner, explore some of the "ways in which conditions of power, authority, freedom, and social justice are deeply embedded in technical structures," is largely ignored by bioethicists today.[141]

Even though this literature has intense relevance to nursing, it does not appear in the nursing bioethics literature, which largely focused on direct patient care issues and, at the time, slow codes and definitions of futility, extremely troubling issues for nurses. In an affirmation of Winner's position, technological issues at the end of life were addressed, politically, when the President's Commission published its report *Deciding to Forego Life-Sustaining Treatment* (1983).[142] Nursing is, of course, intimately involved in care at the end of life—and its technologization. If we accept Winner's thesis that human agency has the power to redirect the misuse of technology or its untoward consequences through the political process, it argues for nursing and nurses' participation in the political processes that can set boundaries and guidelines for the use of domains of technology that affect nursing practice, patient well-being, and society's health.

Conclusion

These social movements and events did not in themselves cause the development of bioethics; rather, they helped to shape the concerns it would choose to address as it emerged as a discipline. In these loosely related social movements and events, there is a specific constellation of concerns and social pressures that reflect the core questions of the discipline. The equation is something like this:

- [(Medical sovereignty, authoritarianism, and paternalism, (especially in relation to women) and litigation against physicians) ✚
- (Consumer disenchantment and mistrust of institutions, including medicine, and concern for patient rights) ✚
- (The skyrocketing and uncontrolled medical costs) ✚
- (The rise of technology and its medical excesses)] ▶
- Specific questions that arise in the emerging bioethics, including:

medical paternalism, medical misogyny and sexism, opacity and whistleblowing, patient self-determination, futile treatment, withholding and withdrawing treatment, access to and costs of care, cost-containment.

Questions of the structural health disparities, androcentrism, and the male body as normative would take longer to emerge, and certainly the concerns of nursing were not deemed worthy of attention except insofar as they pertained to the implementation of medical orders. It was, after all, nurses who were responsible for implementing medical orders, even where nurses deemed them futile. But the more specific nursing concerns were not in evidence in the new bioethics. Why is nursing, the largest single health-care workforce, not adequately represented on presidential commissions when veterinarians and dentists are? Why has the US always refused to create a sustainable nursing workforce? Why among the National Institutes of Health (founded 1887) was the National Institute for Nursing Research (1997) the rump end of institutes, succeeded only by those devoted to emerging sciences such as mapping the genome. On the whole, bioethics as a field does not tend to address the larger, structural issues, or the more granular clinical or institutional concerns of nurses, unless nurses take it upon themselves to press for their attention.

The emergence in the 1960s and 1970s of bioethics as a discipline, and the questions it chose to address as core concerns, was conditioned by the social context from which it arose. Those concerns are not the result of some rational calculation, or a survey of patient concerns to determine their preponderance, or deterministically foisted upon bioethics. Choices were made. But those choices were responses to both the social pressures upon physicians as well as the demands of scientific progress, technological innovation, and governmental involvement. Unlike bioethics, however, the ethical concerns of nursing emerge from the tradition and history of nursing and its values, ideals, and aspirations; the notions of good within nursing; and the lived experience of nursing, which hears the ethical concerns of patients in the process of caregiving. It is a continuous, renewing, and ongoing ethical tradition of over 150 years of modern nursing. Nursing's ethical concerns are not specifically or solely those of medicine nor of a medically normative bioethics; they are its own species.

Notes

1 Peggy Chinn, text message. Nov. 24, 2022.
2 Tom Beauchamp and James Childress, *The Principles of Biomedical Ethics* (New York: Oxford University Press, 1979).
3 The National Commission for the Protection of Human Subjects of Biomedical and Behavioral Research, Department of Health, Education and Welfare, *The Belmont Report: Ethical Principles and Guidelines for the Protection of Human Subjects of Research* (Washington, DC: USGPO, 1979).
4 John H. Zammito, *Kant, Herder, & the Birth of Anthropology* (Chicago: University of Chicago Press, 2002).
5 Ibid., 121–122.
6 Karl Vorländer, *Immanuel Kant: Der Mann und Der Werk*. 2nd ed. (Hamburg: Meiner, 1977).
7 Ibid., 194.
8 Zammito, *Kant, Herder*, 125.
9 Immanuel Kant, *Observations on the Feeling of the Beautiful and Sublime*, John Goldwait trans. (Berkeley, CA: University of California, 1960).
10 Immanuel Kant, *Bemerkungen in den "Beobachtungen über das Gefühl des Schönen und Erhabenen,"* Marie Rischmüller trans. (Hamburg: Meiner, 1991). Original, 1764.
11 Immanuel Kant. *Observations on the Feeling of the Beautiful and Sublime and Other Writings*. Patrick Frierson and Paul Guyer, trans. (Cambridge, MA: Cambridge University Press, 2011), 39.
12 Zammito, *Kant, Herder*, 129.
13 Zammito, *Kant, Herder*, 133.
14 Michael Walschots, "Hutcheson and Kant: Moral Sense and Moral Feeling," in *Kant and the Scottish Enlightenment*, Elizabeth Robinson and Chris W. Surprenant (eds.) (London: Routledge, 2017), 36–54.
15 Immanuel Kant, *Groundwork of the Metaphysics of Morals*, Mary Gregor (ed.) (New York: Cambridge University Press, 1998).
16 *Nuremberg Code, 1947, "Trials of War Criminals before the Nuremberg Military Tribunals under Control Council Law No. 10"* Vol. 2 (Washington, DC: US Government Printing Office, 1949), 181–182.

17 *World Medical Association, Declaration of Helsinki: Ethical Principles for Medical Research Involving Human Subjects, JAMA* 310, no. 20 (2013): 2191–2194. DOI:10.1001/jama.2013.281053. PMID 24141714.
18 Albert Jonsen, *The Birth of Bioethics* (New York: Oxford University Press, 1998), 133–140.
19 United States Public Health Service, The USPHS Syphilis Study at Tuskegee. https://www.cdc.gov/tuskegee/index.html
20 Henry K. Beecher, "Ethics and Clinical Research," *New England Journal of Medicine* 274, no. 24 (June 1966): 1456–1460.
21 Ibid.
22 Maurice Henry Pappworth, "Human Guinea Pigs: A Warning," *Twentieth Century Magazine* (1962): 66–75.
23 Maurice Henry Pappworth, *Human Guinea Pigs: Experimentation on Man* (London: Routledge & Kegan Paul, 1967).
24 M.H. Pappworth, "'Human Guinea Pigs'—a History," *British Medical Journal* 301 (December 1990): 1456–1460.
25 Ibid., 1456.
26 Mary R. Walsh, *Doctors Wanted: No Women Need Apply* (New Haven, CT: Yale University Press, 1977), 176–193.
27 Paul Starr, *The Social Transformation of American Medicine: The Rise of a Sovereign Profession and the Making of a Vast Industry* (New York: Basic Books, 1982).
28 American Medical Association, *Code of Medical Ethics of the American Medical Association* (Chicago: AMA, 1847).
29 Ibid., 84.
30 Ibid., 84.
31 Ibid., 86.
32 Ibid., 106.
33 Terence J. Johnson, *Professions and Power* (Cambridge, MA: University of Cambridge Press, 1972), 57.
34 AMA *Code.*, 100.
35 Ibid., 106.
36 Ibid., 95.
37 Ibid., 96.
38 We will not, here, examine professionalization or professionalism.
39 "Adumbration of a code of ethics" (James Luther Adams) means to describe in outline or state a code of ethics.
40 George Kimmich Beach (ed.), *The Essential James Luther Adams: Selected Essays and Addresses* (Boston: Skinner House Books, 1998).
41 Abraham Flexner, "Is Social Work a Profession?" *School and Society* I (1915): 901–911.
42 A.M. Carr-Saunders and P.A. Wilson, *The Professions* (Oxford: Clarendon Press, 1933).
43 Genevieve K. Bixler and Roy W. Bixler, "The Status of Nursing as a Profession," *American Journal of Nursing* 45, no. 9 (1945): 730–735.
44 American Nurses Association, "A Tentative Code, for the Nursing Profession," *American Journal of Nursing* 40, no. 9 (1940): 977–980.
45 Marsha Fowler, "Nursing and Social Ethics," in N.A. Chaska (ed.), *The Nursing Profession: Turning Points* (St. Louis, MO: C.V. Mosby, 1989), 24–30.
46 Genevieve K. Bixler and Roy W. Bixler, "The Professional Status of Nursing," *American Journal of Nursing* 59, no. 8 (1959): 1142–1146.
47 Terence Johnson, *Professions and Power* (London: Macmillan, 1972).
48 Ibid., 23.
49 Fowler, "Social Ethics," 25.

50 Joseph D. Stamey, "The Emerging Ethic: Religious, Non-Religious, or Anti-Religious?" (Unpublished paper, 1971), 15.

51 Paul Deats, Jr., "The Quest for a Social Ethic," in Paul Deats, Jr. *Toward a Discipline of Social Ethics: Essays in Honor of Walter George Muelder* (Boston: Boston University Press, 1972), 39.

52 Johnson, *Professions and Power*, 79, 82, 83.

53 Ibid., 83.

54 Starr, *Transformation*, xv.

55 Ibid., 21–22.

56 Johnson, *Professions and Power*, 41.

57 H. Jamous and B. Peloille, "Professions or Self-Perpetuating Systems? Changes in the French University-Hospital System," in J.A. Jackson (ed.), *Professions and Professionalization* (Cambridge, MA: Cambridge University Press, 1970) (section includes 109–152), 111–120.

58 Jamous and Peloille, *Professions*, 112.

59 Johnson, *Professions and Power*, 42–43.

60 Jamous and Peloille, *Professions*, 138.

61 President's Advisory Commission on Consumer Protection and Quality in the Health Care Industry, *Consumer Bill of Rights and Responsibilities: Executive Summary* (Washington, DC: US Government Printing Office, 1997). https://web.archive.org/web/20050404034905/http://www.hcqualitycommission.gov/final/append_a.html

62 Robert N. Mayer, *The Consumer Movement: Guardians of the Marketplace* (Boston: Twayne Publishers, 1989), 1.

63 Allan J. McDonald and James R. Hansen, *Truth, Lies, and O-Rings: Inside the Space Shuttle Challenger Disaster* (Gainesville, FL: University Press of Florida, 2009).

64 D. Birsch and J. Fielder, *The Ford Pinto Case: A Study in Applied Ethics, Business, and Technology* (Albany, NY: State University of New York Press, 1994).

65 Mark Dowie, "Pinto Madness," *Mother Jones* (Sept./Oct. 1977), 18. https://www.motherjones.com/politics/1977/09/pinto-madness/

66 Matthew T. Lee and M. David Ermann, "Pinto 'Madness' as a Flawed Landmark Narrative: An Organizational and Network Analysis," *Social Problems* 46, no. 1 (1 February 1999): 30–47.

67 Brent Fisse and John Braithwaite, "The Impact of Publicity on Corporate Offenders: Ford Motor Company and the Pinto Papers," in M. David Ermann and Richard J. Lundman (eds.), *Corporate and Governmental Deviance: Problems of Organizational Behavior in Contemporary Society*, 3rd ed. (New York: Oxford University Press, 1987).

68 Lawrence, William. *Of Acceptable Risk: Science and the Determination of Safety* (New York: William Kaufmann, 1976).

69 Baruch Fischoff, Sarah Lichtenstein, Paul Slovic, Ralph Keeney, and Stephen Derby, *Approaches to Acceptable Risk: A Critical Guide* (Washington, DC: Division of Technical Information and document Control US Nuclear Regulatory Commission, 1980). https://www.nrc.gov/docs/ML0716/ML071650351.pdf

70 Ibid., i.

71 Ibid., ii.

72 Albert O. Hirschman, *Exit, Voice, and Loyalty: Responses to Decline in Firms, Organizations, and States* (Cambridge, MA: Harvard University Press, 1970).

73 N. Perry, "Indecent Exposures: Theorizing Whistleblowing," *Organization Studies* 19, no. 2 (1988): 235–257.

74 "rat fink, n. and adj." OED Online. Oxford University Press, December 2022, https://www.oed.com/view/Entry/158438?isAdvanced=false&result=1&rskey=GdHKiw& (accessed January 18, 2023).

75 Judith P. Swazey and Stephen R. Scher (eds.), *Whistleblowing in Biomedical Research: Policies and Procedures Responding to Reports of Misconduct. Report*

of the President's Commission for the Study of Ethical Problems in Medicine and Biomedical and Behavioral Research (Washington, DC: US Government Printing Office, 1981).

76 Ibid., 173–192.

77 Ibid., 178.

78 Alan F. Westin, Whistle-Blowing! Loyalty and Dissent in the Corporation (New York: McGraw-Hill, 1981). Quoted in Swazey and Scher (eds.), Whistleblowing in Biomedical Research, 179.

79 C. Fred Alford, Whistleblowers: Broken Lives and Organizational Power (Ithaca, NY: Cornell University Press, 2001).

80 Swazey, Scher, Whistleblowing, 179–180.

81 https://www.whistleblowers.org/how-to-stop-retaliation/

82 D. Banisar, "Whistleblowing: International Standards and Developments," in I. Sandoval (ed.), Corruption and Transparency: Debating the Frontiers between State, Market and Society (Washington, DC: World Bank-Institute for Social Research, UNAM, 2011). http://ssrn.com/abstract=1753180

83 Charles Graeber, The Good Nurse: A True Story of Medicine, Madness, and Murder (New York: Twelve, 2013).

84 Edward H. Clarke, Sex in Education or, A Fair Chance for Girls (Boston: James R. Osgood and Company, 1873).

85 Rachel Gross, "Please Don't Call My Cervix Incompetent: There's No End to the Weird Ways Medicine Describes Women's Bodies," The Atlantic, Jan. 25, 2023. https://www.theatlantic.com/health/archive/2023/01/geriatric-pregnancy-old-outdated-medical-terms/672834/

86 Susan Molinari and Beth Brooke, "Women Are More Likely to Die or Be Injured in Car Crashes. There's a Simple Reason Why," The Washington Post, Dec. 21, 2021. https://www.washingtonpost.com/opinions/2021/12/21/female-crash-test-dummies-nhtsa/

87 First-wave feminism, 1880s–1920, was associated with the women's suffrage movement and the removal of the legal strictures to women's freedom and full enfranchisement.

88 Ruth Rosen, The World Split Open: How the Modern Women's Movement Changed America, Revised Edition (New York: Penguin Books, 2000), 175.

89 Mary Frances Berry, The Pig Farmer's Daughter and Other Tales of American Justice: Episodes of Racism and Sexism in the Courts from 1865 to the Present (New York: Penguin, 1999).

90 Henning Sjöström, Thalidomide and the Power of the Drug Companies (New York: Penguin, 1972).

91 Taher Al Jishi and Consolato Sergi, "Current Perspective of Diethylstilbestrol (DES) Exposure in Mothers and Offspring," Reproductive Toxicology 71 (2017): 71–77.

92 R.N. Hoover, M. Hyer, R,M, Pfeiffer, E. Adam, B. Bond, A.L. Cheville, T. Colton, P. Hartge, E.E. Hatch, A.L. Herbst, B.Y. Karlan, R. Kaufman, K.L. Noller, J.R. Palmer, S.J. Robboy, R.C. Saal, W. Strohsnitter, L. Titus-Ernstoff, and R. Troisi, "Adverse Health Outcomes in Women Exposed In Utero to Diethylstibestrol," New England Journal of Medicine (Oct. 6, 2011). https://www.nih.gov/news-events/news-releases/women-exposed-des-womb-face-increased-cancer-risk

93 Pilar Zamora-León, "Are the Effects of DES Over? A Tragic Lesson from the Past," International Journal of Environmental Research 18, no. 19 (Sept. 30, 2021): 10309.

94 Paula S. Johnson, Therese Fitzgerald, Alina Saiganicoff, Susan Wood, and Jill M. Goldstein, Sex-Specific Medical Research: Why Women's Health Can't Wait (Boston: Brigham and Women's Hospital, 2014). https://www.brighamandwomens.org/assets/bwh/womens-health/pdfs/connorsreportfinal.pdf

95 Tracy Bale and C. Neill Epperson, "Sex as a Biological Variable: Who, What, When, Why, and How," Neuropsychopharmacology 42 (2017): 386–396.

96 Matthew E. Arnegard, Lori A. Whitten, Chyren Hunter, and Janine Austin Clayton. "Sex as a Biological Variable: A 5-Year Progress Report and Call to Action," *Journal of Women's Health* 29, no. 6 (June 2020): 858–864.

97 Rebecca M. Shansky and Anne Z. Murphy, "Considering Sex as a Biological Variable Will Require a Global Shift in Science Culture," *Nature Neuroscience* 24 (2021): 457–464.

98 J.B. Delston, "When Doctors Deny Drugs: Sexism and Contraception Access in the Medical Field," *Bioethics* 31, no. 9 (Nov. 2017): 703–710.

99 Laila A. Gharzai, Kent A. Griffith, Whitney H. Beeler, Heather L. Burrows, Maya M. Hammoud, Phillip E. Rodgers, Michael S. Sabel, John M. Carethers, and Reshma Jagsi, "Speaker Introductions at Grand Rounds: Differences in Formality of Address by Gender and Specialty," *Journal of Women's Health* 31, no. 2 (Feb. 2022): 202–209.

100 National Institutes of Health Office of Research on Women's Health. Policy on Sex as a Biological Variable, January 2016. https://orwh.od.nih.gov/sex-gender/nih-policy-sex-biological-variable

101 Candace Tingen, Joan D. Nagel, and Janine A. Clayton. "Monitoring the Implementation of the National Institutes of Health Strategic Plan for Women's Health and Sex/Gender Differences Research: Strategies and Successes," *Global Advances in Health and Medicine* 2, no. 5 (September 2013): 44–49.

102 National Institutes of Health (NIH) Central Resource for Grants and Funding Information, *Policy Inclusion of Women and Minorities as Participants in Research Involving Human Subjects,* 2017. https://grants.nih.gov/policy/inclusion/women-and-minorities.htm

103 Ruth Rosen, *The World Split Open: How the Modern Women's Movement Changed America*, Tantor eBooks, 2000.

104 Sheryl B. Ruzek, *The Women's Health Movement: Feminist Alternatives to Medical Control* (New York: Praeger, 1979).

105 Boston Women's Health Book Collective's *Our Bodies, Ourselves: A Book by and for Women* (New York: Simon & Schuster, 1973).

106 Barbara Ehrenreich and Dierdre English, *Witches, Midwives, and Nurses: A History of Women Healers* (New York: The Feminist Press, 1973). https://www.feministes-radicales.org/wp-content/uploads/2012/06/Barbara-Ehrenreich-and-Deirdre-English-Witches-Midwives-and-Nurses-A-History-of-Women-Healers.-Introduction.pdf

107 Heta Häyry, *The Limits of Medical Paternalism: Social Ethics and Policy Series* (London: Routledge, 1991), 5–11.

108 Helen Reddy, "I Am Woman" from *I Don't Know How to Love Him*, Capital Records, 1972. https://www.abc.net.au/news/2020–09–30/i-am-woman-helen-reddy-blazed-a-trail-then-left-it-all-behind/10496882.https://www.abc.net.au/news/2020–09–30/i-am-woman-helen-reddy-blazed-a-trail-then-left-it-all-behind/10496882

109 Star, *Transformation*, 391.

110 Albert Jonsen, *The Birth of Bioethics* (New York: Oxford University Press, 2003), 133–140.

111 Ivan Illich, "Medical Nemesis," *The Lancet* 303, no. 7863 (1974): 918–921.

112 Donald S. Burke, "Lessons Learned from the 1954 Field Trial of Poliomyelitis Vaccine," *Clinical Trials* 1, no. 1 (2004): 3–5.

113 I acknowledge a vested interest here as my brother received one of these vaccines at school in San Francisco. In addition, having become one of the first MS prepared respiratory clinical nurse specialists in 1974, I cared for several patients in iron lungs, by that point in their late teens.

114 Neal Nathanson, and Alexander D. Langmuir, "The Cutter Incident. Poliomyelitis following Formaldehyde-Inactivated Poliovirus Vaccination in the United States

during the spring of 1955. II. Relationship of Poliomyelitis to Cutter Vaccine," *American Journal of Hygiene* 78, no. 1 (1963): 29–60.

115 Paul A. Offit, *The Cutter Incident: How America's First Polio Vaccine Led to the Growing Vaccine Crisis* (New Haven, CT: Yale University Press, 2005).

116 Paul A. Offit, MD, "The Cutter Incident, 50 Years Later," *The New England Journal of Medicine* 352, no. 14 (Apr. 7, 2005): 1411–1412. https://www.proquest.com/scholarly-journals/cutter-incident-50-years-later/docview/223931729/se-2.

117 R.A. Berenson, "Evolution, Distribution, and Regulation of Intensive Care Units." In R.A. Berenson, *Intensive Care Units (ICUs): Clinical Outcomes, Costs, and Decision-making* (Health Technology Case Study 28), prepared for the Office of Technology Assessment, US Congress, OTA-HCS-28, Washington, DC, November 1984, 11–20.

118 David A. Morrow, James C. Fang, Dan J. Fintel, Christopher B. Granger, N. Katz, Frederick G. Kushner, Jeffrey T. Kuvin, Jose Lopez-Sendon, Dorothea McAreavey, Brahmajee Nallamothu, Lee Page II, Joseph E. Parrillo, Pamela N. Peterson, and Chris Winkelman, "Evolution of Critical Care Cardiology: Transformation of the Cardiovascular Intensive Care Unit and the Emerging Need for New Medical Staffing and Training Models," *Circulation* 126, no. 11 (September 11, 2012): 1408–1428.

119 Ake Grenvik and M.R. Pinsky, "Evolution of the Intensive Care Unit as a Clinical Center and Critical Care Medicine as a Discipline," *Critical Care Clinics* 25, no. 1 (Jan 2009): 239–250.

120 J.L. Vincent, M. Singer, J.J. Marini, R. Moreno, M. Levy, M.A. Matthay, et al., "Thirty Years of Critical Care Medicine," *Critical Care* 14 (2010): 311.

121 Stefano Bambi, "Evolution of Intensive Care Unit Nursing," In Irene Comisso, Alberto Lucchini, Stefano Bambi, Gian Domenico Giusti, and Matteo Manici, *Nursing in Critical Care Setting* (Dordrecht: Springer Nature B.V., 2018), 489–524.

122 J.L. Vincent, "Critical Care—Where Have We Been and Where Are We Going?" *Critical Care* 17 (2013): S2.

123 Jacques Ellul, *La Technique ou l'Enjeu du Siècle* (Paris: Armand Colin, 1954).

124 Jacques Ellul, *The Technological Society*, John Wilkinson trans. (New York: Knopf, 1964).

125 Ibid., xxv–xxvi; italics in original.

126 Ibid., 325.

127 Ibid., 21.

128 Ibid., 73.

129 Ibid., 73.

130 Ibid., 74.

131 Sam Matlack, "Confronting the Technological Society," *The New Atlantis* 43 (Summer/Fall 2014). https://www.thenewatlantis.com/publications/confronting-the-technological-society

132 Langdon Winner, *Autonomous Technology: Technics-out-of-Control as a Theme in Political Thought* (Cambridge, MA: MIT Press, 1977).

133 Mary W. Shelley, *Frankenstein, or the Modern Prometheus* (1818), ePublished Feb. 23, 2022. https://www.gutenberg.org/files/84/84-h/84-h.htm

134 David Mechanic, "The Growth of Medical Technology and Bureaucracy," *Milbank Memorial Fund Quarterly: Health and Society* 55, no. 1 (1977): 61718.

135 Winner, *Autonomous Technology,* 323.

136 Winner, *Autonomous Technology,* 323; italics in original.

137 John Weckert, "Is There a New Technological Imperative?" in Marcel Van de Voorde and Gunjan Jeswani (eds.), *Ethics in Nanotechnology: Emerging Technologies Aspects* (Berlin, Boston: De Gruyter, 2021), 21–40.

138 David Chandler, "Technological or Media Determinism," 1995. http://visual-memory.co.uk/daniel//Documents/tecdet/tdet07.html

139 Jay Weinstein, Review of *Feeling Helpless: The Idea of Autonomous Technology in Social Science*, by Langdon Winner, *Theory and Society* 10, no. 4 (1981): 567–578.
140 J. Fielder, "Autonomous Technology, Democracy, and the Nimbys," in Langdon Winner (ed.), *Democracy in a Technological Society, Philosophy and Technology*, vol. 9 (Dordrecht: Springer, 1992), 105–121.
141 M.L. Tina Stevens, "History and Bioethics," in Franklin Miller, John C. Fletcher, and James M Humber (eds.), *The Nature and Prospect of Bioethics: Interdisciplinary Perspectives* (Totowa, NJ: Humana Press, 2003), 192.
142 President's Commission for the Study of Ethical Problems in Medicine and Biomedical and Behavioral Research, *Deciding to Forego Life Sustaining Treatment* (Washington, DC: US Government Printing Office, 1983). Full text available at: https://repository. library.georgetown.edu/bitstream/handle/10822/559344/deciding_to_forego_ tx.pdf?sequence=1

6

NURSING'S NESCIENT EMBRACE OF A NASCENT BIOETHICS

The acceleration of technological and scientific development in the mid-nineteenth century affected every aspect of day-to-day modern life and was not limited to advances in medical science and technology. Some changes more directly affected, and somewhat exclusively affected, bioethics and set the field on track eventually to develop a bioethical–medical industrial complex; that is, an authority and power that gave it a commanding social presence and facilitated its movement into nursing. The Seattle dialysis case would bring medical decisions regarding rationing into public consciousness, and the plight of children born with diminished cognitive ability would poke a stick at medicine. Both would facilitate the development of the field, as would the development of a range of bedside-care and hospital technologies. The "creation" of bioethics is not unlike the creation of a star, where a hazy cloud of gas and dust form a nebula that undergoes pressure, so that their nuclei undergo fusion, exerting an outward pressure forming a star. As the enormous cloud of the gas and dust of science, technology, medicine, and specific needs for health care form a nebula, squeezed by social pressure, the nuclei are joined by fusion, and a star—bioethics—is born and new galaxies seeded. A star is a luminous ball of gas held together by its own gravity, with a core of fusion energy that prevents it from collapsing in on itself. A star, in turn, has a gravitational force that attracts other bodies into its orbit. Bioethics has weight (gravitas), utility (attractive force), and authority (outward pressure), and …

Dust and Gas Fuse: Six Cases Illustrate This Fusion

The Seattle Hemodialysis Case

In 1962, Shana Alexander, a writer for *Time* magazine, roused public awareness and precipitated a national debate with the publication of her poignant article "They

DOI: 10.4324/9781003262107-7

Decide Who Lives, Who Dies: Medical Miracle Puts Moral Burden on Small Committee."[1] Her article focuses on a case at Swedish Hospital in Seattle, Washington, a case about the allocation of a scarce life-saving resource, the "artificial kidney" machine, of which Swedish Hospital had five in a clinical trial. A choice had to be made: which one of 50 patients would receive treatment using the artificial kidney (hemodialysis machine)? A committee of seven persons had been formed to make this decision and consisted of an attorney, a banker, a housewife, a minister, a government official, a labor leader, and a surgeon.[2] They were given no decisional guidelines. It is here that Alexander (who was Jewish) quotes a portion of the *Unetanah Tokef* Hebrew prayer, "Who shall live and who shall die; who shall attain the measure of man's days and who shall not attain it; who shall be at ease and who shall be afflicted."[3] On rather specious grounds, the nephrologists urged the committee to pass rules to exclude persons over 45, and children, which the committee did. The committee then composed a list of factors that they would use to make their decisions. These factors included:

> Age and sex of patient; marital status and number of dependents; income; net worth; emotional stability, with particular regard to the patient's capacity to accept the treatment; educational background; nature of occupation, past performance and future potential; and names of people who could serve as references.[4]

They also limited candidates to Washington state residents. The committee members were thrown in the deep end of the pool, with little guidance, and no guidelines. The guidelines that they did formulate, that is the weighted factors that they did devise, were problematic. It was 1962. Married women did not have an independent net worth and, then as now, did not have pay equity. Women and minority persons could arbitrarily be excluded from higher education or professions. In terms of occupation, professions existed in a hierarchy of social esteem, for example, physicians over auto mechanics. Overall, the criteria favored white, married, male, professionals, with higher education, with children, and with a committee guesstimate as to their capacity to accept treatment, and their future potential. These factors fall within the category of *social worth criteria*. Such criteria are based in the values, biases, and prejudices of those formulating them and are manifestly unjust.[5,6] While criteria are here being used to apply to a specific experimental technology, the question of criteria would later surface regarding experimental HIV drugs, and even later to solid organ transplants.[7,8]

Following Alexander's evocative article, there was extensive media coverage of the case, and the larger issue of the allocation of scarce medical resources that roused a public furor. It is important to note that the Seattle dialysis center was the only such center nationally that had appointed a decisional committee, with lay members, and that, more importantly, utilized social worth criteria.[9] Nationally, other centers had no similar committee and utilized traditional medical triage criteria. The Seattle case resulted in federal legislative action that, in 1972, created the National End-Stage Renal Disease (ESRD) Program. The program extended Medicare coverage to persons with ERSD for medical expenses for hemodialysis and for renal transplant.[10] It is perplexing, but perhaps a testimony to the power of Alexander's writing, that Congress resolved the issue in this way. Rather than creating a more just means of choosing patients than that of social worth criteria that only the Seattle center was using, and to embrace an alternative means such as the medical triage system that all other centers were using, Congress instead effectively said "we won't choose," and made everyone with ESRD eligible for hemodialysis or transplant by underwriting costs. It was a maneuver that avoided addressing the ethical questions. Admittedly, by doing so, it avoided creating other ethical questions that arise within the existing health-care system and its disparities of access to basic, emergency, and hospital care.

Social worth criteria (also known as social utility, social value, or social contribution criteria) had been roundly rejected within bioethics by both theologians and philosophers. Social worth criteria do not take account of the various structural oppressions of society that disadvantage various groups within society. Such criteria are blind, and sometimes willfully blind, to who has power and privilege, or to who and how persons are harmed by the structures of society by, for example, loculating them in lower-paying jobs or denying them access to higher education.

The Karen Ann Quinlan Case

There were a number of legal cases, all poignant, that turned on moral as well as legal issues (see Appendix IV in Chapter 6). In general, the law would customarily take five years to catch up with the moral deliberations in medicine. The Quinlan case also became a public case with considerable media coverage.

Karen Ann Quinlan was the adopted daughter of a devout Roman Catholic couple. In 1975, she was 21 when she collapsed at a birthday party after reportedly having taken a mix of alcohol and diazepam. She felt ill, so was taken home by her roommates. About 15 minutes later, when her friends checked on her, she had stopped breathing. An ambulance was called. Mouth-to-mouth resuscitation was attempted but she did not regain consciousness. She was admitted to a hospital in a coma. She was subsequently transferred to a larger hospital. She had irreversible brain damage and periods of respiratory failure and was placed on a ventilator. She was determined to be in a persistent vegetative state (PVS). In the UK, the more precisely defined terms continuous vegetative state and permanent vegetative state are preferred.[11] Quinlan's condition deteriorated over several months. The parents filed a lawsuit asking that, in accord with the Papal determination, extraordinary means of treatment, specifically the ventilator, be discontinued. Within the Roman Catholic tradition, in relation to the duty to preserve life, a distinction is made between ordinary and extraordinary means. Ordinary means must be taken to preserve life, while morally extraordinary means can be refused or terminated.[12,13] Court battles ensued as did divisive public commentaries. The parents stated that they did not want their daughter to die but also did not want her to have to live on a ventilator. The courts granted permission to withdraw the ventilator and it was removed. Karen Ann lived for just over nine additional years, in a PVS, before dying (in 1985) of pneumonia and respiratory failure. Her case both captured public attention and moved the medico-moral discussion of treatment withdrawal forward.

The Tony Bland Case

A similar medico-moral case made its way through the courts in the UK. Tony Bland was an 18-year-old fan of Liverpool Football Club. At a match (1989), he was caught in a crush on the football ground in Hillsborough; 94 people died with a 95th dying in hospital a few days later. The crowd was negligently mismanaged by the police who were subsequently, though many years later, held responsible. In the crush, Tony suffered crushed ribs and punctured lungs and a resultant hypoxia. Bland was initially resuscitated and survived but had sustained devastating brain damage that left him in a persistent vegetative state. Four years later, he remained in a PVS, never having regained consciousness. EEG and CT scans showed no cortical activity. His body was being sustained by artificial hydration and nutrition and nursing care. The physicians and family determined that treatment should be withdrawn. The then current UK law had only previously allowed selective nontreatment of infants. The case was to wend its way through the legal process and courts. Eventually, the case was decided affirmatively on behalf of the physicians, family, and Tony himself. Treatment was withdrawn and he died in 1993, four years after the Hillsborough disaster, the worst disaster in British sports history.[14,15,16,17]

The Yale–New Haven Cases

In 1973, Raymond Duff and Alastair Campbell published an article in the *New England Journal of Medicine*, "Moral and Ethical Dilemmas in the Special Care Nursery."[18] This article details the wrenching nature of treatment and nontreatment decisions for neonates. It gained considerable traction in bioethics circles. The authors write:

> Of 299 consecutive deaths occurring in a special-care nursery, 43 (14 percent) were related to withholding treatment. In this group were 15 with multiple anomalies, eight with trisomy, eight with cardiopulmonary disease, seven with meningomyelocele, three with other Central-nervous-system disorders, and two with short-bowel syndrome. After careful consideration of each of these 43 infants, parents and physicians in a group decision concluded that prognosis for meaningful life was extremely poor or hopeless, and therefore rejected further treatment. The awesome finality of these decisions, combined with a potential for error in prognosis, made the choice agonizing for families and health professionals. Nevertheless, the issue has to be faced, for not to decide is an arbitrary and potentially devastating decision by default.[19]

At issue here were nontreatment decisions specifically. Decisions had to be made for infants with a range of disabilities and likelihood of meaningful life, or even survival with treatment. Also at issue was the question of parental decisions that refused surgery for repairable congenital defects, and what were to be regarded as legitimate and sufficient grounds for nontreatment. Questions arose about the calculus parents may use in their determination, and whether considerations for the burden of raising a disabled child, the perceived effect it would have on siblings, and the issue of stigma should be considered morally licit. Duff and Campbell write:

> Families had strong but mixed feelings about management decisions. Living with the handicapped is clearly a family affair, and families of deformed infants thought there were limits to what they could bear or should be expected to bear. Most of them wanted maximal efforts to sustain life and to rehabilitate the handicapped; in such cases, they were supported fully. However, some families, especially those having children with severe defects, feared that they and their other children would become socially enslaved, economically deprived, and permanently stigmatized, all perhaps for a lost cause.... In some cases, families considered the death of the child right both for the child and for the family.[20]

One particular case was especially troubling:

> An infant with Down's syndrome and intestinal atresia, like the much publicized one at Johns Hopkins Hospital, was not treated because his parents thought that surgery was wrong for their baby and themselves. He died seven days after birth.[21]

Physicians acquiesced to the parental decision. The Johns Hopkins case was among a number of what were pseudonymously termed "Baby Doe Cases."

The Baby Doe Cases

A number of medical-legal cases arose in the early 1980s that were collectively referred to as the *Baby Doe Cases*.[22] In 1982, an infant, "Baby Doe," was born with a surgically reparable trachea-esophageal fistula. However, the infant had Down Syndrome. The parents refused permission for surgery specifically because of Down Syndrome. The hospital asked the Juvenile Court to appoint a guardian for the infant to determine whether or not the fistula should be repaired, which it did. However, the court subsequently upheld the parents' right to refuse surgery for the infant. The infant died five days later of dehydration and pneumonia. There was a public outcry, particularly from disability rights advocates and pro-life groups and the case came to the attention of President Reagan, the Attorney General, and the US Department of Health and Human Services (HHS). Treatment regulations were formulated in 1983 and were novel in that they intervened in the physician–patient relationship. They engendered significant opposition from physicians, physician groups, and the courts which forced their revision. They were to be tested in the *Baby Jane Doe* case.

Infant Jane Doe was born with multiple, significant but treatable congenital defects: spina bifida and hydrocephalus. The parents elected not to consent to surgery and to opt instead for conservative therapy.[23,24,25] When the infant was discharged, the parents took her home. There was a succession of legal battles, a raging national debate over selective nontreatment of infants, medical associations opposing intrusion into clinical practice, pro-life advocates demanding full treatment of all neonates, and more. In addition, a hotline had been established for anonymous reporting of nontreatment; it generated a number of officious meddlers who invoked government intervention, often to the harm of the suffering parents who had carefully and reasonably decided for nontreatment. The issue was incendiary; the debate was public and heated.[26] Final regulations were approved in 1984 and with those regulations came the creation of hospital Infant Care Review Committees (ICRCs). Court cases continued even after the regulations were finalized. The creation of ICRCs set in place yet another formal structure for bioethics.[27]

The Celluloid Case: *Who Should Survive?*

In 1972, the Joseph P. Kennedy, Jr. Foundation (the Foundation) sponsored the creation of the film *Who Should Survive?* The film is moving, poignant, frustrating, angering, and more, though it does not record the extremity of distress the nurses experienced in the case. Its official description is:

> Summary. [The film] Examines the true case of a mongoloid baby born with an intestinal blockage which could be repaired surgically but whose parents do not want the burden of a retarded child and refused to permit the operation. [The film] explains that the surgeon agrees not to challenge the decision of the courts, the hospital does not overrule him, and the infant is put in a side room and dies 15 days later. [It] recreates the situation with the actual doctors and nurses playing their true roles. [It] discusses the ethical, legal, and scientific dilemmas with a panel including Mrs. Sydney Callahan, mother, psychologist, author, and columnist; Robert E. Cooke, M.D.; Reverend John Fletcher; William Curran, Ph.D., professor of legal medicine; and Renee Fox, Ph.D., professor of sociology.[28]

The mother of the infant, incidentally, was a nurse. The film is publicly accessible online. It was widely viewed in bioethics circles and in academic courses in bioethics in the 1970s and 1980s before falling out of use. It remains, however, an important and useful film even though it is now dated.

Moving away from clinical cases, not all pressure on medicine was external; internal pressures could make medicine's star collapse more than it had during the consumer movement and the loss of social trust. Failures of self-policing and the distancing from the patient were two such forces.

Failure of Medical Self-Policing, a Reminder

The horrors of Nazi experimentation on human subjects, and the failure of medicine in the US and UK to prevent or stop ethically repugnant experimentation has already been addressed (Chapter 5). It was included in the section on the social context of the rise of biomedical ethics as an international movement, yet it is important to recall that it had consequences for American, British, and Canadian medicine, and indeed research globally. One of the more important consequences was the creation of research review ethics committees. These committees serve as a pre-implementation review board for research proposals and have become one of the components of the bioethical structures that grew in the 1970s and 1980s. In the US they are referred to as Institutional Review Boards (IRBs) and as Research Ethics Committees (RECs) in Canada and the UK.[29,30,31] The overall aim of such committees is the protection of human and animal subjects, but also as a means of assuring the quality of the research itself, and the integrity of its conduct.

What the Patient Says, What the Machine Says

Stanley Reiser's text *Medicine and the Reign of Technology*,[32] though in the strain of our prior discussion on technology, differs from other approaches in that it examines individual medical technologies and the ethical dimensions of each. It is, thus, a book directed principally toward physicians and subsidiarily toward those interested in biomedical ethics. Reiser examines various dimensions of the use of dissection, the stethoscope, the ophthalmoscope, X-rays, the microscope, the sphygmograph, the galvanometer, blood chemistries, bacteriology, and more. The book is heavily historical in nature, chronicling the development of various implements of medicine, from stethoscopes to lab analysis of bodily fluids and tissues. It is his meta-analysis and commentary that nourished early conversations in bioethics. He writes:

> Since the nineteenth century, physicians have moved through a series of stages: from communication with their patients' experiences... to direct communication with their patients' bodies through techniques of physical examination, to indirect connection... through machines and technical experts. After each... new stage... skills in using old techniques have declined, with the resulting sacrifice of the insights they provided. Insofar as technological evidence occupies the time and commands the chief allegiance of both doctor and patient, it diminishes the possibility that a close personal relationship will develop between the two.... The physician in the last two centuries has gradually relinquished his unsatisfactory attachment to subjective evidence—what the patient says—only

to substitute a devotion to technological evidence—what the machine says....
These circumstances tend to estrange him from the patient and from his own
judgment.[33]

From the perspective of nursing ethics, the important contribution that Reiser
makes is to align clinical technology with the loss of relationship. Others have
written about the physician–patient relationship, notably Paul Ramsey in *The
Patient as Person*[34] and William May in *The Physician's Covenant*,[35] though they
have not linked it with technology as Reiser does, using physical distance as both
a metaphor and an explanation for the loss of the relationship or, using Reiser's
own term, estrangement. Nursing too must be wary of technological distance.
Semanticist Alfred Korzybski once wrote "the map is not the territory." Or in
Alan Watts, inimitable rephrasing, "the menu is not the meal."[36,37] By extension,
the telemetry readings are not the patient. The lab results are not the patient.
Only the patient is the patient. It is the patient with whom the nurse must have a
relationship.

In some ways, Reiser's estimation of technology's effects upon the physician–
patient relationship collaterally presages the effects of bioethics. Nursing ethics
was developed as intimately tied to the classes of nurse relationships, especially
that of the nurse–patient relationship as the relationship of primacy. Nursing ethics
also developed as expressive of the tradition's values, virtues, and the good intrinsic to nursing within the nurse–patient relationship. As Patricia Benner's chapter
(9) will show, nursing ethics in the nurse–patient relationship is a situated, contextual, responsive, attuned ethics that cannot be done without knowing the patient,
cannot be done as if a case study, cannot be done by committee, and cannot be
done at a distance. Abstract, decontextual, *a priori* principles are the telemetry of
bioethics.

The Religiogenesis of Bioethics

While bioethics, as an interdisciplinary field, is a new discipline, bioethical decisions have been the domain of clergy and theologians for centuries. There is,
indeed, nothing new under the sun. Only this newfangled interdisciplinary field is
new; "bioethics" as the domain of pastoral care and theological analysis is ancient.

Arthur Caplan has written that bioethics is "the bastard child of philosophy and,
truth be told, of theology as well."[38] That is not accurate. Bioethics is the child
of theology who was kidnapped by philosophy. The origins of bioethics reside
in religion, or more specifically among the clergy who had to address the moral
questions of the faithful surrounding questions of life, health, and illness. In this
sense bioethics is millennia old and is the domain of the religious leaders and their
congregants—the people—not physicians only. Those who rendered definitive decisions on moral questions for their tradition were clergy-theologians and scholars.
An example (and there are much older examples as well) is the discussions of

the care of *goses* (terminally ill persons judged to be within three days of death), in terms of hastening death that is found in the *Shulchan Aruch*, dating from the 1500s, a scant 400-something years before the emergence of bioethics.

> One in a dying condition is considered a living being in all respects. We may not tie up his jaws, nor may we anoint him with oil, nor wash him, nor stop off his organs of the extremities, nor may we remove the pillow from under him, nor may we place him on sand, clay-ground or earth, nor may we place on his stomach a dish, a shovel, a flask of water or a globule of salt, nor may we summon the townspeople on his behalf, nor may we hire pipers and lamenting women, nor may we close his eyes before his soul departs. And whosoever closes [the dying person's] eyes before death is regarded as one who sheds blood. One may not rend garments, nor bare the shoulder in mourning, nor make a lamentation for him, nor bring a coffin into the house in his presence before he dies, nor may we begin the recital of *Zidduk Haddin* before his soul departs.[39]

This is to say that a person who is dying is a living being and must be treated only as such. Death may be neither hastened, nor impeded, and the *goses* may not be subject to distressing actions.

Day-to-day questions of the moral life—such as divorce, usury, health, illness, childbirth—as well as the duties of physicians specifically are discussed in detail in the theological literature of the Abrahamic, Buddhist, and Hindu traditions. Some of these writings are ancient.[40] In a religious context, members of the community would seek moral advice on their personal lives from the clergy, and the community could seek guidance for the tradition itself. This is to say that the faithful, out of their lived experience, would ask specific normative questions of clergy, not the kinds of questions common to philosophers. While *bioethics* is generally an ethics for physicians primarily, and other health and human services professionals, it is nonetheless regarded as a professional ethics and philosophical enterprise. Religious ethics makes it clear that moral concerns relative to health and illness are the domain of the ordinary person, and the issues that assault their lives. Questions such as "Imam, may I put my mother in a nursing home?" is a question about adult child-to-parent obligations, and is a concern of religious ethics that does not receive attention in professionalized bioethics. These are laypersons questions that reach and become clergy questions, and even theologian questions,[41] but are not questions of bioethics. The everyday ethical concerns of ordinary persons that impinge upon life, health, and illness are the domain of religious, theological—and, yes, nursing—ethics.

The religious literature on normative ethical questions related to health and illness is an unbroken line from ancient times to the present. Thus, as the field of bioethics emerged, the most prominent voices were those of theologians or, because early bioethics education was often situated in religious seminaries, those who were theologically trained but may or may not have had a religious affiliation.

The Waxing and Waning of Religion in Bioethics

Paul Ramsey (1913–1988) is pivotal in systematizing ethics in health care and laying a foundation for bioethics. Ramsey, a Methodist minister, theologian, and Christian ethicist, was among those regarded as a *public intellectual*. It is important to understand the role and position of *public intellectuals* to understand Paul Ramsey's import, but perhaps also to point nursing toward fostering our own public intellectuals.

Public Intellectuals

At its simplest, a public intellectual is a person whose recognized achievements and authority, in one domain of learning or creativity, provides the basis for a broader social authority. She or he may have a capacity to interpret the world, or make connections, explicate issues, critique the status quo, or help others make sense of a range of issues or questions to a wider national or international public. The best among them do not generalize expertise; that is, they do not stray into areas in which they are ill-equipped to speak, and do not presume omnicompetence. While they have a public position, they call for debate and are not polemicists. Instead, they foster authentic, thoughtful, public exchange and debate on perplexing social issues or questions and may represent a loyal opposition to things the way they are. They come from a variety of fields or disciplines. The list is long, but these persons, for example, would be regarded as public intellectuals:[42,43,44,45]

> Amartya Sen, Paul Farmer, Michael Foucault, Hannah Arendt, Gloria Steinem, Edouard Said, Jürgen Habermas, Vine Deloria, Jr., Northrop Frye, W.E.B. DuBois, Ida B. Wells Barnett, Cornel West, Toni Morrison, Patricia Williams, bel hooks, Joan Didion, Marshall McLuhan, Antonio Gramsci, Isaac Asimov, Margaret MacMillan, C.S. Lewis, Susan Sontag, Lionel Trilling, John Ralston Saul, Lawrence Tribe, George Will, Patrick Devlin, H.L.A. Hart, Onora O'Neill, Jean Vanier, Jonathan Saks, Stephen Hawking, Peter Singer, Albert Bandura, Vaclav Smil, Reinhold Niebuhr, and Paul Ramsey.

Public intellectuals such as John Dewey, William James, Marie Stopes, John S. Mill, and John Rawls have deeply influenced nursing ethics.

Paul Ramsey was such a public intellectual who taught Christian ethics at Princeton. Ramsay is credited with laying the intellectual foundations of bioethics with the publication of his book *The Patient as Person*[46] (1970) which is a compilation of Ramsey's invited Lyman Beecher Lectures at Yale University in 1969. Albert Jonsen writes that:

> Those lectures and the book that resulted from them can rightly be called the founding preaching and scriptures of the field of bioethics. Bioethics did not exist when Paul Ramsey stepped to the podium on April 14, 1969. The word

itself first appeared a year later in an article by Dr. Van Rensselaer Potter... So, when Paul Ramsey took up the general topic of medical ethics in an era of rapid technological advances, he was addressing an audience that had heard rumors of problems. No one had yet attempted to articulate these problems in a systematic and comprehensive fashion. Ramsey, then, was not the first to speak of these questions as ethical, but he was the first to take a synoptic view.[47]

Incidentally, Ramsey's book *Basic Christian Ethics*[48] was reviewed by the 30-year-old John Rawls.[49] Paul Ramsey was a public intellectual who spoke both to professions and the public, but also to legislators. He operated within the tradition of *public theology*.[50,51,52] Public theology, within Christian theology, is the engagement of the church with society and its social issues, particularly with regard to issues of social justice; human well-being, welfare, and flourishing; and the common good.[53,54] Public theologians (not unique to Christianity but also including the Jewish, Islamic, and Buddhist traditions) present their theological position for debate and critique over matters of common concern, not as a matter of polemics.[55,56] Thus, issues in medical ethics would fall within the domain of public theology.[57,58,59,60]

Individual theologians such as Paul Ramsey, Richard McCormick, James Gustafson, Joseph Fletcher, John Fletcher, and others were among the vanguard in the emergence of bioethics. Centers such as the Park Ridge Center for the Study of Health, Faith and Ethics furthered religious deliberation on medical and health issues. The Park Ridge Center was founded by historian Martin Marty, also a public theologian and historian; he served as its first president. Special note needs to be made of the stunning publications written under the aegis of the Park Ridge Center. These include *Healing and Restoring*,[61] *Caring and Curing*,[62] the journal *Second Opinion, The Park Ridge Center Bulletin,* and a remarkable series on health and medicine in 22 faith traditions. Each book (with a title template) addressed one tradition such as *Health and Medicine in the Hindu Tradition*,[63] *Health and Medicine in the Catholic Tradition,* also Christian Science, Jewish, Methodist, Reformed, Evangelical, Lutheran, Anglican, Islamic, Anabaptist, Buddhist, and Shamanic traditions.

The Secularization of Bioethics

By the 1990s, bioethics shifted from theological and medical voices predominating to an increasingly interdisciplinary field led by philosophers. Daniel Callahan makes note of this shift:

> The most striking change over the past two decades or so has been the secularization of bioethics. The field has moved from one dominated by religious and medical traditions to one now increasingly shaped by philosophical and legal concepts. The consequence has been a mode of public discourse that

emphasizes secular themes: universal rights, individual self-direction, procedural justice, and a systematic denial of either a common good or a transcendent individual good.[64]

Albert Jonsen makes a similar observation in reference to Paul Ramsey:

If [Paul Ramsey] examined the vital field of bioethics today, he would be dismayed to see that it remains conflicted about its ethical foundations. He would decry the wavering about principle and cases,... He would be appalled to see the intricate structure of ethical argument, with its exceptionless principles, collapse into a principle of autonomy, which, as he once said, merely "enthrones arbitrary freedom."... He would probably be sad to discover that the strong religious voices of early bioethics are now drowned out in an essentially secular discourse.[65]

As bioethics secularized, religious voices were silenced in part because they felt unwelcome, in part because of a secular presumption that religious voices are sectarian and do not come with shared values, and partly because religious persons would shift to a common language. Unlike religiously affiliated laypersons, theologians remained moderately welcome as one among peers and were expected to speak in their theological language. Philosophical theologians are "bilingual" and could code switch between theological and philosophical/secular language. Certainly, as the legal and regulatory structures around bioethics developed, the language was resolutely secular. There is a cost to this secularization. Courtney Campbell's worthy essay notes that:

The tensions between religious discourse and bioethics pose dual challenges of *accessibility* and *meaning*. Insofar as the incorporation of moral claims from a specific religious tradition or community is deemed to undermine the possibilities for a generally accessible bioethics discourse, the significance of religious perspectives may be very limited. Yet the criterion of accessibility may limit the moral richness of bioethics, for the costs of conformity to public discourse requirements may be the loss of meaning and content about ultimate concerns embedded in a particular tradition, whether religious or professional.[66]

Bioethics analyzes but does not resolve questions and is ill-equipped to address issues of meaning—it provides tools for analysis of the question but does not specify answers and does not address some of life's core questions that are addressed by religion (or even nonreligious existential reflection).

Theological bioethics was never solely limited to medical treatment quandaries, or even to persons in hospitals. Theology (like nursing) is concerned for the whole person, so the whole of life is considered in theological (bio)ethics.

Religion addresses different questions. Philosophical theology still employs the tools of philosophy but draws upon sources from the tradition as well as from non-religious philosophy, and sometimes from religious traditions outside its own. Theology is neither nonrational nor irrational; it argues both from and within its own domain. In some instances, its view of particular questions will be distinctive of its own sources and speak mainly to those within the tradition. At other times, its response to other questions corresponds closely with the views of other traditions or of those who do not embrace a religious tradition. For example, on the question of abortion, the view of Roman Catholics may be shared by evangelical or fundamentalist Protestants and be rejected by mainline Protestants—an "extended-family" dispute. The view of abortion among mainline Protestants (Lutheran, Methodist, Presbyterian, et al.) and Jews more closely aligns with that of nonreligious persons. However, on the issue of euthanasia, there is significant correlation between positions of Christianity, Judaism, and Islam, though differing in sources and at the metaphysical level of interpretation. Here, all three traditions may differ from the positions taken by non-religious philosophers. On issues such as, for example, the treatment of those with a disability as still possessing dignity, the theological and philosophical positions will walk together.[67]

The Compulsory Apostasy of Nursing

When asked whether there is a place for religion in the discourse of bioethics in practice and policy domains, the response is an unequivocal "ummm." Bioethicists or ethicists who are not aligned with religion, or who disavow religion entirely, customarily draw upon the notion that in a pluralistic society religious perspectives are not universally shared, so their answer is "no." There are also arguments that the arena of ethical discourse needs to be accessible, rational, and value neutral, or more specifically free of particularistic personal (religious) values and affirmation. This is, of course, a corollary to asserting that science is neutral and value free. Bioethicists or ethicists within a faith tradition, that is, moral theologians, often adopt the *lingua franca* of the discipline and its manifestation in committees. Callahan writes that:

> The discipline of medicine is now as resolutely secular as any that can be found in our society. It is a true child of the enlightenment…, nicely epitomized in the two federal commissions established during the 1970s, the National Commission for the Protection of Human Subjects in 1974, and the President's commission in 1979. Both professional staffs of the two groups and those called upon to give testimony before them were drawn mainly from medicine, philosophy, and health policy sciences, and the law. The approaches and concepts commonly employed in their reports, moreover, showed not the least visible trace of religious influence. An ethic of universal principles—especially autonomy, beneficence, and justice—was given a place of prestige in the 1978 *Belmont Report* issued by the National Commission.[68]

In its various forums, Campbell writes, "bioethics discourse is prominently shaped by an ethic of principles—autonomy, beneficence, and justice—that seems well-suited as a method of conflict resolution because such norms are deemed to command general acceptance."[69] Persons with a religious commitment often adopt the prevailing language of biomedical-ethical principlism, or bioethics more generally, and leave their religious concepts and lexicon at the boarding gate "mettle detector" (please forgive the lexical humor).

Beyond eschewing religious perspectives, for nurses the discourse is rigged. The methodology of bioethics, the privileging of specific ethical theories (Kant & Mill & Rawls), the preferred principles of principlism, the issues and questions that are addressed, the quandaries that are chosen for resolution, all have antecedently been selected. Nurses and nursing did not choose the methodology, theories, principles, issues, or quandaries, and for the most part had no part in their determination. Bioethics essentially demands that nurses leave their nursing identity, values, and the goods intrinsic to nursing at the door. Though Callahan is actually writing of the secularization of bioethics and the loss of religious perspectives, his words are also true of nursing perspectives. Nurses on ethics committees are

> Forced to pretend that we are not creatures both of particular moral communities and the more sprawling, inchoate general community that we celebrate as an expression of our pluralism. Yet that pluralism becomes a form of oppression if, in its very name, we are told to shut up in public about our private lives and beliefs and talk a form of what Jeffrey Stout has called moral esperanto. The rules of that language are that it deny the concreteness and irregularities of real communities, that it eschews vision and speculation about goals and meaning, and that it enshrines the discourse... especially that of rights as the preferred mode of daily relations.[70]

Nurses are creatures of a particular moral community called nursing, a community of an ongoing, living tradition and narrative of its own, with distinctive relationships, obligations, duties, values, virtues, ideals, goods, and ends. Whether commission or committee, nurses were largely excluded or had only token representation in the bioethical community of moral discourse and were forced to adopt its *Esperanto*.

What would bioethical discourse or the proceedings of ethics committees be like if, instead, they had proceeded on the basis of nursing discourse, of feminist ethics, or an ethics of caring; or focused on issues of dignity, respect, holism, and suffering; or emphasized a principle of beneficence (if principles at all), or relationship, character, and community? How would a virtue ethics base have changed the kinds of questions asked? How would bioethical discourse change if it were guided by nursing concerns, values, ends and goals? This is where collective and individual moral courage is called for, from nurses, a prophetic voice of nursing that critiques the status quo, its privilege, its blind spots, and the ways in which they harm all recipients of care. At every level, nurses and nursing organizations need vigorously to intrude nursing values into biomedical ethical and policy discourse, to demand their due consideration among the prevailing and competing values.

Religious Ethics and the Nurse

The religious origins of health-care ethics are important to nursing on at least five counts. First, the ethical questions that arose came from the laity, from ordinary persons, facing a question or crisis in life, health, or illness. The questions did not start with the scholars and theologians, who identified them on their positional own terms, but were placed in their hands by ordinary persons seeking guidance. Only then would the philosophical and practical theologians of the day undertake analysis of the ethical issue, not simply for speculative analysis but with an end of practical guidance. Many of the issues in nursing ethics come from patients themselves, or nurses. A second reason that the religious base of ethics is important is that nurses often care for persons who embrace a particular faith tradition, and express concerns for how their formal tradition or its culture might provide guidance. That guidance may or may not be accepted in whole or in part. Third, these ethical questions are often broader, unrelated to technology, and are not addressed within the field of bioethics. Fourth, religiously based ethics takes account of the whole person, her or his situatedness; the person's values, value structure, and aims; their relational network, and all the lifeworld and values-affirming factors that are as, or more, important to the patient than a purely rational decision making. Nursing shares with religion a concern for the totality of the patient-as-person. Fifth, some nurses profess a specific faith tradition themselves and knowledge of the tradition's resources and guidance can be helpful to the nurse's own self-understanding and guidance, and to patient care.

 This examination of the religiogenesis of bioethics is not a tangent but is some of the gas and dust of the nebula that will undergo fusion. It figures into the movement of bioethics into nursing as we shall see momentarily. But first, it is necessary to look at additional context in the rise of bioethics, before returning to the religious commitment that led to the founding of several structures that promoted both the rise and coalescence of bioethics, and its movement into nursing.

The Bioethics Empire

While bioethics begins as an academic discipline, it becomes attractive to a constellation of disciplines, evolving into an interdisciplinary endeavor, or field, that addresses from bottom to top clinical practice, research, social medicine, and health policy. To accomplish this, it is necessary for *power structures* to be created. Power structures are meant to stand in balance (and perhaps tension) with *meaning and value structures*.[71]

Meaning and value structures are the ethical norms, values, ideals, ethics, and moral ethos embedded within practices, in this case the practice of medicine, nursing, and health care. This would include the ethical literature, oaths, codes, and ethical position statements of a profession, as well as the norms embedded in the tradition and narrative of the practice. These may be carried forward and asserted by the profession itself and through the field of bioethics. For bioethics, this would include a range of ethical declarations such as those on human rights. It is the function of meaning and value structures to guide, inform, and restrain a profession as a whole or its members in their practice, research, scholarship, and social action. *Power structures* are the enabling structures that include any and all sources of social and political power (e.g., social prestige, autonomy of the profession, moneys, and authority). It is a profession's power structures that enable the realization of its meaning and values, without which the meaning and value structures are impotent. However, it is the *meaning and value structures* that guide the use of power and prevent its excesses or ill uses. For example, guidelines for the use of human subjects in research (in the *meaning and value structure*) are of no effect unless they are enforceable through, for example, regulations, sanctions, and oversight (in the *power structure*). In the obverse, meaning and value structures hold power structures to account, such as in the studies of misogyny in medical practice; or racism in nursing structures such as nursing education, research, and organizations. For the interdisciplinary field of bioethics to realize its goals of addressing moral issues in medicine, it became necessary to create, or co-create, a range of structures including think-tanks, networks, and educational, authoritative, and regulatory bodies.

"Beating Up Bioethics"—Tina Steven's Argument about the Origin of Bioethics

For a different interpretation of the rise of bioethics than is found in the standard works, we can look to Tina Stevens' *Bioethics in America: Origins and Cultural Politics*.[72] The received interpretation of the history of bioethics is that it arose in a period of social ferment in the 1960s, reactions to medical paternalism, and concerns that surrounded the innovations in medical technology and its clinical deployment. Questions, both medical and public, arose about the appropriate use (or not) of technology, and its overuse, particularly at the end of life; bioethics is alleged to have developed to assist in navigating the murky waters. This view would situate bioethics within the realm of *meaning and value structures*. Historian Stevens, however, interprets the rise of bioethics in a way that would instead situate it within social *power structures*. Her critique follows on from those of Lewis Mumford, Jacques Ellul, Herbert Marcuse, and Theodore Rozak and their concerns for the technological society that America had become. Stevens' book makes a three-part argument. First, she argues that social dis-ease with innovation in American society is persistent and Americans were particularly disquieted by the unleashing of the atomic bombs on Japan and the extraordinary devastation and loss of life that they caused. Mumford himself was said to have been left speechless for days after the news broke. Scientifically, value-neutral nuclear fission was hardly socially value neutral. This, Stevens argues, became a public skittishness about scientific and medical advances that then gave rise to a *bioethics movement*. It was not the turmoil of the 1960s and 1970s, or the Beecher and Tuskegee research disclosures, that generated bioethics. The second argument is that the Hastings Center sought to remain independent in order to have its opinions remain pristine, free of the pressures of funding sources. It also sought to maintain a nonideological, neutral, and irenic posture, and this, while avoiding any activism. Recall that the Hastings Center, founded in 1969, followed years of the biting social critique of society, science, and medicine (by Mumford, Marcuse, Ellul, Rozak, and many others). It did not take up that mantle. Rather, Callahan sought to steer the Center away from the critique of science and from conflictual positions. Instead of challenging medical scientific advances and their use, the Center moved in the direction of producing guidelines for their ethical use. Based on the Center's own archival documents, Stevens writes that the Center adopted characteristics "that were necessary for mutually assured survival—of both the bioethics community and the continued ideological trajectory of science and medicine."[73,74] Her final argument brings together the redefinition of death (1968) and the Karen Ann Quinlan case. Her argument is that the Quinlan case, which helped kickstart bioethics, was cast as a pivotal "right to die." It was, more accurately, a right to withdraw treatment; Quinlan was not brain dead. Stevens writes that "the definition was adopted, after all, not because of an exigent need to deal with the nature of death on its own terms but over the interest in facilitating organ procurement."[75] She continues, writing that bioethics served

> as a broker of exotic biotechnologies. In 1968, when researchers fretted that the new need for finding transplantable organs would alarm a public unaccustomed to viewing organs as fungible, the concept of brain death was a necessary balm, sanctioned by bioethicists.[76]

After a review of several legal cases regarding the end of life, she discusses the transmogrification of a right to die into a right to assisted suicide, and perhaps eventually a duty to die. But, more salient to nursing, she writes:

> Remembered wrongly, the [Quinlan] case has served to constrain the national discourse surrounding our expectations for humane treatment during chronic or terminal illness, for this discourse now is contorted by a jurisprudence wedded to the strange oxymoronic slogan that we have a right to die.... instead of developing the obligations of the healthy—the compassionate obligation to seek ways to ease and end suffering.[77]

It is, of course, nursing that provides humane and compassionate care and the relief of suffering at the end of life. For a while, a countervailing voice could be heard in the nursing literature, expressing concerns that the race to authorize assisted suicide could result in the exclusion of nurses from the discussion (as the decisions were made by physicians without consulting nurses), and could have the potential to undercut compassionate end-of-life care that ameliorated the symptoms of dying, or more specifically, nursing care of dying patients and the grieving family. That voice faded to a whisper and failed to challenge the trajectory of the issue. Palliative care did, however, coalesce and grow into a medical specialization, and hospice care, promulgated by nurse-become-physician Cicely Saunders.

Tina Stevens' assessment of the history of American bioethics is an outlier take, to the degree that Albert Jonsen referred to her as a "tuffy" and "bully" and accused her (and Wesley Smith's *Culture of Death*)[78] of "Beating Up Bioethics."[79] Certainly her historian's view that bioethics arose as a means, not of challenging medicine's scientific and technological advances, but to manage the public trepidation that such issues caused, and to pave the way for their adoption and implementation unhindered by public dis-ease should not be so pejoratively dismissed. Her assessment would, of course, dismay bioethicists. Just as medicine became a sovereign power in the US, with its industrial and governmental arms, perhaps bioethics has as well.

Retrodictive Histories of Bioethics

Retrodiction, also known as *postdiction*, is most frequently applied to scientific theories. Retrodiction, like diagnosis, looks backward to find a cause. It moves backward from the present, looking longitudinally at historical stages and events, stage-by-stage, to establish the causal genesis of an event. Once so established, a return to the present will potentially allow for prediction, (that is, prognosis in our analogy), and the realization of a desired end.

Tod Chambers, in "Retrodiction and the Histories of Bioethics," [80] takes aim at the extant histories of bioethics, using literary genre to categorize them as tragedy, satire, comedy, or romance. He writes that:

> The initial problem of these historical frames is that they suggest to the reader that the philosopher is responding to particular historical forces and, thus, that the moral paradigm he or she proposes provides the necessary resolution to the historical cause of the present ethical quandaries.[81]

Chambers sees Tristram Englehardt's *The Foundations of Bioethics*[82] as tragedy in that Engelhardt sees a secular bioethics as a tragic and inevitable response to an increasingly secularized and pluralistic society. Albert Jonsen and Stephen Toulmin's *Abuse of Casuistry* is cast as satire. Chambers writes that:

> The historical frame that Jonsen and Toulmin construct is essentially a satiric one that connects casuistry, social protest, and the bioethics movement. Jonsen and Toulmin do not see the rise of bioethics as something that requires closure;

instead bioethics is a radical revision of moral philosophy and of philosophy's participation in society.[83]

Ezekiel Emanuel's *The Ends of Human Life*[84] is assigned the genre of comedy. Chambers says:

> Emanuel's resolution to the problems faced in medical ethics is communitarian. Medicine's ends cannot be isolated from the larger moral fabric of society. The ends of the medical profession must be balanced against the ends of the larger society... in liberal political philosophy there is not even a theoretical way of resolving the pressing medical ethics issues. Emanuel possesses a "liberal communitarian vision of health care," a utopian vision of American society where people belong to different community health programs.[85]

In the genre of romance, Edmund Pellegrino and David Thomasma's *The Virtues in Medical Practice* fits that bill.[86] "For Pellegrino and Thomasma, medicine is engaged in a battle against the forces of self-interest. They believe that the profession of medicine can triumph over self-interest by reinstating virtue as the foundational value."[87]

Chamber's conclusion is important for our understanding of histories of bioethics, as well as for our own work. He writes:

> histories of bioethics are driven by what the literary critic Frank Kermode referred to as "the sense of an ending." Ethicists begin with an imagined ending, be it a new political structure for health care or a return to virtue, and trace a historical beginning that leads to this ending, be it political liberalism or the dominance of self-interest in the medical culture. The historical narratives of the rise of the bioethics movement make the ethicist's chosen paradigm appear self-evident, but we must understand this historical reflection as retrodictive rather than causal. In the final analysis this battle over the past is a contest for the future.[88]

Chambers ends with a cautionary note regarding the agenda that may underlie historical accounts, but also for work going forward:

> I believe that a single or "universal" history does not exist. Instead I propose that self-doubt should itself serve as a safeguard in the use of such historical frames. If we were less certain of the "objectivity" of our particular history of bioethics, we might in turn be less certain of the moral solution being promoted; that is, Engelhardt's procedural morality, Jonsen and Toulmin's revival of casuistry, Emanuel's liberal communitarianism, and Pellegrino and Thomasma's restoration of virtue. If there is anything that connects all of the histories,... it is the extraordinary certitude the authors seem to possess concerning their particular "take" on the true nature of our moral ills. I believe that the ability to be aware of the rhetoric of one's arguments in turn promotes a hermeneutics of self-doubt, which in turn will foster sounder arguments in the field.[89,90]

In a retrodiction of nursing ethics through its literature and social context, there is, admittedly, an end in sight for nursing itself: the reclamation of nursing ethics and its auxiliary incorporation of the useful aspects of bioethics, in better service of nurses, nursing, and health of individuals and society.

Building a Bioethics Industrial Complex

Bioethics became a bioethical–medical complex with a number of structures that supported its agenda, work, and social authority. These include the development of the Hastings Center and its journal, the *Hastings Center Report*; the several President's Commissions and Council on bioethics, the Institutional Review Boards for surveillance of research proposals; the Infant Care Review Committees, and Institutional Ethics Committees in hospitals nationwide, the American Society for Bioethics and Humanities, the International Bioethics Committee and Commission on the Ethics of Scientific Knowledge and Technology (COMEST) of UNESCO and others. The American Academy of Nursing has an Expert Panel on Bioethics, and the American Nurses Association has a Center for Ethics and Human Rights, and an Ethics Advisory Board. These bioethics structures are capably addressed in a number of books on the history of bioethics and need not be repeated herein. It is more germane here to note that, with the exception of the nursing organizations, nursing was generally excluded from these structures, except in token representation.

The Perplexity of Nursing Exclusion

Despite the fact that nursing is the largest health-care profession in the nation (and globally) nurses and nursing as a profession have largely been excluded, or permitted only token representation, from the determinative echelons of bioethics. Whether the successive President's Commissions on bioethics, the Callahan years of the Hastings Center, The Belmont Report Commission, bioethics doctoral faculties, and so forth, issues such as sexism, devaluing of women's labor, and devaluing of intimate caring function might have some power of explanation, but not fully so. However, if Tina Steven's perspective on the rise of bioethics is correct, it provides a stronger rationale for nursing's exclusion.

If the function of bioethics is *not* that of a critical voice calling for an examination of questions, issues, and trends; and if the function of bioethics *is* that of greasing the wheels of technological advance; and if the function of bioethics is to make social change through medicine and science more palatable; then, nursing is an aberrant and nettlesome voice as it represents values that diverge from and may be at odds with prevailing, corporatized health-care delivery. To return to Ellul, the efficiencies of the technological society and the machine, including medicine, mitigate against the inefficiencies of nursing values: comfort, care, presence, dignity, altruism, integrity, social justice, and more. Even efficient nursing, when not reduced to *techne*, embraces goods and ends that are inimical to the efficiency of corporatized health care. The best nursing, expert nursing, is an impediment to any status quo that undermines the values and goods at the heart of nursing in the service of patient care and the health of society—when nursing takes a stand. Patients and society are better served when nursing is an activist, vocal, needling, nettlesome, meddlesome, uppity, challenging loyal opposition.

Religious Faith Kickstarts Bioethics and Its Movement into Nursing

It is not possible to overestimate the effect that the faith commitment of the Kennedy family, and Eunice Kennedy Shriver in particular, had upon not only the development of the field of bioethics, but its institutions, and the movement of bioethics into nursing. Mrs. Shriver (1921–2009) was a member of the Joseph P. and Rose Kennedy clan, sister of President John F. Kennedy, and Senators Robert and Edward "Ted" Kennedy. She was the fifth of nine children in a devoutly Roman Catholic family. Relevant to what follows, Mrs. Shriver's older sister, Rosemary, was intellectually disabled, and became incapacitated and unable to speak intelligibly following a failed prefrontal lobotomy for seizures and mood swings; she was subsequently institutionalized.[91] Her parents essentially abandoned her, though in later years Rose arranged for Rosemary to visit the surviving family members. Meryl Gordon writes:

> The heroine of this story is Eunice Kennedy Shriver, now best known as one of the founders of the Special Olympics. Horrified by what had been done to her sister, Eunice became a passionate champion for people with disabilities. She persuaded her father to use his fortune to fund research, and after John F. Kennedy was elected president, she successfully lobbied him to establish such government entities as the National Institute of Child Health and Human Development. She later assumed responsibility for Rosemary's care. The family's youngest member, Ted, was only 9 years old when Rosemary vanished from family life with minimal explanation, a frightening and puzzling loss. As a senator, he also took up her cause, citing Rosemary as his inspiration when he sponsored bills like the groundbreaking Americans with Disabilities Act.[92]

Mrs. Shriver earned a degree in sociology and worked as a social worker. She worked in juvenile delinquency, and later in a women's shelter. She had first-hand experience of addressing human need. Upon her death, the Shriver family released this statement:

> The amazing Eunice Kennedy Shriver went home to God this morning.... She... taught us by example and with passion what it means to live a faith-driven life of love and service to others.... Inspired by her love of God, her devotion to her family, and her relentless belief in the dignity and worth of every human life, she worked without ceasing.... She was a living prayer, a living advocate, a living center of power. She set out to change the world and... She founded the movement that became Special Olympics, the largest movement for acceptance and

inclusion for people with intellectual disabilities in the history of the world. Her work transformed the lives of hundreds of millions of people across the globe, and they in turn are her living legacy.[93]

Eunice's devotion to her faith tradition and to her sister were formative in what would become the motif of her life. It would, in addition, deeply affect the emergence of bioethics, the creation of its power structures, and its movement into nursing.

The Influence of Eunice Kennedy Shriver and the Joseph P. Kennedy, Jr. Foundation on the Development of Bioethics and Its Inclusion of Nursing

Eunice Shriver became the executive vice president of the Joseph P. Kennedy, Jr. Foundation and its driving force in 1957. Ted Kennedy served as its president. The patriarch of the family, Joseph P. Kennedy, Sr., had (at Eunice's behest) established the Foundation in memory of his eldest son. The focus of the Foundation was and is on research, programs, bioethics, and policies that benefit persons with intellectual disabilities, and the welfare and well-being of the intellectual disabilities community. As a part of that focus, Mrs. Shriver started Camp Shriver for children with intellectual and physical disabilities, held annually at her home. The success of Camp Shriver led Mrs. Shriver to award grants through the Kennedy Foundation to universities and community recreation departments and centers to hold similar camps for local children.[94] The Kennedy Foundation held symposia and sponsored research on the recreational, activity, nutritional, and support needs of children with intellectual disabilities. In 1966, Mrs. Shriver proposed nationwide sports contests for teams of persons with intellectual disabilities. In 1968, her efforts would culminate in the first International Special Olympics Summer Games, held in Chicago. The Special Olympics grew internationally, and now "the sun never sets on the Special Olympics."[95]

Mrs. Shriver, through the Foundation, provided initial (and some ongoing) funding for a number of bioethics endeavors that served to grow the field. The Foundation endowed two faculty chairs[96] and established the Kennedy Institute of Ethics at Georgetown University.

> In the founding of the Institute, the Kennedy family's commitment to the rights of those whose voices are too-easily silenced, especially those of the intellectually disabled, united with Georgetown University's core Jesuit commitment to ethical reflection engaged with the real world.[97]

In exercising their philanthropy through Georgetown University, the Foundation brings together Mrs. Shriver's and the Kennedy family's passion for aiding persons with intellectual disabilities and for their Catholic faith and its Jesuit tradition.

Initially created as the Joseph and Rose Kennedy Institute for the Study of Human Reproduction and Bioethics, it became the Kennedy Institute of Ethics (KIE); the goal was to create an ethics think-tank that was "truly ecumenical and catholic [universal]." In 1973, with $1.35 million in seed money from the Foundation, the Bioethics Research Library was established and is now the world's premier library for bioethics literature. The library "has grown to over 300,000 books, journal articles, and other archival materials, and it is a destination library with special collections of Jewish, Christian, Islamic, and Secular bioethics texts that draws scholars from around the world."[98] In addition, the KIE offers summer intensive courses in bioethics (now in its 50th year, 44th session), sponsors the *Kennedy Institute of Ethics Journal*, sponsors and hosts resident and visiting scholars, sponsors international and national symposia on bioethical topics, collaborates with the academic programs in bioethics and with the Pellegrino Institute for Clinical Ethics at Georgetown, and more.[99] Its involvement is fulsome and its reach is extensive. Beyond the foundation's engagement with Georgetown University bioethics, it funds Public Policy Fellowships and continues to fund programs, research, and more to benefit persons with intellectual disabilities, their families, and communities.

The foundation made two early contributions to the developing field of bioethics that require specific mention. In 1972, the Kennedy Foundation produced the film *Who Shall Survive?* (see above). Additionally, in 1971, the Foundation convened the *Choices on Our Conscience: The Joseph P. Kennedy Jr. Foundation International Symposium on Human Rights, Retardation, and Research* (1971). A breathtaking array of luminaries from ethics, law, policy, theology, science, medicine, sociology, and more, including Nobel laureates, were invited as presenters and panelists.[100] However, by the early 1970s, when the symposium was convened, bioethics had not yet taken hold in nursing.

Horror Vacui: *The Loss of Nursing Ethics*

To steal from Aristotle, and then bend his words: (human) nature abhors a vacuum (*horror vacui*). Following the 1965 ANA position statement on nursing education,[101] nursing moved into colleges and universities, leaving behind its hospital libraries—ethics books—and was shorn of any content not deemed *nursing* by the colleges. If it were taught at all, ethics education in nursing moved to schools of philosophy or theology at the same time that we see the emergence of bioethics as a discipline. The loss of nursing ethics created a vacuum in nursing that the philosophers and theologians are delighted to fill. Stephen Toulmin, in his article "How Medicine Saved the Life of Ethics,"[102] writes that the

theoretical analyses of moral philosophers concentrated on questions of so-called metaethics. Most professional philosophers assumed that their proper business was not to take sides on substantive ethical questions but rather to consider in a more formal way what kinds of issues and judgments are properly classified as moral in the first place.[103]

In issues or instances of perplexity people turned

> to the philosophers for guidance. Hoping for intelligent and perceptive comments on the actual substance of such issues, they were offered only analytical classifications, which sought to locate the realm of moral issues, not to decide them.[104]

The analytical classifications about which Toulman writes, that frustrated that those seeking tangible guidance from philosophers interested in rationalist analysis, were *a priori*, noncontextual, (allegedly) universal principles (such as Kant's Categorical Imperative), versus a case-based, "real-life" (casuistic) method, the method Toulmin and Jonsen advocated. Toulmin asserts that when medicine and its quandaries, embedded in the physician–patient relationship, were brought to philosophy, there were

> vexed topics raised by particular cases, [that] have obliged philosophers to address once again the Aristotelian problems of *practical reasoning*, which had been on the sidelines for too long. In this sense, we may indeed say that, during the last 20 years, medicine has "saved the life of ethics," and that it has given back to ethics a seriousness and human relevance which it had seemed... to have lost for good.[105]

Nursing too saved the life of philosophy by filling its bioethics classes with cohorts of nursing students. Nursing might have shared its quandaries with philosophers, had there been an interest in the quandaries that vexed and perplexed nurses and nursing rather than medicine. But rather than meeting physicians and nurses at the bedside, philosophy met them in the ether of the Categorical Imperative, and did so with no particular interest in nursing. Still, within nursing's own century-old ethical corpus it had managed to find its way through the quandaries that arose in nursing practice—and had it not been lost, nurses could have drawn upon and extended it. In the 1970s, nurses were being introduced to bioethics, taught by philosophers, but nursing had not developed a cadre of faculty who could teach it. Rescue came from an unexpected source.

The Joseph P. Kennedy, Jr, Fellowships in Medical Ethics

In 1976, The Joseph P. Kennedy, Jr. Foundation began offering annual fellowships in medical ethics, two for physicians and two for nurses. In some years, fellowships were not offered when the qualifications of the candidates did not meet expectations. The last nurse fellowship was awarded in 1984. The fellowship could be taken at either Georgetown University or Harvard University, or at another university if there were special circumstances.[106] A total of 19 nurse fellowships were awarded. The fellowships were specifically in *medical ethics*, not bioethics as the discipline of bioethics had not yet coalesced. Fritz Jahr, a Protestant pastor, theologian, and educator is credited with the first use of the term bioethics, in the form Bio-Ethik, in 1927.[107,108] Biochemist and oncologist Van Rensselaer Potter used the term bioethics, the first known appearance in English, in 1970. His use of the term is not used precisely as it is today.[109] At the time of the early fellowships, *medical ethics* had not shifted to *biomedical ethics* (the interim term) or *bioethics*.

The insistence that the fellowships be awarded to nurses came at the behest of Eunice Kennedy Shriver, the executive vice president of the Foundation.[110] The fellows could, to some extent, craft the fellowship in accord with their own goals. These included acquiring a formal knowledge of ethics, learning about the integration of ethics into nursing curriculum, writing for publication in ethics and nursing, and practical experience in clinical ethics. Fellows could audit or take courses at their fellowship university, as well as engage in an ethics project or research. Fellows were expected to address ethical issues related to persons with intellectual disabilities. After the fellowship year, over half of the nurse fellows became leaders in bioethics in nursing, some did not stay engaged in ethics, and some were relatively close to retirement at the time of the fellowship. The fellows, their year, and site of fellowship are given below.

TABLE 6.1 List of Kennedy Nurse Fellows

Kennedy Nurse Fellow	Year	Site
Aroskar, Mila, EdD, RN, FAAN	1976	Harvard
Davis, Anne, PhD, RN, FAAN	1976	Harvard
Lumpp, Sr. Francesca, CSJ, MSN	1976	Georgetown
Payton, Rita, DA, MS, RN	1976	Notre Dame
Stanley, Sr. Teresa, CCVI, DNSc, RN	1976	Georgetown
Mahon, Kathleen, DNSc, RN	1977	Harvard
Fowler, Marsha, PhD, MDiv, MS, RN, FAAN	1978	Harvard
Gadow, Sally, PHD, RN	1978	Georgetown
Siantz, Mary Lou, PhD, RN	1978	Georgetown
Martin, Cheyenne, PhD, RN	1979	Georgetown & Rice
Mitchell, Christine, MS, MTS, RN, FAAN	1979	Harvard
White, Gladys B, PhD, RN	1979	Georgetown
Fry, Sara T. PhD, RN, FAAN	1981	Georgetown
McCarty, Katherine, MS, RN	1981	Harvard
Ryan, Mary Pat, PhD, RN	1981	Harvard
Silva, Mary Cipriano, PhD, RN, FAAN	1983	George Mason
Moroney, Sarah, MS, MTS, RN	1984	Harvard
Davis, Megan Murphy, PhD, RN	1984	Georgetown
Cady, Patricia, PhD, RN	1988	Boston College

In her ten-year follow-up report on the fellowship outcomes, Sara Fry writes:

The majority of Fellows worked on degree requirements and participated in institutional programs related to mental retardation or the treatment of individuals with disabilities. Others attended courses and seminars; also, the Intensive Bioethics Course and Tuesday Luncheons at Georgetown University. Almost one half of the Fellows taught classes on ethics and produced manuscripts or books during the fellowship period.[111]

The report included a review of the curriculum vitae of ten former fellows. Their post-fellowship productivity included over 500 journal articles, book chapters and books at that point, a rather prodigious output in the early years of bioethics. *Ethical Dilemmas and Nursing Practice* (1983) by Anne Davis and Mila Aroskar was the first book to be published among the fellows.[112] It went to five editions, the last in 2009.[113] The first edition emphasized, though not exclusively, ethical principlism. The second and subsequent editions included a chapter on the history of nursing ethics, and the book moved toward a less principlistic approach. It was the Foundation's expectation, or more specifically Mrs. Shriver's expectation, that the nurse fellows would take medical ethics (yes, still medical ethics at this point) back to their respective universities and integrate it into the nursing curriculum, teach ethics in schools of nursing, and engage in research and scholarship in ethics in nursing. Her expectations were well met as bioethics came to be widely adopted within nursing. It is my contention that the Kennedy Fellowships were pivotal in turning nursing toward bioethics. Nurses' ethical concerns, women's health issues (with the exception of abortion), and the social structures of health disadvantagement and disparities had not and have not figured prominently in bioethics until more recent years. This is not "sour grapes"; instead, it is intended to point out that bioethics was (and remains) medically centric, and a discipline largely generated and dominated, at least in its first 30-plus years, by white, male, upper-middle-class academics.

In the decade report on the Kennedy nurse fellows, Fry et al. write:

Kennedy Nurse Fellows have made significant contributions to nursing ethics during the past 20 years. Although the term, "nursing ethics"—first used by Isabel Hampton Robb in the title to her 1900 book, *Nursing Ethics: For Hospital and Private Use*—has always been considered important in nursing practice, it was not until Kennedy Nurse Fellows began their work that the term began to mean more than merely following certain rules of conduct in attending the sick. As a result of the scholarship of Nurse Fellows, nursing ethics is now recognized as a field of inquiry within health care ethics that specifically explores the nursing role and ethical questions as they affect patient outcomes.... The benefit of Foundation funding to the Nurse Fellows... gave Fellows an opportunity to take time out from professional life to study, think, and undertake a specific project related to health care ethics. They learned from the "masters" in medical ethics at major academic institutions. Each Nurse Fellow described how the fellowship period focused their academic and professional career in relation to health care ethics.[114]

This is an unfortunate mischaracterization of Robb and the early nursing ethics. The report also misidentifies the pre-existing 100-year tradition of nursing ethics and places it within the then emergent bioethics. However, the report is correct in noting that the Kennedy nurse fellows did make a 20-year contribution to bioethics and were pivotal in its adoption into nursing and its ongoing development. While nurses recognize bioethics in nursing as "a field of inquiry within health care ethics," it is unclear that those outside nursing recognize it at all. The 1993 historical reflection supplement to the *Hasting's Center Report* contained 13 articles on the birth of bioethics written by six philosophers, two theologians, two historians, one sociologist, and one journalist. Women were underrepresented; nurses (and persons of color) were not represented in the mix. Indeed, one is hard pressed to find mention of nursing in any of the leading textbooks on bioethics. Where nurses are mentioned, it is customarily either in passing or in a single chapter written by a nurse.[115]

There was another vehicle that facilitated the movement of bioethics into nursing. The gift from the Foundation that underwrote the Kennedy Institute of Ethics (KIE) also supported its summer Intensive Course in Bioethics (ICB). Early nurse fellows situated at Georgetown attended the IBC as did some of us who took our fellowship at Harvard. The IBC, now in its 45th session, has become more clinically and less theoretically focused. It provides an intensive bioethics education to physicians, nurses, clergy/chaplains, dentists, and policy makers. At this point it has been offered to hundreds of health professionals, many from outside the US, thereby exporting US bioethics to other nations. The first years of the ICB were laden with ethics theory, specifically deontology and Kant, utilitarianism and John S. Mill, and principles of biomedicine. It was at that time in a small group setting, sessions were given by Tom Beauchamp, James Childress, LeRoy Walters, Edmund Pellegrino, Andre Hellegers, and others engaged with bioethics in its formative years. Today, there is little awareness that the Kennedy Foundation nurse fellowships, the inclusion of nurses in the ICB, and more specifically the involvement of Mrs. Shriver played a pivotal role in the development of nursing faculty to teach bioethics, the broader development of bioethics in nursing—and the retention of religious voices in bioethics.

Conclusion

Discussing data from the new Webb Space Telescope, Hanna Devlin, quoting astrophysicist Emma Chapman, writes:

Explaining the existence of such massive galaxies close to the dawn of time would require scientists to revisit either some basic rules of cosmology or the understanding of how the first galaxies were seeded from small clouds of stars and dust.[116]

Little has been remembered, or even known, about the dawn of nursing ethics and how its transition into bioethics was seeded. Eunice Shriver, not bioethics, was the true star whose gravitational pull attracted the very men who are credited with creating bioethics into a galaxy itself. Who knew that the woman at the heart of bioethics, who is not acknowledged as such, is the very person who stood with nursing and mandated its inclusion in bioethics. Nursing owes a debt of gratitude to Eunice Kennedy Shriver, of blessed memory.

Appendix IV: Legal Cases That Contributed to US Medico-Moral Law

This is a selection of legal cases that contributed in one way or another to US medico-moral law. Each of these cases played an important role in clarifying legal and moral questions in bioethics and in some cases made it clear that the courts were meant to address the law (or lack thereof) and that the courts were not the appropriate venue for specifically moral questions. Still, the law lagged behind the moral questions that arose in medical care, at times placing clinicians in legal limbo, if not jeopardy. These cases are readily available on the web, along with their media coverage. The full text of the US Supreme Court case decisions can be found at: http://www.law.cornell.edu/supct/supremes.htm

TABLE 6.2 Selected landmark legal cases in bioethics and their legal citations

1927	Buck v. Bell	274 U.S. 200 (1927); (No. 292) 143 Va. 310, affirmed.
1973	Roe v. Wade	410 U.S. 11; (No. 70-18) 314 F.Supp. 1217
1976	Karen Ann Quinlan	(70 N.J. 10, 355 A.2d 647 (NJ 1976))
1976	Tatiana Tarasoff	17 Cal. 3d 425, 551 P.2d 334, 131 Cal. Rptr. 14 (Cal. 1976)
1977	Joseph Saikewicz	373 Mass. 728
1980	Chad Green	1978 Mass. Adv. Sh. 2002, 379 N.E.2d 1053 (1978), reviewed and aff'd, 1979 Mass. Adv. Sh. 2124, 393 N.E.2d 836 (1979)
1981	Brother Fox	423 N.Y.2d 580 (N.Y. Sup. 6 Dec. 1979) also 454 U.S.858 (5 Oct. 1981)
1982	Baby Doe	re Infant Doe, No. GU8204-004A (Monroe County Cir. Ct., Apr. 12, 1982). See also: USCA Title 42, chapter 67, Sec 5106a
1983	Clarence Herbert	195 Cal.Rptr. 484, 491 (Cal. App.2 Dist. 1983)
1985	Claire Conroy	486 A.2d 1209, 1224, 1226 (N.J. 1985)
1986	Paul Brophy	N-4152 (Mass Sup Ct, Sept. 1986)
1986	William Bartling	209 Cal.Rptr. 220, 225–226 (Cal.App. 2 Dist. 1984) and Cal.Rptr. 229:360–367; 1986.
1986	Elizabeth Bouvia	179 Cal. App. 3d 1127; 225 Cal. Rptr. 297; 1986 Cal. App.
1987	Nancy Jobes	In re Jobes, 108 N.J. 394, 419, 529 A.2d 434 [N.J. 1987])
1990	Nancy Cruzan	497 U.S. 261 (1990) 497 U.S. 261
2004	Ewing	Ewing v. Northridge Hospital Medical Center (2004) 120 Cal. App. 4th 1289. See also: (2004) 120 Cal. App. 4th 807
2004	Terri Schiavo	SC FL No. SC04–925, Sept. 23, 2004

Notes

1 Shana Alexander. "They Decide Who Lives, Who Dies: Medical Miracle Puts Moral Burden on Small Committee," *Life* 53, no. 19 (Nov. 9, 1962): 102–125. Text available at: http://www.nephjc.com/news/godpanel (or at) https://books.google.com/books?id =qUoEAAAAMBAJ&lpg=PA102&as_pt=MAGAZINES&pg=PA102#v=onepage&q &f=false

2 Ibid., 106.

3 *Unetanah Tokef.* https://www.sefaria.org/Unetaneh_Tokef.1?lang=bi

4 Alexander, "Who Lives," 106.

5 Veatch, Robert, Allocating Health Resources Ethically: New Roles for Administrators and Clinicians, *Frontiers of Health Service Management*, 1991 Fall;8(1):3–29, 43–4. See also: Bell, Nora, "Triage in Medical Practice: An Unacceptable Model?," *Social Science and Medicine*, 1981 Dec;15F(4):151–6.

6 Center for Disease Control, Ethical Considerations for Decision Making Regarding Allocation of Mechanical Ventilators during a Severe Influenza Pandemic or Other Public Health Emergency. 1 July 2011. https://www.cdc.gov/about/advisory/pdf/VentDocument_Release.pdf

7 HIV drugs rationing criteria.

8 Criteria and solid organ transplants.

9 Robert Baker, "Review of Albert R. Jonsen, 'The New Medicine, the Old Ethics,'" *Medical History* 37, no. 1 (Dec. 1992): 112–113.

10 "Fact Sheet: Medicare End-stage Renal Disease (ESRD) Network Organization Program." https://www.cms.gov/Medicare/End-Stage-Renal-Disease/ESRDNetworkOrganizations/Downloads/ESRDNWBackgrounder-Jun12.pdf

11 B. Jennett and Fred Plum, "Persistent Vegetative State after Brain Damage: A Syndrome in Search of a Name," *Lancet* 1, no. 7753 (Apr. 1, 1972): 734–737. DOI: 10.1016/s0140–6736(72)90242-5. PMID: 4111204.

12 Pope Pius XII, *Address to an International Congress of Anesthesiologists* (Nov. 24, 1957). https://www.vatican.va/roman_curia/congregations/cfaith/documents/rc_con_cfaith_doc_20070801_nota-commento_en.html

13 Pope John Paul II, *Evangelium Vitae*, § 65. https://www.vatican.va/content/john-paul-ii/en/encyclicals/documents/hf_jp-ii_enc_25031995_evangelium-vitae.html

14 David Conn, "Hillsborough Inquests: Teenager 'Thrown' on Top of Man in Ambulance," *Guardian* (Oct. 16, 2015). https://www.theguardian.com/uk-news/2015/oct/16/hillsborough-inquests-teenager-thrown-on-top-of-man-in-ambulance

15 David Conn and Robyn Vinter, "Liverpool Fan's Death Ruled as 97th of Hillsborough Disaster," *Guardian* (July 28, 2021). https://www.theguardian.com/football/2021/jul/28/liverpool-fans-death-ruled-as-97th-victim-of-hillsborough-disaster

16 Sheila A.M. McLean, "Permanent Vegetative State and the Law," *Journal of Neurology, Neurosurgery & Psychiatry* 71 (2001): i26–i27. https://jnnp.bmj.com/content/71/suppl_1/i26

17 Owen Bowcott, "Court Decision Not Required in Life-Support Withdrawal Cases, Judge Rules," *Guardian* (2017). https://www.theguardian.com/lifeandstyle/2017/sep/20/right-to-die-court-decision-severe-illnesses-life-support

18 R.S. Duff and A.G. Campbell, "Moral and Ethical Dilemmas in the Special Care Nursery," *New England Journal of Medicine* 289, no. 17 (Oct. 25, 1973): 890–894.

19 Raymond S. Duff and A.G.M. Campbell, "Moral and Ethical Dilemmas in the Special-Care Nursery," *New England Journal of Medicine* 289, no. 17 (1973): 890–894. DOI: 10.1056/NEJM197310252891705

20 Ibid., 892.

21 Ibid., 891.

22 Michael White, "The End at the Beginning," *The Ochsner Journal* 11, no. 4 (2011): 309–316. https://www.proquest.com/scholarly-journals/end-at-beginning/docview/2157946829/se-2

23 Marcia Chambers, "Baby Doe: Hard Case for Parents and Courts," *The New York Times* (Jan. 8, 1984). https://timesmachine.nytimes.com/timesmachine/1984/01/08/153680. html?pageNumber=328

24 Nat Hentoff, "Whatever Happened to Baby Jane Doe?" *Washington Post* (Dec. 11, 1990). https://www.washingtonpost.com/archive/opinions/1990/12/11/whatever-happened-to-baby-jane-doe/29aef321-10d4-45a6-86c1-ced107248b20/

25 George J. Annas, "The Case of Baby Jane Doe: Child Abuse or Unlawful Federal Intervention?" *American Journal of Public Health* 74, no. 7 (July 1984): 727–729.

26 George F. Will, "The Killing Will Not Stop," *The Washington Post* (April 22, 1982). https://www.washingtonpost.com/archive/politics/1982/04/22/the-killing-will-not-stop/7e69c6b7-b3fd-401c-8344-9a7d24c994d2/

27 Robyn S. Shapiro and Richard Barthel, "Infant Care Review Committees: An Effective Approach to the Baby Doe Dilemma?" *Hastings Law Journal* 37, no. 5 (May 1986): 827–862. PMID: 11655857.

28 The Joseph P. Kennedy, Jr. Foundation, *Who Should Survive?* Publicly available at Indiana University Media Collections Online. https://media.dlib.indiana.edu/media_objects/m613nf22j

29 Fedir Razumenko, "The Genesis and Development of Research Ethics Committees in Canada, 1960–1978," *European Journal for the History of Medicine and Health* 78, no. 2 (2021): 330–352, DOI: 10.1163/26667711-bja10008

30 The National Commission for the Protection of Human Subjects of Biomedical and Behavioral Research, *The Belmont Report: Ethical Principles and Guidelines for the Protection of Human Subjects of Research.* (Washington, DC: US Department of Health and Human Services, April 18, 1979). https://www.hhs.gov/ohrp/regulations-and-policy/belmont-report/read-the-belmont-report/index.html

31 Margaret Moon, "The History and Role of Institutional Review Boards: A Useful Tension," *Virtual Mentor* 11, no. 4 (2009): 311–316. DOI: 10.1001/virtualmentor.2009.11.4. pfor1–0904.

32 Stanley J. Reiser, *Medicine and the Reign of Technology* (Cambridge, MA: Cambridge University Press, Feb. 27, 1978).

33 Ibid., 227, 230.

34 Paul Ramsey, *The Patient as Person: Explorations in Medical Ethics* (New Haven, CT: Yale University Press, 1970).

35 William F. May, *The Physician's Covenant: Images of the Healer in Medical Ethics* (Louisville, KY: Westminster/John Knox Press, 1983).

36 Alfred Korzybski, *Science and Sanity: An Introduction to Non-Aristotelian Systems and General Semantics* (United States: International Non-Aristotelian Library Publishing Company, 1933), 747–761.

37 Alan Watts, *Alan Watts – in the Academy: Essays and Lectures* (New York: State University of New York Press, 2017), 348.

38 Arthur L. Caplan, "Done Good," *Journal of Medical Ethics* 41 (2015): 25–27.

39 Sepharia: A Living Library of Torah Texts Online. *Shulchan Arukh Yoreh De'ah* 339, Chaim N. Denburg translation (Montreal, 1955). https://www.sefaria.org/Shulchan_Arukh%2C_Yoreh_De'ah.339?lang=bi&with=Halakhah&lang2=en

40 I am dodging the question of what constitutes religion, and religion as a Western construct, and using *religion* in the common understanding.

41 In centuries past, religious leaders were often both clergy and theologian. Today theologians are often but not necessarily clergy, and clergy tend not to be theologians. Bear in mind that in some traditions, persons may be drawn out of the life of a congregation, and designated clergy, and may not have any formal ministry or theological education.

42 Richard A. Posner, *Public Intellectuals: A Study of Decline, With a New Preface and Epilogue* (Cambridge, MA: Harvard University Press, 2003).

43 Nelson Wiseman, *The Public Intellectual in Canada* (Toronto: University of Toronto Press, 2013).

44 Michael C. Desch (ed.), *Public Intellectuals in the Global Arena: Professors or Pundits?* (Notre Dame, IN: University of Notre Dame Press, 2016).

45 Tom Nichols, *The Death of Expertise: The Campaign against Established Knowledge and Why it Matters* (New York: Oxford University Press, 2017).

46 Paul Ramsey, *The Patient as Person: Explorations in Medical Ethics* (New Haven, CT: Yale University Press, 1970).

47 Albert Jonsen, "The Birth of Bioethics: Who Is Paul Ramsey?" in Paul Ramsey, *The Patient as Person*, 2nd ed. (New Haven, CT: Yale University Press, 2001).

48 Paul Ramsey, *Basic Christian Ethics* (Louisville, KY: Westminster/John Knox Press, 1950).

49 John Rawls "Ramsey's 'Basic Christian Ethics'," Typescript for *Perspective: A Princeton Journal of Christian Opinion* (May 1951). Pusey Library. Harvard University, Cambridge, MA.

50 Max Stackhouse, "Civil Religion, Political Theology and Public Theology: What's the Difference?" *Political Theology* 5, no. 3 (2004): 275–293. DOI: 10.1558/poth.5.3.275.36715.

51 Max L. Stackhouse, "Public Theology and Ethical Judgment," *Theology Today* 54, no. 2 (1998): 165–179. DOI: 10.1177/004057369705400203.

52 Duncan B. Forrester, "The Scope of Public Theology," *Studies in Christian Ethics* 17, no. 2 (2004): 5–19. DOI: 10.1177/095394680401700209.

53 Sebastian Kim, *Theology in the Public Sphere: Public Theology as a Catalyst for Open Debate* (London: SCM Press, 2011).

54 Hak Joon Lee, "Public Theology," In Craig Hovey and Elizabeth Phillips (eds.), *The Cambridge Companion to Christian Political Theology* (Cambridge, UK: Cambridge University Press, 2015), 44–65. DOI: 10.1017/CCO9781107280823.004.

55 David Tracy, *The Analogical Imagination: Christian Theology and the Culture of Pluralism* (London: SCM Press, 1981).

56 Kim, *Theology in the Public Sphere*.

57 Robert Benne, *The Paradoxical Vision: A Public Theology for the Twenty-first Century* (Minneapolis, MN: Fortress Press, 1995).

58 E. Harold Breitenberg, Jr., "To Tell the Truth: Will the Real Public Theology Please Stand Up?" *Journal of the Society of Christian Ethics* 23, no. 2 (2003): 55–96.

59 Max L. Stackhouse, "Public Theology and Ethical Judgment," *Theology Today* 54, no. 2 (1998): 165–179. DOI: 10.1177/004057369705400203.

60 Katie Day and Sebastian Kim, "Introduction," In Sebastian Kim and Katie Day (eds.), *A Companion to Public Theology: Brill's Companions to Modern Theology* Vol. 1 (Leiden, Netherlands: Brill, 2017), 1–21. DOI: 10.1163/9789004336063.

61 Lawrence E. Sullivan. *Healing and Restoring: Health and Medicine in the World's Religious Traditions* (New York: Macmillan Publishing, 1989).

62 Ronald L. Numbers and Darrel Amundsen, *Caring and Curing: Health and Medicine in the Western Religious Traditions* (The Lutheran General Health Care System/Macmillan Publishing, 1986).

63 Prakash N. Desai. *Health and Medicine in the Hindu Tradition* (New York: Crossroads Publishing, 1989).

64 Daniel Callahan. "Religion and the Secularization of Bioethics," *The Hastings Center Report* 20, no. 4 (July/August 1990), S2.

65 Albert R. Jonsen, "Paul Ramsey, The Beecher Lectures, and the Birth of Bioethics," in Paul Ramsey, *The Patient as Person*, 2nd ed. (New Haven, CT: Yale University Press, 2002).

66 Courtney Campbell, "Religion and Moral Meaning in Bioethics," *The Hastings Center Report* 20, no. 4 (July/August 1990): S5.

67 Daniel Callahan, "Bioethics and the Culture Wars," *Cambridge Quarterly of Healthcare Ethics* 14, no. 4 (2005), 42431.
68 Callahan, "Religion and the Secularization of Bioethics," S3.
69 Campbell, "Religion and Moral Meaning," S9.
70 Daniel Callahan, "Religion and the Secularization of Bioethics," *The Hastings Center Report* 20, no. 4 (July/August 1990), 4.
71 M.D.M. Fowler, "Nursing and Social Ethics," In N.A. Chaska (ed.), *The Nursing Profession: Turning Points* (St. Louis: C.V. Mosby, 1989), 24–30.
72 M.L. Tina Stevens, *Bioethics in America: Origins and Cultural Politics* (Baltimore, MD: Johns Hopkins University Press, 2000).
73 Daniel Callahan, "Calling Scientific Ideology to Account," *Society* 33 (1996): 14–19. DOI: 10.1007/BF02700300
74 Stevens, *Bioethics*, 54.
75 Ibid., 152.
76 Ibid., 153.
77 Ibid., 156–157.
78 Wesley J. Smith, *Culture of Death: The Age of Do Harm Medicine* (New York: Encounter Books, 2016).
79 Albert R. Jonsen, "Beating Up Bioethics," *Hastings Center Report* 31 (2001): 40–45. DOI: 10.2307/3527703
80 Tod T. Chambers, "Retrodiction and the Histories of Bioethics," *Medical Humanities Review* 12, no. 1 (Spring 1998), 10–22.
81 Chambers, "Retrodiction," 19.
82 H. Tristram Engelhardt, *The Foundations of Bioethics*, 2nd ed. (New York: Oxford University Press, 1996).
83 Chambers, "Retrodiction," 16.
84 Ezekiel J. Emanuel, *The Ends of Human Life* (Boston: Harvard University Press, 1991).
85 Chambers, "Retrodiction," 17.
86 Pellegrino, Edmund D. and Thomasma David C., *The Virtues in Medical Practice*, New York: Oxford University Press, 1993.
87 Chambers, "Retrodiction," 18–19.
88 Ibid., 19.
89 Ibid., 20.
90 Yuval Steinitz, "Prediction Versus Retrodiction in Mill," *International Philosophical Quarterly* 34, no. 4 (December 1994): 481–483. DOI: 10.5840/ipq199434443
91 Meryl Gordon, "'Rosemary: The Hidden Kennedy Daughter,' by Kate Clifford Larson," *The New York Times* (Oct. 6, 2015). https://www.nytimes.com/2015/10/11/books/review/rosemary-the-hidden-kennedy-daughter-by-kate-clifford-larson.html
92 Ibid.
93 Mike Allen, "Eunice Kennedy Shriver," *Politico* (August 12, 2009). https://www.politico.com/story/2009/08/eunice-kennedy-shriver-1921–2009–026007
94 Special Olympics. https://www.specialolympics.org/about/history?locale=en
95 Special Olympics. https://www.specialolympics.org/about/history/out-of-the-shadows-events-leading-to-the-founding-of-special-olympics?locale=en
96 At the behest of Mrs. Shriver, I was a member for the Foundation's faculty chair selection group.
97 The Kennedy Institute of Ethics. https://kennedyinstitute.georgetown.edu/about/founding/
98 The Kennedy Institute of Ethics at 40: History (Oct. 28, 2011). https://kennedyinstitute.georgetown.edu/news-events/the-kennedy-institute-of-ethics-at-40-history/
99 Ibid.
100 *Choices on our Conscience: The Joseph P. Kennedy Jr. Foundation International Symposium on Human Rights, Retardation, and Research*, 1971. https://repository.library.georgetown.edu/handle/10822/1063021/browse?type=datecreated

101 Rosemary Donley and Mary Jean Flaherty, "Revisiting the American Nurses Associa-tion's First Position on Education for Nurses: A Comparative Analysis of the First and Second Position Statements on the Education of Nurses," *OJIN: The Online Journal of Issues in Nursing* 13, no. 2 (April 30, 2008). DOI: 10.3912/OJIN.Vol13No02PPT04

102 Stephen Toulmin, "How Medicine Saved the Life of Ethics," *Perspectives in Biology and Medicine* 25, no. 4 (Summer 1982), 736–750.

103 Toulmin, "How Medicine," 736.

104 Ibid.

105 Ibid., 749–750.

106 I have no data regarding the physician fellows, other than that there was only one ap-pointed the year I was a fellow. The fellowships significantly predate the creation of the internet, so there is no online data. Neither is there any history of these fellowships on their website. It appears that some years later other fellowships were created.

107 Fritz Jahr, "Bio-Ethik: Eine Umschau über die ethischen Beziehungen des Menschen zu Tier und Pflanze" *Kosmos: Handweiser für Naturfreunde* 24, no. 1 (1927): 2–4.

108 Hans-Martin Sass, "Bioethik – Bioethics," *Archiv Für Begriffsgeschichte* 56 (2014): 221–228. http://www.jstor.org/stable/24361919.

109 Lolas F. "Bioethics and Animal Research: A Personal Perspective and a Note on the Contribution of Fritz Jahr," *Biological Research* 41, no. 1 (2008): 119–123.

110 I regret that I never asked her why she had a special concern for nurses. However, her early work after earning a degree in sociology was with women and women's shelters. She was concerned about the situation of women in society and bioethics at that time was a white, male, upper-middle-class field. Mrs. Shriver actively sought the opinion of nurses in private and in committees.

111 Sara Fry, Katherine Collopy, and Mary Duffy, *The Kennedy Nurse Fellows in Medical and Nursing Ethics, 1976–1996: A Report of Their Professional Accomplishments and Contributions to Health Care Ethics*. Unpublished report for the Joseph P. Kennedy, Jr. Foundation (Feb. 10, 1996, 1–23). pp 7, 11.

112 Anne J. Davis and Mila A. Aroskar, *Ethical Dilemmas and Nursing Practice* (New York: Appleton-Century-Crofts, 1983).

113 Anne J. Davis, Marsha D. Fowler, and Mila A. Aroskar. *Ethical Dilemmas and Nursing Practice*, 5th ed. (New York: Pearson, 2009).

114 Fry, Collopy, Duffy, *Kennedy Nurse Fellows*, 13.

115 Based on an informal review of the leading 20 books on bioethics.

116 Hannah Devlin. "James Webb Telescope Detects Evidence of Ancient 'Universe Breaker' Galaxies," *Guardian*, Feb. 22, 2023. https://www.theguardian.com/science/2023/feb/22/universe-breakers-james-webb-telescope-detects-six-ancient-galaxies?utm_term=63f6f2d47f14d686e3069c1830e0a079&utm_campaign=GuardianTodayUK&utm_source=esp&utm_medium=Email&CMP=GTUK_email

7

NURSING ETHICS IN THE UNITED KINGDOM, 1888 TO THE 1960S (WITH A NOD TO CANADA)

Introduction

Early nursing leaders were visionary women. Individually, they were resolute, scary bright, erudite, politically savvy, indomitable in the face of resistance, intractable in the face of patriarchy; there *would* be nursing, a modern nursing, scientific, educated, and professional. Together, they became a formidable international alliance. Their bonds were individual and organizational as they came to create national associations, and the International Council of Nurses (ICN).

These early nursing leaders were faced with a shared need to establish, secure control of, and standardize nursing education in each of their countries; to create systems of mandatory testing, registration, and licensure; and to unify the profession under national and international representative bodies for effective social authority, power, and voice that would further the ends of both health and nursing. These leaders also established vehicles of national and international communication, for the dissemination of a broad range of information, through journals such as *The Nursing Record* (1888, UK), *The Nursing Times* (1905, UK), *The Trained Nurse and Hospital Review* (1886, US), and *The American Journal of Nursing* (1900, US), the *Pacific Coast Journal of Nursing* (1910, US), and the *Canadian Nurse* (1905, Canada). However, they understood that they could not effectively bring about the organization and advance of nursing unless they could achieve women's suffrage across and among the nations that they represented. Early nursing leaders collaborated in national and international women's suffrage movements as well as in the creation of nursing and the architecture that it would need to establish and sustain it. They worked together to create a consistency and uniformity of nursing education and practice within and among nations. With the International Council of Nurses (ICN) as a vehicle, approximately quadrennial ICN Congresses furthered their collaborative work, and were

DOI: 10.4324/9781003262107-8

held in the capitals of various nations to further facilitate national efforts at their highest levels, and potentially secure political or aristocratic patronage. The unity and close collaboration continued until World War I. Aeleah Soine writes about "the collaborative and interrelated nature of nursing reform prior to World War I," focusing on the contribution of German nurses in this collaboration. She writes that:

> German, American, and British nurses... organized national and international nursing associations to realize state registration as a stepping stone to other markers of professional recognition, such as collegiate education, full political citizenship, social welfare, and labor legislation. However, the consequent reliance of these strategies on nation-states as arbiters of citizenship and professional status undermined the shared ideological foundation of international and national nursing leaders. [Her] article contributes to a more multinational understanding of how these international nursing leaders transcended and were confined by the limits of their nation-states in the years leading up to World War I.[1]

Nursing leaders across Europe, Canada, the US, Anglophone nations, and others held a uniform ideology and shared values, and faced similar sociopolitical issues. However, as Soine points out, the requirements for establishing education, registration, and more in the separate nations frayed a degree of unity, while World War I disrupted their collaboration. However, prior to World War I, collaboration between US, UK, and Canadian and European nursing leaders was particularly dense with letters, face-to-face organizational meetings, shared ICN committee work, collaborations, and visits; nurse, matron, faculty, and superintendent exchanges, student exchanges, and more. Given the extensive collaboration among nursing leaders internationally, especially the US, UK, Canada, and Western Europe, it would not be unreasonable to hypothesize that US and UK nursing developed similarly in terms of the development of the profession's ethics.[2] That hypothesis generally holds, though not in relation to the nature of the codes of ethics and the production of nursing ethics textbooks. Here we will examine the early UK journals for ethics content, in an effort to identify and examine its enduring themes.

Sources for This Study[3]

This study entailed a paged physical review and content analysis of the earliest UK nursing journals, nursing textbooks, and nursing ethics books, dating from the 1880s. It was necessary to review these print materials page-by-page; most of this material is not digitalized and in those few instances where it is (*The Nursing Record/British Journal of Nursing*), changes in vocabulary and concepts make it unsearchable. The rhetorical style of the period and its vocabulary differs from that of today. The vocabulary for ethics and ethical concepts, especially, is different and variant, making it impossible to use a computerized word search to locate nursing ethics content.

The Nursing Record (*NR*), which became the *British Journal of Nursing* (*BJN*) in 1902, was published from 1888 to 1956. For the *NR/BJN*, 3,280 issues could be reviewed, which is approximately 91,000 pages that were examined individually. *The Nursing Times* (*NT*) began publication in 1905, of which approximately 4,250 issues (years 1905–1965, and for comparison 1966–1989) were physically examined page-by-page for this research; that is, approximately 126,000 pages were reviewed. As a part of the review, pages containing ethical content were photographed. Approximately 22,450 photos were taken.

Content was determined to be *ethical* if it principally focused on norms of value, both nonmoral values (*goods* and *ends*, i.e. "things" of value to be sought) and moral values (*virtues*, moral character), and ideals of the profession, norms of obligation (*duties*), or goods intrinsic to nursing.[4] Nonmoral values are *ends* to be sought such as health, dignity, and respect. While confusing, *nonmoral values* are "things" and not persons; only persons can be "moral," hence the term *nonmoral values* refers to things, and only *moral values* refers to persons. Moral values refer to norms such as compassion, courage, and patience, and are often referred to as *virtues* or *character* meaning, specifically *moral character* as opposed to personality. Content that was determined to be social-ethical in nature was so designated where it involved a measure of criticism of social structures, disparities, injustices, inequalities, prejudices and the like.

In addition to the early national journals, the early UK general nursing textbooks written by nurses were examined, as the first chapter of these works most often address nursing ethics, even while the remainder of the book's content is clinical. The few pre-1965 UK nursing-ethics-specific textbooks that are extant were read in their entirety.

Some of the nursing textbook publishers were multinational and so nursing ethics books published in the US, or UK, or Canada were also released simultaneously in other English-speaking countries. For example, W.B. Saunders was both a US and UK publisher of early nursing textbooks in the late 1800s and thereafter. Where there is firm evidence that an American nurse's textbook was used in the UK as well as in the US, or that she worked binationally, those authors (Dock, Goodnow) are included among the British works in the development of the themes below. Quotations within the themes below represent a general consensus view within the literature and are not idiosyncratic. They do, however, represent a specific group of nurses—educators, matrons, leaders, and writers who generated the editorials, standing columns, and many of the articles. However, "ordinary nurses" were represented as well; they wrote articles, opinion pieces, personal experiences, letters to the editor, and more.

First, a Plea for Forbearance...

I write what follows with a degree of foreboding. My ancestors may well have fired flintlock muskets at redcoats, even while some mined slate in Wales. I am not academically prepared as a historian; I am not British; I not Canadian. I am American, and I am acutely aware of American hegemony in many realms, including in nursing and in ethics. That hegemony extends to receiving gifted students from other nations and sending them home with an American nursing education and, later, an American bioethics unattenuated by the culture and nursing tradition of their home nations. I trust that the data in this chapter will prove useful to others, even if my interpretation may err (for which I beg the readers' forbearance).

Shared Content, Shared Leaders

Early nursing leaders had a prodigious written output in letters, articles, curricular standards, books, alumnae newsletters, and more. The degree of interchange and exchange between and among nursing leaders internationally is astonishing, even by today's standards. They shared freely—UK journals made regular use of articles, directly lifted (and credited) from the *American Journal of Nursing*, the *Pacific Coast Journal of Nursing*, and the *Trained Nurse and Hospital Review*. While the UK journals devote a considerable amount of attention to concerns for registration, title protection, educational standardization, and so forth, the content of concern in this chapter is that which is specifically ethical in nature. The paged journal review and content analysis indicates several large domains of ethical concern, each with sufficient, substantive, discrete data for its own research. From these domains I derive several, tentative ethical themes. It is recognized that there is some overlap of themes, and that they may circle back upon one another, or be recombined in other ways. As the nursing ethical literature today does not, as yet, address the UK nursing ethical tradition, these themes are proposed as a starting point for further research. At this point, the themes are more descriptive than analytical in order to provide an initial survey of the ethical content of this period literature; neither are they homogeneous. This is simply a starting point. These themes are my invitation to established scholars (and doctoral students) to advance this research, to analyze this literature in greater depth, with a range of critical apparatus, and with greater skill than is demonstrated here.

They Doth Diverge... Seemingly

Nursing ethics in the US and UK have much in common, but they also seem to diverge. The early nursing textbooks, meaning the general medical-surgical nursing textbooks of both nations frequently had a first chapter on the moral character and duties of the nurse; however, when it came to generating ethics textbooks per se, the US nursing leaders went bonkers, and the UK leaders were much more restrained, as were the Canadians. The American books, from Isabel Robb's onward, were reviewed favorably and commended for use in the UK journals, though I was unable to ascertain the extent of their use in the UK. The journals in both the UK and US contain ample and commensurate ethics content, though the UK journals were more consistently attentive to Parliament's machinations than the US journals were to those of Congress. This is, however, simply circling the barn without going in. We need to look at the ways in which the two literatures differed and to possible contributing factors.

Ethics *or not* Ethics

My colleagues in the UK tend to assert that UK nursing ethics has emphasized *character* and *conduct*, and that US nursing ethics has emphasized *ethics*, by which they mean the contemporary understanding of *bioethics*. While it is true that contemporary ethics in nursing takes the shape of *bioethics*, with a heavy reliance upon abstract, *a priori*, noncontextual, rationalistic ethical principles, nursing ethics prior to bioethics never has, and neither has the ANA *Code of Ethics*. One UK colleague proudly pointed out to me that UK nurses have a *code of conduct*, not a *code of ethics*; that is accurate as they serve different purposes, but it does not mean that the UK has neglected ethics. The emphasis on *conduct* is found in regulatory documents, while the moral literature emphasizes *character* and the *values*, *ideals*, and *moral duties* that propel nursing ethics. The most apparent difference between nursing ethics in the US and the UK is that early US nursing was influenced by the leading Pragmatist philosopher John Dewey, who had published a book on ethics.[5] US nursing educators drew from Dewey's ethics, and also utilized a range of philosophical works, such as prominent UK philosopher John Mackenzie's *A Manual of Ethics*[6] (see Chapter 1). These were employed as a skeleton; they then drew upon the nursing ethics literature to give flesh to the philosophical literature in the practice arena. The US approach to ethics is attached, in part, within the development of teacher education for nursing instructors in the early 1900s, and the alliance between nursing and universities in the US and later Canada. These or other philosophical influences are not discernable in the UK nursing ethics literature.

Philosophy, Educational Theory, and Nursing Education

Nursing in the US moved into colleges and universities in the 1960s, largely before that movement occurred in the UK. Up to the publication of the 1965 ANA statement on nursing education, calling for a baccalaureate degree as the point of entry into practice,[7] 80 percent of nursing education took place in hospital-based nursing schools with a strong emphasis on the apprenticeship component of education. After 1965, there was a precipitous decline in hospital-based diploma programs. There were a few university programs prior to 1965, such as the Yale University master's degree nursing program established in 1923. In Canada, the first baccalaureate nursing program was established at the University of British Columbia in 1919. However, nurse historian Lynn Kirkwood observes that in Canada, nursing leaders

> chose to "tread softly" and be satisfied with university education for a small group of nurses, ... creating a two-tiered system of entry into the profession and two cultures for nursing—the professional culture, rooted in education and science, and a craft culture, rooted in domestic skills.[8]

Canadian nursing faced the tensions of workforce demand against the need to increase nursing level of preparation. In her excellent article, Canadian nurse Ina Bramadat speaks to our entangled educational history:

> training schools developed more slowly in Canada, and during the early years, many Canadian women migrated to schools in the United States for their basic training. Later, this migration would continue for post-graduate education, then for master's and doctoral preparation. As a result, the development of Canadian nursing has closely paralleled, and has been strongly influenced by, nursing in the United States.[9]

Canadian nursing education diverged from that of the UK, the Nightingale model, and came to more closely resemble American nursing. In the UK, the University of Edinburgh had established a bachelor's degree nursing program in 1960 and a master's degree program in 1973. Then, in 2008, the Nursing and Midwifery Council determined that pre-registration nursing education should be a baccalaureate degree. Nursing education in the UK retained an apprenticeship focus for many years after the US and Canada had modified its apprenticeship components.

Bramadat speaks to what she terms the *professional model* of nursing education (as opposed to *Nightingale* or *apprenticeship models*). She writes that the professional model had an

> emphasis on uniform educational standards, formation of professional organizations, and registration and licensure of nurses, as a means of achieving autonomy and professional preparation of nurses. At the turn of the century, this was not so much a model for nurse training as a movement among certain nursing leaders to raise the standards of the existing hospital-based schools. This movement was spearheaded by a small group of nursing leaders through the professional organizations: the Society of Superintendents of Training Schools for Nursing, which was formed in 1893 by superintendents from Canada and the United States, and the Associated Alumnae of the United States and Canada, formed in 1897. The impact on nursing education was most evident in three areas: (1) the advanced training of superintendents and teachers, (2) the alliance of nursing and general education, and (3) the development and standardization of nursing curricula.[10]

As the leader of the Superintendents Society, Canadian-born Isabel Robb negotiated with Teachers College Columbia University (New York) to offer a postgraduate course of study to prepare superintendents for training schools in education (teaching), administration, and public health. American and Canadian nursing educators were formally prepared in administration, public health and epidemiology, philosophy, ethics, and educational theory. They were not "winging it" in curriculum development or teaching. Bramadat writes:

> This was the first nursing programme of its kind in the world. It initiated the movement of nursing into the educational mainstream and brought nursing educators into contact with some of the most influential leaders in general education of the day, such as Thorndike, Dewey, and MacMurray [sic].... Not only did it herald the beginning of a move to the educational mainstream, it also initiated a close alliance in North America between nursing and education. Faculty and students at Teachers College kept closely in touch with the leaders in general education. They were strongly influenced by contemporary educational theory and by the education model in which theory was taught in the class-room and practice followed in the clinical setting. By adopting the education model rather than the medical model of training, nursing fostered a split between theory and practice that is still a major source of divisiveness and concern among nurses. Parsons... argues that the alliance with education rather than with medicine also relegated nursing to a second-class rank in university circles.[11]

Edward Thorndike was a foundational psychologist and theorist of education. John Dewey, whom we have met previously, was a pragmatist philosopher, psychologist, and educational theorist. John Macmurray was a Scottish personalist philosopher, critical of rationalist, individualist, cognitivist approaches to philosophy—the "opposite" of contemporary bioethics. His work emphasized humans as persons-in-relationship, with agency. These three figures would, thus, influence the shape of nursing education, the theory–clinical division, Bramadat notes, and the shape of nursing ethics.[12]

There are several points to draw from this. First, Canada and the US have a closer affinity to one another than either has to the UK educational system. The persistence of an apprenticeship model in the UK would preserve nursing ethics in the apprenticeship-for-ethical-comportment and would preserve its emphasis on character. Second, the triumvirate of Thorndike, Dewey, and Macmurray would provide nursing ethics with philosophical content that was relationally sensitive, took account of community and society, was practice oriented, and was sensitive to nursing values, ideals, ends, and aims. Nursing in North America would alloy its ethics with philosophical traditions and educational theory that were harmonious with nursing's way of being in the world, its social concerns, its relational patient care, and its core values. This is to say that nursing in North America would retain its own ethical core yet supplement it with non-rationalist (even anti-rationalist) philosophy. This difference in educational systems and the incorporation of philosophy would account for the more frequent North American use of the term *ethics* over that of *virtue* or *character*, even though the content of North American nursing ethics was relational and character based, not ethics as rationalism.

But Not So Different After All

While US nursing ethics faculty read Kant, Mill, Aristotle, and others, and utilized Dewey, they (like Dewey) resisted rationalist ethics and philosophy. Even so, one will find that there is considerable overlap between the US and UK nursing ethics both in terms of values and topics, but also in relation to the formation of the nursing student into a nurse and nursing identity, with its attendant core values, and on the emphasis on character in that process. The values, ideals, and moral character attributes arose from within the shared (even internationally shared) tradition of nursing and its practice. Early US nursing had a strong clinical apprenticeship that has, over the decades, devolved into an emphasis on *techne* (rational calculation), overshadowing concern for moral character development. My sense is that this was not the case with UK nursing, but I am not certain. As we move to examine some of the ethical themes that I have identified from the UK journals and books, US nurses will nod at their familiarity—and that some of the individuals involved were themselves "shared."

Ethical Themes in Early Nursing Literature of the UK

NURSING AS A PROFESSION, VOCATION, CALLING, OR TRADE

Early nursing leaders intended to create nursing as a true profession, commensurate with other professions in rigor, standing, privileges, and remuneration. Simultaneously they continued to regard nursing as a calling, with the commitment, devotion, altruism, and other qualities associated with a calling. Nursing education was, admittedly, grueling but the conditions of nursing education were "the graving tools which fashion character, stamina, grit, endurance, patience and pluck" and, "if nursing is your vocation, get busy in learning all its arts and sciences."[13] Margaret Fox writes that:

> "Vocation" is a sense of "call," a single heart, the feeling that one *wants* to do the thing undertaken and that nothing else ever can be so congenial. A sense of vocation dignifies the work, magnifies the office; it gives strength, purpose, and the requisite feeling of "aloofness" so that one is less likely to be drawn aside from high endeavor. It deepens the sense of responsibility and sets the feet on sure ground... the spirit of vocation is not incompatible with the professional spirit... It is in perfect accord with a correct professional attitude at all times, and, united with it, magnetises the abilities and irradiates the faculties... Vocation deepens interest, vitalizes every effort, increases adaptability and usefulness, widens the sphere and ennobles life... To attempt to divorce the spirit of vocation from nursing means the plucking out of the very golden heart of the profession: it is cutting off the living root that nourishes the whole tree...[14]

Nursing leaders claimed the status of a *profession*, while recognizing a need to grow fully into being an educated and scientific profession, with full social, regulatory, and legal recognition. And yet, it also wanted nurses to have a sense of *calling* to nursing, specifically a personal and Christian calling, one that would sustain nurses, with honor and dignity, through thick and thin, and for better or for worse in terms of work conditions or environment. Nursing itself was not a calling; it is an individual who is called *to* nursing. The call resides within the individual, and not all who engage in nursing are necessarily called to do so. Some are called to nursing, and some are not, and some enter nursing, possibly for pecuniary reasons, without being called to it. However, the notion of a *calling*, or *vocation* (from the Latin, *vocare, to call*) carried the sense of unpaid service to God, which set up a tension between *profession* and *calling* that had to be navigated.

> Surely it does not matter whether we call nursing a profession, a calling, or a vocation. To me, it seems that in these days it is undoubtedly a profession, but one for which we should have a special vocation. The name is not worth quarreling over so long as the spirit is understood.[15]

This is not hard-and-fast but, in general, *profession* referred to the scientific aspects of theory and practice, *vocation* referred to the ways in which the moral character of the nurse was exemplified in patient care (e.g., kindness, compassion) and other relationships, and *calling* reflected a commitment to the values and ideals of the profession that enabled the nurse "whose mind is cheered by visions of the ideal [to] do the dull routine work best."[16] Nursing leaders retained and protected this uneasy tension. When they discovered that they did not have the political muscle to demand "a living wage" for their educated professionals called to nursing, they sought—against professional norms—to unionize, which then risked casting nursing as a *trade*. A concern about nursing as profession-versus-vocation is typified by Evelyn Pearce's words:

> Nursing, like medicine, is an honourable service and honour will always be accorded to those who follow it. Many take up nursing from altruistic motives: they have a great desire to help others, and it is their innate kindness which inspires the desire to train and become proficient in nursing. Some do it merely to earn a living: to them it is a career, but as nursing is essentially humanitarian, it is doubtful whether it can be as well done when it is taken up simply as a career than when it is inspired by a spiritual ideal.[17]

This is a late (1953) statement in the nursing ethics literature, but it is an ongoing concern in the literature to retain a caring, compassionate, loving, humanitarian nature to the art of nursing, even while nursing scientized and professionalized, and to have devoted practitioners for whom nursing is an inner identity and a calling.[18]

Early nursing was a balancing act between aspiration to recognition as a profession, with the ability to negotiate an adequate and just pay commensurate with education and skill, while retaining the commitment, character, and ideals that were inherent to a calling. The literature reflects a binary, either/or argument, which can be seen as either unresolved or as an enduring both/and tension that is and should be maintained.

Here, the pioneer UK psychologist, philosopher, and nursing educator Beatrice Edgell brings together nursing-as-vocation, character, moral courage, and clinical wisdom. She writes:

> Where there is vocation the nurse... will give of her best, and this best is something for which professional skill and knowledge is not enough. In the thoroughly trained nurse...we may take efficiency for granted. Character supplies that something more which makes the nurse or worker a power for good in the service to which she is devoted. If one looks at the list of excellences set forth by Plato and Aristotle one can recognize two virtues... required by the nurse.... These are courage and wisdom... what is intended here is the fixed habitude of moral courage.... The... nurse who is working outside the walls of the hospital is confronted with many situations that call for the greatest moral courage. She may have to tackle "difficult" people, she may have to track down and show up bold abuses. In much of her work, she may meet with resistance and will need both courage and patience to overcome opposition. With the cultivation of courage should go the cultivation of wisdom. Wisdom... is not knowledge, although it presupposes knowledge; it is rather ability to apply knowledge in the right way and at the right time... wisdom requires experience.... To size up a person or a situation, to realize what can or cannot be done, when it is useful and when it is useless to speak, demands judgment, and such judgment is based on much past experience... [nurses] need to be clear about general principles, to have ideals, a sense of the direction which they wish to go. If they have taken their general bearings well, they will be more able to judge correctly the significance of any particular episode.[19]

Edgell was the first UK woman to earn a PhD in psychology, and to become a professor of psychology, and the first woman president of the Aristotelian Society. She also held a degree in philosophy. Though not a nurse, she served as examiner in psychology for the Royal College of Nursing. Her textbook *Ethical Problems: An Introduction to Ethics for Hospital Nurses and Social Workers* (1929) was widely used by students in both nursing and social work. It is largely Aristotelian in perspective, meaning that it utilized Aristotle's virtue theory of ethics and its development in ethics. Aristotle's virtue theory emphasizes the kind of persons we are *to be* as a person of virtue, a nurse of virtue. For Aristotle's virtue theory, *being* is prior to *doing*; that is, *being good* is prior to *doing right*.[20]

THE IMPORTANCE OF MAINTAINING IDEALS IN NURSING PRACTICE AND EDUCATION

This is a minor but important theme that reiterates the notion that nursing is a profession and a "high calling." It is generally a thread that is incorporated into other articles, rather than being discussed as a separate topic. There is sufficient material to identify this either as a theme on its own, or as a sub-theme. This theme emphasizes the importance of ideals, and maintaining and reinforcing those ideals, and their role in practice, teaching, and student learning.[21] The discussion surrounding this theme is that of the tension between the ideals espoused by teachers and the profession, that then come into contact with the gritty reality of nursing practice, and the spartan or meager, and sometimes dire, conditions under which nurses lived and worked.[22,23,24] Recall that hospital nurses lived in a nursing residence (sometimes dormitory) within or adjacent to the hospital. This tension between the ideal and the real can be seen as an early precursor to today's discourse on moral distress.

"CLASSES OF RELATIONSHIPS" AND THEIR ETHICAL DUTIES

This theme is less a theme than a structural template that is not itself argued or discussed but is a constant. Early nursing ethics was based on a set of relationships that were reconfigured and recombined over the decades, but in the American literature included nurse-to-family, nurse-to-patient, nurse-to-physician, nurse-to-self, nurse-to-nurse, nurse-to-her school of nursing, nurse-to-nursing, and nurse-to-society.[25] While the UK literature itself has a relational structure, it also picks up the relational ethics found in the American literature and reprints it.[26] UK physician Humphrey Rolleston uses a relational template to examine the threefold duties of a nurse: (a) duties to the patient, (b) to the doctor, (c) the nurse's duties to herself.[27] Citing work at Johns Hopkins (US), an 1896 *Nursing Record* article notes the relationships in the Johns Hopkins work as (a) the duty of the nurse to physicians, (b) the duty of the nurse to the patient, (c) the duty of the nurse to her school, (d) the duty of nurses to each other, (e) the duty of the nurse to the public, (f) the duty of the physician to the nurse, and (g) the duty of the public to the nurse.[28] This specification is interesting in its deviation from other such specifications: it places the physician first, whereas all others put the patient first, and it includes the duties of the physician and society (public) to the nurse.

The moral duties and values of nurses were generated from within each of these relationships, as were the desired moral qualities (virtues) of the nurse. Virtues and values did not stand apart from relationships or practice but were enacted within them in accord with the demands of the fluctuating patient situation. The virtues, though taught in lecture classes (see Edgell above), were modeled, and formed in the apprenticeship element of education, in the clinical settings. This relational nexus of nursing ethics persists into the 1990s. In the late 1990s and 2000s, we begin to see a new literature, taken from American principle-based bioethics, surface in the UK journals and books.[29]

The first relationship that is specified is always nurse-to-family, sometimes nurse-to-patient (and in the home setting, nurse-to-family, friends, and servants). Early nursing, until after World War II, took place predominantly in the home so that nurses dealt with the individual only as a part of a family and were privy to the quiddities and goings-on of family life in the home. It is within the context of these relationships that ethical duties arise.

PROFESSIONAL SECRETS IN THE NURSE TO PATIENT RELATIONSHIP

The first relationship identified is always nurse-to-family and later (as nursing moved out of homes and into hospitals) nurse-to-patient. Nurses in the home were privy to all the machinations, misbehavior, idiosyncrasies, blessings, and hardships of the family's life. As a consequence, and commensurate with the ethical obligation of devotion (fidelity) to the patient, the literature reflects a duty of *professional secrets*.[30,31] By *professional* is meant the *nursing* profession, not medicine. The nurse had to decide what to tell or not tell the physician, so she made a judgment about information she acquired. Whatever the physician's interest, prurient or not, in non-medically relevant observations or knowledge obtained by the nurse, the nurse simply would not disclose this information. Another and related duty was that of not "talking out-of-school," to other nurses, friends of the patient's family, even some nosy relatives. In contemporary times, this came to be called *confidentiality*. However, confidentiality is significantly narrower in scope than is professional secrets, and *confidentiality* is generally *rights* or law based, not relationally based. At this point in its history, nursing generated its own and fulsome set of moral norms, based on these classes of relationships.

The obligation to professional secrecy takes an interesting turn in the literature. Because they were privy to household (and perhaps neighborhood) secrets, apparently the local constabulary attempted to employ nurses as detectives to secure those secrets for their investigations.

> The nurse enters the house of the patient in the guise of a friend, and at once assumes the most confidential and intimate relationships with both patient and household, relations, which are only possible, because she is a member of an honorable profession, and can be trusted not to abuse the confidence placed in her loyalty and discretion. We do not believe the nurse is to be found who would so prostitute her calling, as to play the part of confidential attendance and friend, while in reality making use of the exceptional facilities, which she enjoys to act as a detective in the interest of a criminal department. If she did so act, she would certainly lay herself open to the epithet that applied to the nurse-detective by the accused woman in the case under consideration, "Judas Iscariot."[32]

The norm of professional secrecy in the nurse–patient relationship was inviolable, even under color of law. Nurses were not to be detectives for the police; professional secrets were to be maintained and the "police must find other means of bringing criminals to justice."[33]

Probationers were exhorted to *sealed lips* and to *professional reticence* in speaking about patients and their affairs.

> Whatsoever knowledge you make of a patient's personal and private affairs, by reason of your attendance upon him, what's up where he or his friends may confide in you, should be sacred and inviolable. Knowledge thus gained is no more yours to be discussed with, or mentioned to other persons, than are his possessions

yours to take and spend or appropriate for your own use. You should not dream of stealing from a patient but remember that most patients would rather you should do this than that you should be so dishonorable as to gossip about their private affairs.[34]

"CONDUCT IS THE OUTCOME OF CHARACTER": VIRTUE ETHICS

Early nursing ethics, up until the rise of bioethics in the mid-1960s in the US (later in the UK), emphasized the moral character of the nurse. This was a *virtue ethics* emphasis, though alternative terms of *character, qualities, personality, tempera-ment*, and *attributes* were used, though *character* was the most common. The term *character ethics* would be more faithful to this literature's terminology. Nursing leaders and educators were concerned to recruit women of the right character, preferably educated women of the right character, though recruiting educated women to nursing, early on, was a slog. Once recruited, in the process of nurs-ing education instructors would work toward the formation of a nursing identity and the interiorization of nursing values, ideals, and duties in probationers and nurses (students). This involved classroom education and clinical apprenticeship (and tutor modeling). It was furthered and reinforced through the various relation-ships that were a part of nursing, but especially the nurse-to-patient relationship.[35] Within the clinical apprenticeship portion of nursing education, the moral quali-ties of the classroom teaching were brought to life and enacted within the several "classes" of relationship. These moral qualities included patience, compassion, honor, moral courage, and devotion. *Moral courage* was specifically termed as such. These were attributes that were to be *habituated* (internalized and formed through habit) so that they would emerge within the various relationships, within the practice setting, as the occasion demanded. That is to say that they were an-chored in the expectations of the community of practicing nurses to manifest in clinical practice, and its immediate, fluctuating context. It was understood that moral character was essential to the acceptance and guidance of the moral val-ues and ideals of nursing and to right conduct. E. Margaret Fox (1914) elegantly writes:

> In many relationships in life people are inclined to take themselves too seri-ously; with regard to the profession of nursing you can hardly do so... In no other field of work, save that of medicine, are you brought into a succession of close and delicate intimacies with others. You are admitted where the patient's nearest and dearest relatives are excluded. You are told what is never breathed even in confidence to wife, mother, or son; your hasty, lightly-expressed opinion may depress or exalt some yearning spirit in a manner out of all proportion to your knowledge or experience. It is also true that what seems to you a trifling error may prove a fatal mistake, dragging after it a never-ending train of tragic consequences. Is it not, then, important that you should at once begin to realise

the responsibilities you have taken upon yourselves in becoming nurses? This sense of responsibility should influence all you say and do, for your words and actions will show what you are.

Therefore, as conduct is the outcome of character, so character is more important in a nurse than mere cleverness. How necessary it is then, that such attributes as reverence, gentleness, discretion, and uprightness should enter into every nurse's character, and be continually cultivated by the earnest practice of good habits and patient continuance of well-doing.[36]

There is no one, definitive, list of the virtues to be desired in nurses though most lists greatly overlap with one another and include tact, courtesy, honor, moral courage, devotion (to the patient), loyalty (to one's school and hospital), selflessness, kindness, punctuality (in patient care, e.g., medications), honor, discipline, and sympathy. The lists compiled by those in nursing ethics differed from the less well-informed lists of some instructors, which tended toward socially conditioned *womanly virtues*. Such lists present two problems that subject them to significant misinterpretation. First, words in English can undergo a sense evolution in which their denotation changes over time. For example (as noted previously), the adjective *naughty* originally referred to persons who had *naught*; that is, persons who were poor or needy, not to someone wicked.[37] In terms of these lists of desirable moral attributes of the nurse, *sympathy*, in these lists, is closer to today's *empathy*.[38] A second problem is that the lists are extracted from the historical contexts that shaped their meaning for nurses. For example, the characteristics of *discipline*, which included *obedience, neatness*, and *punctuality*. Discipline and obedience make today's nurses bristle and connote patriarchy, hierarchy, subordination, and subservience. Neatness seems frivolous or silly. However, understanding that early modern nursing adopted a modified military structure within hospitals conditions the meaning of these attributes. The discipline and obedience were understood in *military* terms where one stood for a superior officer; was obedient in following orders, yet not blindly, not compliant with unlawful orders. Neatness, also patterned after military dress code. Of neatness, Minnie Goodnow[39] writes that "the nurse must make her personal appearance the subject of extreme care. Every moment of her time on duty she is on dress parade."[40] Neatness, then, also represents an element of the quasi-military ethos of the hospital, not a womanly notion of femininity, perfection, or cleanliness. *Punctuality* referred to the delivery of medications and treatments on time, and only rarely to start-of-shift tardiness. Nurses of that day would have understood what we might today misinterpret. Miss Mollett is the first to expound systematically on specific virtues, at length in the UK nursing literature.

Collaterally, brief mention should be made of the tension that existed between nursing and medicine that may (or may not) have affected the individual nurse–physician relationship (loyalty, obedience): medicine's resistance to and attempts to hamstring the advance of nursing education, from the later 1800s and for over a century thereafter. A 1957 editorial in *The Nursing Times* cites a series of *Lancet* articles from the 1850s:

> In 1857 Mr. J.F. South resisted Miss Nightingale's endeavors to introduce training for nurses holding the opinion that all was well in the nursing world and that "as regards the nurses and ward maids... these require little teaching beyond poultice making". In the *Lancet* (December 15), Dr. Ritchie Russel writes "it would be advantageous in the national interest to downgrade the level of training of the State-registered nurse and to make the assistant nurse become the national standard."[41]

One physician proposes "a new *Lancet* Commission to allow the medical profession to redefine the kind of nurse this country requires."[42] In rebuttal, the editorial responds:

> Referring to the kind of nurse the country requires would the doctors not agree with the statement made by the World Health Organization working conference on Nursing Education, that the kind of nurse needed in all parts of the world is "one who is prepared, through general and professional education, to share as a member of the health team in the care of the sick, the prevention of disease and the promotion of health? This is a very much wider definition than that of the Nurses Act of 1949, which states that "a nurse means a nurse for the sick and nursing shall be construed accordingly."... this does not mean that the nurse should be the person 'the doctor wants' but the person the patient and the medical profession need to ensure success of the work of the team in helping that patient retain or regain his health.[43]

Throughout the journal literature there are indications that between nursing and medicine, the attribute of *loyalty* was not a two-way street.

Virtues—Miss Mollett's Six Necessary Nursing Characteristics

Virtues are what makes a *good* nurse, *good* in a moral sense, but also good in a clinical sense as the two are fused. So, what makes for a good nurse? In 1888, Miss Mollett (1882–1885 certificate from Barts and subsequently Matron, Chelsea Infirmary) identifies six necessary (and interdependent) nursing characteristics: honor, purity, courage, discipline, culture, and love, though later *sympathy*[44] is substituted for *love*. She wrote a series of articles for *The Nursing Record*, one on each virtue.

Honor

She begins with honor, a characteristic that combines integrity, truthfulness, and rectitude (which is morally sound behavior or thinking). Describing *honor*, Mollett writes:

> Nursing is the woman's share of medical work, and it is a profession that no one who has not the keenest sense of honour should ever undertake. A nurse's honour

consists essentially in always acting with entire truthfulness and rectitude, at all times to do the best work of which she is capable, to bring to bear upon that work in all its details her best energies, her highest faculties and fullest powers; so alone will she be worthy of the responsibility that rests in her hands.[45]

Honor is in effect irrespective of the burden of work conditions.

Purity

Purity entails performing duties decently and in order, without any impropriety, being an influence for good, and shunning all coarseness, including coarse levity. It also includes a perspective that threads throughout the early nursing ethics and general literature:

> It has been said "there is one great and dangerous peculiarity of nursing, espe-cially of hospital nursing, mainly that it is the only case, queens not excepted, where a woman is really in charge of men;" but that "great peculiarity" ceases to be "dangerous" if a high-minded woman unite the boundless tact, courage, and patience necessary to restrain male patients to a perfect and stainless purity in every thought, word, and deed."[46]

Throughout the nursing ethical literature, nurses are at risk when in contact with men both as patients, but more especially as physicians and internes. Though a bit abstruse, Mollett is here referring to the potential for *sexual harassment* by male patients (and physicians) or what today are termed *boundary violations*. For Mollett, purity was subject to a slippery slope. If the nurse lets her cleanliness slide, or begins to use opiates or stimulants, all could be lost in short order. Mollett sum-marizes purity in this way:

> Living away from the protection of her home, a nurse... is still mainly depend-ent on her own strength and character, on the thoroughness of her own self-discipline, for the power to resist self-indulgence and laxity of moral courage. Conscious of the immense influence for good or evil her example must have on those entrusted to her care, a nurse's life should not only be truly blameless in thought, word, and deed, but, in its singleness of purpose, above even the suspi-cion of evil; she should avoid even the semblance of frivolity or a flippant dis-regard for perfect purity; and it is in the sustaining power, the refining influence of that utter purity that she will find her most perfect safeguard against many of those temptations, difficulties and trials that must beset her path.[47]

Courage

Courage is "the backbone of honour and purity," and the last of the three absolutely essential characteristics (virtues) of the nurse. Courage enables the nurse to "carry into practice unflinchingly those principles she knows to be right."[48] Its absence renders honor and purity of no effect. Courage is essential for nurses

> to live the higher, purer life as well as dream it, to do the good they feel to be right, and to abstain from the evil they know to be wrong; not to be afraid of telling a lie, but with higher courage and without fear to choose to be truthful, to dare to take their stand on what they know and feel to be the right ground, and having chosen, to stand firm.[49]

She notes that courage and other qualities should be supplemented "with that essentially English quality of 'pluck.'" *Pluck* appears throughout this literature, often paired as *pluck and determination*. Part of what is interesting about her discussion of courage is that she specifically identifies courage as *moral courage,* which finds its way into contemporary nursing ethics as if it were a new concept. Mollett sees courage as an essential part of the practice environment. She writes that "no quality is more communicable than courage, and the sister infuses some of her own courage into her nurses by showing them what to do, and where their fear can be attacked."[50] Courage is physical as well as moral as nurses risk exposure to dread diseases, conditions of squalor, and sexual harassment.

Incidentally, courage as *moral courage* appears in both the UK and US literature. American nurse educator Charlotte Aikens, in *Studies in Ethics for Nurses* (1923), uses the terms *courage* and *backbone*. She writes that executive ability in the nurse requires "these two striking and important traits of character—moral courage and self-reliance. These two might be combined in the well-understood quality known as back-bone."[51]

Three More Characteristics

Honor, *purity*, and *courage* are essential. Mollett identifies three additional necessary, but not absolutely essential, characteristics: *discipline*, *culture*, and *love*. These three qualities are

> rare qualities and highly prized—most highly in nursing; but they are not essential. A nurse may faithfully and truly fulfill her life's work, though not a loving woman; but she can never do so if she be dishonourable, impure, or cowardly."[52]

Discipline

At every level, *discipline*, Mollett maintains, is essential to the well-working of the hospital. And yet, "discipline should never retain the form without the spirit. True living discipline is founded on loyalty; the obedience to a discipline that has its root in fear and not in loyalty is dead and mechanical, not alive."[53] She defines *true discipline* as "the obedience loyally given to rules and laws that have been voluntarily accepted."[54] There is an element, then, of free will and self-determination in accepting the organizational discipline; that is, its rules and structures as part of life in nursing service. She regards discipline as among the rarest of virtues: "Cheerful obedience to discipline, the idea of accepting restraint in any spirit but a hostile one, loyalty to superiors, faithful submission to subordination are the very rarest virtues among them." Such discipline is, however, dependent upon self-discipline. Neither institutional discipline, nor self-discipline, were to extend to the suppression of individuality or personal moral or intellectual growth. Both forms of discipline invite and support loyalty, freely given—including loyalty to one's nursing school.

Culture

Culture would seem an odd virtue, but ought not to be understood as it might be used today. By *culture*, Mollett does not mean tea and dainty biscuits. By *culture*, she means "performing one's work as a skilled artist who loves his creations."[55] Culture combines devotion to one's nursing work, a broadly educated mind, and equalitarian treatment of patients. She writes:

> But while her work should be her chief aim and interest in life, a trained sick nurse, to be able to enter fully into it, should have the breadth of understanding, freedom from prejudice, and refinement of manner that spring from a cultured mind—a mind that has had a liberal and not a narrower education, largely gained by contact with educated men and women, and a refined home training, for she is brought into connection with people of every class and train of thought, whom it is her duty to understand, to be able to sympathise with, and whose various peculiarities she must therefore be able to appreciate, if she is to be equally in touch with the lowest of her patients, and the most highly trained and scientifically educated medical men.[56]

Sympathy

Mollett's final "necessary characteristic" is changed from *love* to *sympathy*, for which she gives no explanation. Her understanding of *sympathy* is closer to what today would be called *empathy*, a word not yet in use in her day. Mollett writes in 1888; *empathy* does not appear in English usage until 1903.[57] She states that "sympathy should be *with*, not *for* its object," by putting yourself in the other person's place, viewing her or his situation from their viewpoint rather than your own.[58] She notes, however, that in the absence of genuine sympathy there should be no pretense to it and instead a demonstration of kindness, courtesy, and consideration—and never condemnation or denigration. She does link sympathy to love, originally one of her six virtues:

> The root of all the highest and truest sympathy, is pure love, the noblest of all human qualities, and yet hardly to be ranked as one. For the true and honest

love of humanity, in its highest sense, is as a vast reservoir, from which all the streams of compassion, sympathy, and kindness to others are fed.[59]

Oddly, but very interestingly, Mollett concludes her series on the virtues necessary to nurses with these words: *homo sum, humani nil a mihi alienum puto* (I am a man, no man is alien to me).[60]

Though couched in a late 1800s language, Mollett's attributes of honor, purity, courage, discipline, culture, and sympathy encompass a remarkable range of contemporary attributes. In sum, they include: truthfulness, rectitude, integrity, doing one's work decently and in order, avoiding impropriety, being a force for good, maintaining self-discipline and shunning personal laxity, unflinchingly standing firm on what one knows to be morally right, exercising moral pluck, observance of institutional rules and standards and the exercise of self-discipline in ways that (both) affirm individuality and personal moral and intellectual growth; loving one's nursing work, being liberally (that is broadly) educated, embracing an equalitarian respect for all regardless of social station or economic status; genuine compassion, empathy, kindness; and a love for humanity. This is a remarkable list of necessary and essential virtues or moral attributes that really are as important today as they were 130 years ago when Miss Mollett wrote of them. These are not the *womanly virtues* but rather the virtues that we want of the nurse who cares for our wealthy uncles, our dissolute and drug-addicted prodigal sons, our poor and frail pensioner aunt Violet, and all those we love and worry about—and all those in society in need of nursing whom we have yet to serve.

The understanding of virtue in this period rests on an Aristotelian virtue theory where virtues are habituated, interiorized through practice, reflection, and habit. They would be attributes of the person's character, something that the person was as a person. More contemporary virtue theory does not see virtue as something of a possession, but understands virtue more dynamically. Virtue today is seen as embedded within the tradition and narrative of communities of practice; that is, the tradition and narrative and practice of nursing itself generates norms of moral value, virtue that is then internalized as one becomes and practices as a nurse. There are things that a nurse ought not do, *because* she or he is a nurse; there are things that a nurse ought to do because she or he is a nurse—it is in the DNA of nursing itself and commonly held within the value structure of the tradition. These virtues emerge in changing situations as the occasion arises but are given boundaries and direction by the community narrative and tradition. (See Chapter 9 for a fuller discussion.)

Etiquette *or* Ethics?

A word needs to be said about etiquette. There are a number of early publications, in both nursing and medicine, titled either *Ethics and Etiquette* or *Manners and Morals*, that covered the same ground. The two, ethics and etiquette, were seen as inextricably linked in that etiquette was the outward expression of one's ethics. This early nursing ethics must not be wrongly dismissed as "primarily feminine etiquette,"[61] or sentiment, or class-driven behavior. To do so is to misunderstand both this literature and etiquette.[62]

Etiquette refers to the canons of behavior, such as courtesy, civility, and tact, that would allow diplomacy, negotiation, and relationships to proceed with a common relational understanding, where participants know what to expect of one another. Courtesy, civility, and tact were three bi-directional attributes expected of the student, sister, matron, and physician that formed the interstices of relationships and communication, and even allowed for disagreement to be resolved. The etymology of *etiquette* notwithstanding, there were some less qualified authors simply looking for a paragon of Victorian womanhood and manners. *The Nursing Times* provides an amusing statement of the expected attributes of a morally good nurse:

> **Recipe for making a good nurse**: Mix together equal parts of pluck and good health with well balanced sympathy, stiffen with energy and soften with the milk of human kindness. Use a first-class training school as a mixer. Add the sweetness of a smile, a little ginger, and generous amounts of tact, humor and unselfishness, with plenty of patience; pour into the mouth of womanhood, time with enthusiasm, finish with a cap and garnish with ambition. The sauce of experience is always an improvement to this recipe, which, if followed closely, should be very successful and exceedingly popular.[63,64]

Almost as much as lemon-drizzle cake, this recipe was well liked: it appeared in *The Nursing Times* (1931), *The British Journal of Nursing* (1930), *The Canadian Nurse* (1921), and *The Pacific Coast Journal of Nursing* (1919); in the records of the London Hospital, Whitechapel; in numerous training school yearbooks, and elsewhere. The earliest use seems (so far) to be the *Pacific Coast Journal of Nursing* in 1919, which credits it to the Buffalo [NY] General Hospital Alumnae Record. There were other such recipes, sometimes set in verse, but of the same sentiment.[65] In the 1980s, and thereafter, it is picked up by feminist nursing literature[66] and nursing historians for opprobrium rather than approbation.

Discussions of *the good nurse* were always discussions of the *morally* good nurse that contained a prior assumption of knowledge, skill, and wisdom; that is, clinical expertise. *Good nursing* was always technically, scientifically, and morally good nursing, inseparably. The attributes of moral character were often linked to the nurse's duties to self; indeed, Fox's chapter is titled "The Ethics of Nursing and the Care of the Nurse's Own Health."[67]

Nursing's sequestered education and living situation, and ethos, resulted in a perpetuation of character ethics beyond the time society had begun its shift to a duties-based morality. Initially, it looked like nursing simply caught up in the 1970s and 1980s. However, there is a transitional element that helps to propel and facilitate the change. In the later 1950s, the nursing schools were experiencing a high rate of *wastage*; that is, student attrition. Wastage could also refer to sister tutors, or graduate nurses. The chief causes of student wastage, approximately one-third of all students (32 percent) were: theoretical inability (50 percent); home troubles (25 percent); marriage (12.5 percent); and misbehavior (12.5 percent).[68] There was wrangling over whether wastage of students was due to the quality of the student, the residential conditions, oppression by the nurse overseeing the residence, or the structure of the education. Various approaches were taken to resolve issues in each of these. However, great attention was given to how students were recruited and what *ability* and *psychological temperament* (i.e., intellect and personality) were needed for success in retention to graduation.[69,70] There is, in this period (1940s through the 1960s), considerable communication between US and UK educators and leaders, particularly on testing applicants for nurses' training.

Personality *or* Moral Character/Virtue?

In order to halt the wastage of nursing students, in both the UK and US, psychologists conducted studies on nursing students and identified a set of psychological and intellectual attributes—independent of moral character—that correlated with those students who would remain for the full course of education. Nursing schools began employing a range of psychological tests that culled prospective students who did not possess the requisite attributes. Note that these psychological qualities were independent of the nursing community ethos; that is, not derived from nursing community, tradition, values, or practice.[71,72,73,74,75] Questions arose about exactly who was choosing new students—psychological tests or nursing educators, and how that fit with nursing values. I had originally thought the psychological testing approach facilitated nursing's transition into the ambient social ethos that had relinquished virtue ethics in favor of a duty-based ethics, but I now believe that to have been in error. As late as 1962, Hillary Way, in *Ethics for Nurses*, retains a relational structure to ethics with a strong virtue element.[76] Her work is divided into sections: sense of duty, duty to ourselves, the nurse's virtues, duty to others, authority and discipline, and unwritten laws of nursing. It is not a strong work, and contains a hodge-podge of topics, but it does continue the ethical tradition of relationships, virtue, discipline, duty, and relationships.

DUTIES TO SELF

Throughout the early nursing literature nurses were enjoined—commanded—to care for themselves. *Duty* (or *duties) to self*, as it was termed, was an extensive, aggregate duty that included maintaining and promoting one's own physical, mental, and spiritual well-being. Specifically, it included the basics of sleep, nutrition, keeping warm, exercise, recreation, and ongoing learning. However, the recommendations in this domain were extensive and address every aspect of the nurse's life and world. Entire articles are devoted to recommendations for reading for pleasure and for learning. Columns are devoted to reading recommendations for both medical and nursing books as well as health books for patients who might need nursing attention (e.g., mothercraft books). Articles and columns cover economical places and ways to travel for holidays,[77,78] the joys of a tent holiday,[79] how to watch an eclipse,[80] a 12-part series on table tennis, patterns for sewing and knitting, recipes for all occasions including Shrove Tuesday pancakes,[81] recipes for "Tasty Tid-bits and Dishes Dainty for Invalids and Convalescents," including *consommé aux choufleurs*, lobster pudding with anchovy sauce, and *marrons à la vanille*;[82] recommendations for how to set up a home in one's lodgings, how to purchase furniture for a reasonable price, how to engage in birdwatching from the hospital windows,[83] how and when to retire; information on a range of sciences such as geology, astronomy, the movement of glaciers,[84] the birth of a cuckoo,[85] how bees make honey,[86] or wax, or swarm;[87] and whether there is life on other planets;[88] local wildflowers in bloom; how to enjoy or write poetry,[89] how to act in a drama or skit, how to speak in public; recommendations for spiritual development, a range of legal advice (e.g., rental contracts), and much more. There were crossword puzzles, bits of poetry, humorous anecdotes, and nurse-written poems. Recommendations were given for plays to see, museums and exhibits to visit, and places to go trekking, and how to take a bicycle trip around Norway. All of this was not simply for the nurse's well-being, but for her enjoyment of life and understanding of the natural world around her.[90] For decades, the journals themselves sponsored multiple competitions including lawn tennis,[91] table tennis,[92] needlework competitions,[93] fancy-work competition,[94] essay contests on a range of nursing and non-nursing topics, first person stories, and more.[95]

It is worth one's time to spend a few feel-good hours with the dust mites of these old journals. An extraordinary amount of journal space in every issue is given to fostering the well-being of the nurse, for the nurse's own sake. It was recognized that a nurse's health and well-being also benefit the patient and employer, but the emphasis of this literature is upon the nurse for the nurse's own sake. This literature promotes a very broad, liberal education; world awareness, political awareness, knowledge of the physical world, well spent leisure and recreation, broad reading; ongoing learning about the natural and social world around the nurse, ongoing learning in nursing; maintaining sound friendships and social relations within nursing; the health of the nurse, including rest, recreation, nutrition, hygiene, foot care, going to plays and concerts, clothing, travel, hobbies, and sports; financial, housing, and legal advice; and much more. This is an extensive, resolutely positive, helpful, and charming literature that cares for the nurse as a whole person.

"INTERNATIONALISM AND THE ONENESS OF THE NURSING SISTERHOOD"[96]

Perhaps *oneness* is a stretch, but certainly a degree of *unity* and *common cause* is accurate. Nursing leaders had shared concerns across national boundaries that ensured a degree of cooperation and mutual support for issues of the social location of women (e.g., suffrage and enfranchisement, education, employment), the health of the public broadly conceived (e.g., poverty, urban squalor, child labor), specific forms of contagion (e.g., venereal diseases, tuberculosis), and the work conditions and wages of nurses. This theme calls all nurses to have a broad interest in women and nursing worldwide. Minnie Goodnow (1938) writes:

> The nurse should be able to trace the fact that her profession is a part of the whole "woman" movement, of the struggle of women down through the ages to free themselves from the domination of men and to take their places in the world as individuals, with the liberty and responsibility which that involves. The progress of nursing has gone hand in hand with this struggle; and it is in the countries where women are freest to live their own lives that it has made its greatest successes. It is important also, in these days when all questions are becoming international ones, that nurses should know what is taking place on the other side of the world.[97]
>
> The woman movement is not yet complete... there are enormous numbers of women still untouched by it. It involves problems of early marriage versus late—which usually means education or lack of it; and of marriage versus career, a still more fundamental question. Another huge world-problem is nationalism versus responsibility for other nations... shall we, can we live in splendid isolation and develop ourselves and our own country? Or must we perforce accept the responsibility of seeing that the countries of the world progress more or less together? Nurses... easily see their duty to community, to their nation. Can they, through education through travel, through contacts of any sort, come to see their duty to other nations? Nursing history answers that they have. For many years they have gone out to the ends of the earth to help other countries develop good nursing... the world lies before nurses... shall we prepare for the challenge of humanity and then go to its help?[98]

In a list of facts that "trained nurses should note and remember," the second is "The Internationalism of Nursing":

> That there is no nationality in Nursing. That the preservation of Health, and comfort in sickness, is the Nurse's Duty. Hence, her sphere is worldwide, and her colleagues the nurses of all nations. It follows that her sympathies must be universal. To foster this depth of feeling, and breadth of views, the International Council of Nurses was founded in 1899... [it] meets in Conference and intimate social intercourse once in three years.[99]

The thread of "Internationalism" (for some reason, often capitalized) persists into at least the 1960s. In 1961, Irish nurse Mona Grey writes of the "healthy infection" of internationalism among nurses. "It is a healthy infection since it both cures and prevents isolationism, insularity, and ignorance... In nursing and health affairs we are not 'foreigners' but 'internationals'—as citizens of the world of nursing we have a right to the enjoyment of the healthy infection of internationalism."[100] By 1962, there is a new twist to Internationalism as a concern arises for the standardization of nursing education, role terminology and more, as the UK moves to join the European Union.[101,102]

As with the issue of unity in the early 1900s, it began to loosen as different nations regulated nurses and nursing education differently so that common approaches no longer held. By the 1960s, the considerably disparate development of nursing, and significant differences in the social location of women across nations, as well as differences in national economies, made and still make international unity of nurses difficult, the ICN notwithstanding.[103] It tends to be forgotten that while there is little uniformity in nursing across nations, there can still be unity. A 1961 *Nursing Times* editorial notes that "Unity is fairly easily achieved in terms of agreement on abstract ideals. Uniformity is far less easy to reach... the problems of nursing could only be solved by each national nursing association working within its own culture."[104]

While UK nurses are prodded to international engagement, there were levels at which this was expected. At the very least foreign travel and reading were encouraged. While some of that travel was for holiday purposes, it was often a "busman's holiday" that entailed visits to hospitals, nursing schools, and nurses in other countries. There are first-person journal articles from nurses reporting on nursing or hospitals in Europe, South America, Africa, North America, and in obscure corners of the world, as well as in some countries that no longer exist. Nurses could see evidence of international collaboration through the reports of various leaders, and had the opportunity themselves to participate in the international nursing congresses of the International Council of Nurses (ICN). The ICN was founded in 1899 by English nurse Ethel Gordon Fenwick and others. The *International Nursing Review* (INR) commenced in 1953 but followed a less formal predecessor publication (*ICN Calling*; *International Nursing Bulletin*). The journal, ICN's international congresses, and publications helped to coalesce the international nursing community to the present day. The ICN is the largest, oldest, and widest continuing women's organization in the world (though today not women only!).

CITIZENSHIP, CIVIC PARTICIPATION, AND POLITICAL ENGAGEMENT

At the turn of the 20th century, nursing leaders were dedicated to the suffrage movement. Some were arrested, some brutally beaten, some force fed, and some died for their participation in protests. It wasn't all "jam and Jerusalem": some of the horrors of the movement were depicted in the 2015 centennial film *Suffragette*.[105] The nursing leaders who struggled for women's rights, in part so that they could create a profession for women, enjoined all early trained nurses to vote, to be informed voters, to follow the machinations of Parliament, to support any nurse who would stand for MP, and perhaps to become that nurse-MP. Every issue of these journals reports on Parliament with regard to women's suffrage, the Poor Law, midwifery, nursing, children, factories, and all things that touched upon health. These journals also printed verbatim various reports or minutes of sessions of Parliament. These leaders and educators had no truck with nurses who were not politically informed.

Nursing ethics textbooks, as well as early nursing history textbooks, gave considerable attention to the nurse-as-citizen theme, as did professional associations. The 1909 ICN congress[106] devoted one of its nine sessions to "The Nurse as Citizen" and another to "The Nurse as Patriot." The Nurses' Social Union, formed in 1908, had as its purposes networking, continuing education, recreation, mutual help and understanding, and "to foster a true sense of citizenship among nurses and to utilize more completely their special knowledge, experience, and opportunities for the welfare of the community."[107] Citizenship at both a national and international level was echoed by numerous journal articles over the years. In the article "The Ward Sister as Citizen," the "suggestions for a good citizen are, firstly, do your own work well; secondly, study the public affairs of your own country and the world as a whole; thirdly, keep well informed so that your opinion is of real value..."[108]

PATRIOTISM, HEROISM, AND EDITH CAVELL

Throughout the early nursing literature, nurses are called to be patriotic. *Patriotism* was used as a general notion for any concerted service to the country; it was broader than military, auxiliary, or wartime service.

> This is patriotism as we reckon it: that, come weal or woe, come peace or strife, in the training school as on the field of battle, in hospital work, in the district, in the home of the rich as in the one-roomed tenement, in the factory, in the prison, in the workhouse, in the mission-field, we are banded together at all times, and with all our powers of mind and body, not merely to succour the sick in body and the diseased in mind and spirit; beyond and above all that, to undermine the conditions which lie at the root of disease.[109]

District nursing, workhouse or Poor Law nursing, or tenement nursing, were regarded as patriotic forms of nursing service. In a sense, *patriotism* was a reflection of concern for *social justice*.

However, with the advent of World War I and World War II, *patriotism* becomes linked to wartime service and to heroism, particularly following the execution of nurse Edith Cavell. Edith Cavell was a British nurse and director working in Belgium who helped save the lives of both German and Allied soldiers, and helped British, French, and Belgian soldiers and German draft-aged males escape German-occupied Belgium. She was betrayed, tried by court martial, convicted of war treason, and sentenced to death. There was worldwide news coverage and pleas for clemency. She was executed by a German firing squad on October 12, 1915. Her execution was condemned internationally. Nurse Edith Cavell's body was repatriated in May of 1919 in a solemn national event. Her execution also became a part of the war propaganda machine. That notwithstanding, she became a symbol of nursing patriotism, humanitarianism, and heroism in Britain and among nurses around the world. She was canonized as a saint by the Church of England.[110,111,112]

The day before her execution Cavell wrote a tender letter to the nurses of her training school and hospital in which she prays their forgiveness for any error, severity, or grievance they might have against her. She bids them farewell with a call to loyalty to one another and an *esprit de corps*.[113] The literature asks what is it about Edith Cavell that makes her a hero when any number of others have also sacrificed their lives and are not so regarded. Certainly, the words recorded in her last visit with the chaplain are moving. However, it is her final words that were deemed heroic: "Patriotism is not enough. I must have no hatred or bitterness towards anyone."[114] In anticipation, she forgives those who will execute her within hours.

Much as nursing was viewed as a moral endeavor in itself, it was also regarded as intrinsically patriotic as it sought the welfare and well-being of the community. Nurses brought health education, patient and family care, and shared in "tea and sympathy" within the community that they served. In so doing, they were seen as serving the patient, family, community, and nation.

NURSE PAY, JUST REMUNERATION, WORK CONDITIONS, OVERSTRAIN, EQUITY

It is extremely difficult to find a single journal issue that does not contain some material, whether an editorial, a letter to the editor, an article, or even a poem about the inadequacy of remuneration, the exploitation of nurses, deplorable work conditions, the long hours worked per day or week,[115] or nurse overstrain—and what Parliament was or was not doing about it.[116] When nursing wages were compared with scullery maids and porters, nurses did not fare well with what was called their "charwoman pay." Given the extent of the nurses' formal education, both classroom and apprenticeship aspects, nurses were greatly underpaid, not just among educated professions, but even among women's occupational groups. The nature and the hours of the work were difficult, but the conditions of the work setting could be difficult to deplorable.[117] Nurses were required to "live in" (as were students) and their living quarters could be inadequately furnished, shared with many, unheated, and the food inadequate in amount and nutrition. With a customary work schedule, nurses suffered fatigue and illnesses. However, where pressed farther, nurses suffered *over-fatigue*—a kind of fatigue from which one does not bounce back—and *overstrain* which referred to an excess of both physical and emotional stress.[118] In one recorded instance, the Hull board of Guardians acknowledged that a nurse had died of overwork, having "fallen victim to zeal in the discharge of her duties. One Guardian was very much afraid, too, that it was partly on account of the Workhouse being understaffed in the matter of nurses that so much work had fallen on that poor girl."[119] After the acknowledgment, the issue was dropped. The commentator writes:

> It appears to ask that there must be something radically wrong in the management of an institution, when the death of a member of the nursing staff is necessary to ensure to those who remain immunity from the sufferings which she underwent. It is a well-known fact that conscientious nurses will go on working until they can no longer, rather than that the patients under their care should remain untended; but it is, therefore, all the more incumbent upon those responsible for their welfare, that adequate assistance and rest should be afforded to them. We hope that the terrible object lesson afforded to guardians by the death of Nurse Longley is a unique one, and one, moreover, which will not be repeated.[120]

This incident took place about 25 years after the founding of Nightingale's school, when nursing was still attempting to get a grip on education and practice. Some schools were excellent, others deplorable, and everything between. However, overwork was pervasive in the nursing world. The British nursing journals documented reports of overwork in other countries: "Nursing problems are the same the world over. The old question of nursing overwork is now being discussed in the Dutch nursing world... Some are literally 'worked-out' after a few years."[121] Overstrain is so pervasive that in 1912, H. Hecker of Germany delivers an address to the International Council of Nurses on "Overstrain of Nurses."[122,123]

In a period during which any physician (whatever his training) could designate his surgery beds a hospital, he could also declare it a school of nursing. Hapless young women were then recruited as students and cheap labor, to give service yet without receiving a solid nursing education or even a range of patient care experience. Nursing, itself, could not stop this physician practice, but it could and did take a stand on educational quality, curriculum content, the range of patient care, and the minimum number of beds that a hospital must have to become a nursing school.

POVERTY, CLASS, HEALTH DISPARITIES, AND ACCESS TO TRAINED NURSING CARE

This literature expresses a persisting concern for the middle class and their access to nursing care and midwifery, based on "the right of life to health."[124] The primary concern was the health consequences of poverty, for access to care, specifically nursing care and midwifery, which inevitably raised the issue of the cost of care. An editorial calls for "the provision of hospital accommodation for that large class of the community too well off to be properly admitted into the wards of voluntary hospitals and too poor to be able to afford private nursing home fees ..."[125] The concern for access to care was attended by the concern for the cost of care, and that the allocation of hospital beds for middle-class patients was inadequate. Nurses were intimately aware of the health price of poverty:

> We know all too well the difficulty of treating cases of serious illness and complicated surgery in the small private house [the patient's home], and from personal knowledge can supply a mental picture of the inevitable confusion in such homes, often maintained on tiny incomes, allowing of hardly any margin for emergencies of this nature, when father or mother is suddenly struck down by disease or accident; the want of adequate accommodation, the absence of all conditions that must be assured if the patient is to be nursed back to health; and even if, at untold trouble, these are more or less secured, the grinding anxiety attendant upon the weekly addition of expenses which will cripple the family resources for many months to come.[126]

Margaret Breay also raises the issue of middle-class patients and proposes a range of possible solutions for further discussion. She is clear that nurses need remuneration for their services and that some societal arrangements need to be made for those in the middle class for whom sickness requiring payment for trained nursing care would mean financial ruin.

> The difficulty the middle-class experiences in obtaining the same skilled care and illness, as is attainable by both their poorer and richer neighbors, and the means of overcoming the difficulty, are matters over which all those who interest themselves in the nursing problems of the present day must often ponder... The wealthy classes... are able to obtain without difficulty a thoroughly competent nurse, should occasion arise. But with the middle classes it is otherwise, and the trained nurse, who seems a necessity if a life (perhaps that of the bread winner of the family) is to be preserved, seems also an unattainable luxury.[127]

When the National Insurance Act was passed, the minimum qualifications of physicians and midwives were specified under the Act. That was not true for nurses. "In regard to nurses, however, the insured sick have no such protection,... against fraudulent and incompetent nursing care."[128] Breay then presents the substance of her case:

> Take, for instance, the case of the Cumberland Nursing Association, which... apparently contemplates nursing the insured sick. The Association has 50 nurses... 11 of whom are Queen's nurses, 7 have had some hospital training, and 32 are village nurses. Is it proposed that the whole of the nursing of the insured sick throughout the county should be performed by 11 Queen's nurses, or are the sick poor—who it must be remembered... are generally acutely ill when they need to services of a nurse—to be handed over to the remainder of the staff, some of whom have had "some hospital training," and to the village nurses most of

whom are dangerously ignorant of the theory and practice of nursing, but are certified midwives, with some instruction in elementary duties, and who, for purposes of policy, are described as nurses[129] instead of midwives.[130]

Care of the health needs of the poor also took tangible form. Some of the district nurses had patients who lived without heat or electricity. In the nursing community, district nurses listed clothing needs for the destitute among their patients, to be supplied by the nursing community if they could:[131]

Nurse F.L.M. (Tooting): a flannel or flannelette nightshirts, an old blanket or pants, for small man suffering from rheumatism...
Nurse G.M. (Alton): warm coat or sweater for Harry, aged 15, tuberculosis...
Nurse D. (East Ham): (a) a warm overcoat or set of clothes for Freddy, age 6, infantile paralysis...

Nurses were acutely aware of the health consequences of poverty.[132] Nursing concern for those living in poverty extended to those within the nursing family. *The Nursing Times* reports that Mrs. McEvoy, one of Nightingale's first class of 15 probationers, in old age was living in destitution with her husband in the United States. Upon discovering this, prominent US nurse Charlotte Aikens solicited donations for her welfare from younger nurses.[133]

VENEREAL DISEASE

Venereal disease (VD) is a stand-in issue, as an exemplar of a much larger domain of concern—for women generally, poor women specifically, prostitutes, and girl-children trafficked for sex, and unmarried mothers.[134] Much of this has been covered in Chapter 4 in a much fuller exposition, as an example of nursing's social ethics, and need not be repeated here. VD was a vehicle by which nursing leaders could begin with a serious social problem of a medical nature and extend it to many of the deeper concerns for women that needed to be addressed.[135] VD as a theme brings together concerns for public health, for the health status of women, for health disparities and social conditions that create illness, for sex trafficking of young girls (*white slavery*),[136] for international nursing collaboration on shared concerns, for political unity among nurses across international boundaries, and much more.

Both *The Nursing Times* and *The Nursing Record* ran articles on the clinical aspects of VD. Both also ran articles that pointed out the injustices of the socio-medical approach to VD. Here, as elsewhere, the British and American nurses were united. In 1911, the *British Journal of Nursing* weighed in on the proposed Page Bill in New York:

The women, including the trained nurses in America, are conducting their campaign against the obnoxious clause 79 of the Page Bill in New York, by taking the unassailable position that it is not only monstrous but unscientific to compulsorily detain and treat the persons of one sex who have contracted a contagious and communicable disease, and to hope by this means to eradicate the disease, while no control is exercised over the members of the opposite sex, by whom it is originally communicated to the woman compulsorily incarcerated.[137]

The concern for women is spoken aloud, even for women whom society stigmatizes as prostitutes who face social and legal persecution.

MATERNAL–CHILD CONCERNS: WAIF, FOUNDLING, BASTARD, CHILD HEALTH AND WELFARE, UNMARRIED MOMS, SEX TRAFFICKED GIRL CHILDREN, AND ACCESS OF POOR WOMEN TO BIRTH CONTROL EDUCATION

Very early on, nursing diversified into approximately 20 different specialties, two of which were pediatric and district nursing. District nurses (*visiting nurses* in the US), would see patients in their homes—and children in the streets, foundlings abandoned on doorsteps, children of one or both alcoholic parents; destitute, abused, malnourished,[138] unwanted,[139] abandoned infants[140] or children;[141] children laboring in factories; children born out of wedlock (bastards); girl-children pregnant from rape or trafficked for sex;[142] and unmarried mothers (usually young). The nursing journals follow the deliberations of Parliament and its legislation, and the journals have a lot to say about the inadequacies of the legislation and the consequent child suffering that nurses witness.[143] Much of the infant material is seen in the midwifery journal pages (within the larger nursing journals). Attention is given to the actual care of these children, as well as the legislation that affects their welfare and well-being. There is a particular concern for unwed, pregnant girls or young women and their children who fall under the bastardy laws.

The Ancient Statute of Merton (1235), considered to be England's first statute, defined legitimacy: "He is a bastard that is born before the marriage of his parents."[144] The Poor Law of 1576 subsequently became the basis of law regarding illegitimate children. The intent and purpose of the law was to punish the infant's parents and "to relieve the parish of the cost of supporting the mother and child."[145] If the father were known, he could be pressured to pay upkeep. In reality, the law primarily punished the mother and child, often leaving them destitute and stigmatized for life. *The Nursing Times* calls for "greater care of the illegitimate child" and supports the revision of the bastardy laws to require the father's financial support for the pregnancy and for sustaining the child and mother after the birth.[146,147,148] Social stigmatization of an unmarried woman included the stigmatization of the infant or child as well.[149] There was a dispute within the Queen Victoria's Jubilee Institute for Nurses over nurse-midwifery care of unmarried pregnant women that resulted in the issuance of a letter that was, in essence, a policy statement:

It has been brought to the notice of the Council of the Queen's Institute that, owing to the rules of some of the affiliated associations, midwife-nurses have been debarred from rendering much-needed assistance in cases of single women during and after confinement. The Council desires to place on record its opinion that rules which deprive unmarried women of attendance at the time of childbirth are uncharitable in principle and exceedingly harmful in practice. How far the principle of punishing the offences of mothers by neglecting and injuring their unoffending children can be reconciled with the dictates of humanity and the teachings of Christ, must be let to the conscience of individual nursing associations.... The helplessness of this class of children renders the duty of nursing associations towards them the more imperative, and there is no branch of their work in which a breach of their trust would be more deplorable.[150]

This editorial lays claim to nursing care of unmarried, pregnant mothers, largely for the benefit of the infant, but also as a requisite charitable expression of nursing. There is still, in this passage though not everywhere, a negative judgment on unwed pregnancy. That particular judgment has diminished over the decades, but the principle of nursing care for all, regardless of stigma, criminality, or even enemy combatant status, pertains.

Nurses and midwives were also concerned about access to birth control education. A brief article in *The Midwife*, Supplement to the *British Journal of Nursing*, states:

Women of the well-to-do classes obtain by their wealth a scientific knowledge of methods of birth control, which is denied to working-class wives by their poverty. The Ministry of Health, by a stock letter forbidding the Welfare Centers to impart scientific information on this point, shuts in the face of working-class wives, the door between ignorance and knowledge, while it leaves wide open to them the highway between despair and quackery. The consequences are widespread and well-known. The fact is that knowledge of methods of birth control cannot be shut out from special circles by ostracism, or banned for one class by those of another, who practise it themselves.[151]

Many of the issues in this theme relate to the consequences of poverty, one of which is the social stigmatization imposed by the Poor Law. This stigma fell on both impoverished persons and the nurses who served in Poor Law communities.[152]

Nurses also pursued specific infant-related issues such as a clean milk supply (as well as uncontaminated meat and eggs in the food chain)[153,154,155] and fought the use of flammable flannelette (cotton flannel) or flannel (wool mix) in children's wear.[156] These issues required parliamentary action, which was slow and lumbering in the nurses' estimation, and frustrating of their own sense of urgency, yet they persisted in their activism. They also decried the conditions of foundling hospitals: "the Foundling is not the best way, even under the improved conditions of today, of dealing with not-wanted-at-home children."[157,158,159]

These Themes

Each of these themes above could provide sufficient material for a chapter—or a doctoral dissertation. I recognize that the themes overlap, intertwine, and double back on one another (and may be incomplete). They are offered here as a preliminary incursion into the UK nursing ethical issues and concerns, prior to the rise of the field of bioethics, in the hopes that others will take this work deeper and further.

The UK Nursing Ethics Literature—Why So Few Ethics Textbooks?

The relationship between UK, US, and Canadian nursing ethics is a Gordian knot that is perhaps best severed, but I prefer to attempt to untie it. This is the knot: the UK, Canada, and US are intimately tied in their origin stories, in being bound by gender expectations and gender-restrictive laws, by very broad and similar concerns for the shape of society and myriad structures of oppression that generated ill health, by organizational ties, by shared leaders and exchanges, by congresses and work groups, and much more. They worked together to establish international uniform requirements for schools and uniform curriculum, and commensurate practice across nations. All three countries (as well as other nations) shared a concern for the ethics of nursing practice, expressed in relational terms, and rooted in character—virtue—instantiated (*inculcated* in the UK literature) in the process of moral formation in its range of forms. All three nations served together on the standing ICN Committee on Ethics. They even plagiarized each other's articles of incorporation for their national organizations which included "to establish and maintain a code of ethics." Why then is it that the US produces a massive cache of textbooks and journal articles on *ethics*, and neither Canada nor the UK are so excessive? There are some bits and pieces that contribute to loosening the knot but don't quite untie it.

With regard to Canada and the US, geographic proximity trumped cultural and political ties. As noted previously a number of Canadian leaders pursued nursing education in the US. Canadian leader Mary Agnes Snively studied basic nursing at Bellevue (NY), then returned to Canada. Canadian Isabel Robb also pursued a nursing education in the US, but stayed and became a US leader. Many of the Canadian educators received their advanced teacher preparation at Columbia University in the US. Though addressing another matter, an 1899 editorial in *The Nursing Record & Hospital World* opines:

> we hope that one result of the opportunity of intercourse with leaders of the Nursing Profession in America afforded by the coming [ICN] International Congress, will be to inspire British Nurses with the spirit which animates American and Canadian women in their professional affairs. The Canadian nurses have... linked themselves professionally, not with the mother country, as under ordinary conditions would be natural and advisable, but have associated themselves with... the United States, with the result that their Association is speedily becoming a professional force of much importance.[160]

Indeed, the original nursing membership organization that was formed in 1896 was the Nurses Associated Alumnae of the United States and Canada. When it attempted to incorporate in New York, it could not legally incorporate a binational organization and Canada went its own way. Canada, then, does not return to the mothership. Instead, it sails back and forth in the US educational waters—and influence. Canadian and American nurse educators were exposed to Progressivism and Pragmatism, both of which were congruent with nursing ethics, and certainly nursing's social ethics. It would be natural for US and Canadian nursing ethics to bear a resemblance, and they do. However, that does not explain why there is no sizable body of Canadian-authored nursing ethics textbooks. Admittedly, the population of Canada in 1900 was 5.5 million and 76.2 million in the US, and US nurses greatly outnumbered Canadian nurses. In addition, a great majority of nursing publishers had their offices in the US and UK. The shared education and the persistent intermingling of Canadian and US nursing leaders accounts for a similarity in their ethics as well as their shared usage of the term *ethics*, even when referring to moral character, in their literature. Likewise, the population of the UK in 1900 was 41.5 million.[161] Though there are early collegiate-associated programs in the UK, and eventually university degree programs, the US made this move earlier. Given that UK nursing was not uninterested in ethics, this might, possibly, explain the US penchant for writing ethics textbooks and articles. Well, that and possibly the presence of multiple book and nursing journal publishers in the US. It could be that UK schools used US ethics textbooks, but there is not yet hard evidence for this. This is not a question for which I have a satisfactory answer.

As to Journal Articles

The Canadian Nurse, established in 1905, begins as a 50-page quarterly journal that becomes monthly. The first article on ethics was contributed by American nurse Charlotte Aikens.[162] The UK journals reprinted American articles, and the American journals reprinted British articles. There is a general entanglement here. The early discussions of ethics by and among the three nations often followed the speeches given at the ICN—that were reprinted, in whole or in part, in UK, Canadian, and US journals. The ICN had an *ethics* committee, and the ICN speeches consistently use the term *ethics*. The American nursing ethics textbooks are advertised, reviewed, and excerpted in the *Canadian Nurse*, as well as in the UK journals. The general journal literature (not simply for nursing ethics articles) was largely internationally communal.

Nursing Ethics More Generically

While there is an abundance of topical articles, there is also a more generic ethics literature that falls into two categories, based on audience: literature directed toward probationers (students), and literature directed toward graduate nurses. The literature directed toward nursing students was primarily found in the first chapters of the medical-surgical textbooks from the late 1800s into the 1900s when ethics textbooks began to be published. These first chapters taught students what it meant to *be* a nurse as foundational and intrinsic to the succeeding chapters that taught how to *do* nursing techniques.

All this literature is expressive of experience in nursing and its tradition and narrative, and the ethics that it generates. The chapters ooze with the reality of nursing life, practice, demands, and satisfactions. There are commonalities among these chapters that include:

- The patient comes first
- The patient is an individual—who is due loyalty, kindness, compassion, gentleness, sympathy, understanding, courtesy, impartiality as to station in life[163]
- Safeguard patient secrets; build trust and confidence
- The ideal of service: "the nurse is present to serve humanity in the form of the sick person"[164]
- Impartiality: "Nursing knows no barriers; the sick must be cared for regardless of religion, creed, race, colour. This refers to nurses as well as patients..."[165,166]
- The moral character of a good nurse
- The moral environment or milieu—discipline, etiquette, tact, courtesy, respect, obedience to medical and nursing superiors[167]
- The nurse has broad duties to herself in both personal and professional dimensions
- Nurse as team member: courtesy, consideration, respect, forbearance, toward nurse colleagues
- Beware of men: physicians, internes, male patients and family members
- Respect and bring honor to the profession

There are many of these first chapters, but Janet Ross and Kathleen Wilson's chapter is a good representative of this genre.[168]

The journal articles have graduate nurses as their primary audience. The British Medical Association awarded first prize to nurse E.C.N. Wilson, SRN for her essay "The Practical Solution to Ethical Problems," published in the 1955 *Nursing Times.*[169] While this is a curious place to start a discussion of the journal articles, to do so is to begin with what a clinical nurse perceived as ethical issues in practice. At the beginning of the essay, she identifies the ethical problems that confront the nurse. What is important about this essay resides in what she identifies as ethical problems and their practical solutions. She discusses several specific male-patient situations, then that of a woman with an unwanted pregnancy. Her male patients are variously beset by prolonged illness, stroke, conditions for which there is no recovery, and the proximity of death. The ethical problems that she identifies are focused on patient responses to illness, and not the illnesses or their medical treatments. Her ethical problems relating to the specific cases she mentions include:

> long illness as taxing, job loss with impoverishment, fear and nonproductive or futile worry, uncontrolled negative thoughts, envy of healthy persons, patient shrinks from social contacts, loneliness, nuclear family places caregiving burden and stresses on housewife, pain and symptoms of dying, fear of dying, unwanted pregnancy/annual pregnancy, blaming husband for annual pregnancies, attempted self-abortion, domestic violence, friction between nurses and more.

Her practical solutions to these ethical problems are skilled relational interventions tailored to the specific patient—including build trust, safeguard secrets, engage in conversation, encourage visitors, do not destroy hope, support family relationships, engage in discussion where there is co-worker friction, and so on. What she sees as practical solutions, and what she sees as ethical problems—center on good, skilled, attuned, responsive nursing care of patient responses to illness, disability, dementia, dying, and unwanted pregnancy, within a relationship of trust, fidelity, and caring.

In a comment in *The Nursing Times* (1955), an anonymous author writes:

> wherever nurses are at work... nursing has a common denominator, and it is the word 'care'. A Canadian doctor expressed it well when he said, "Two things are necessary in the treatment of patients, their cure and their care. Their cure is the task of the medical profession and their care the responsibility of the nursing profession, and I do not know which is the nobler.[170]

We know.

A frequent ethics author, Catherine Wood wrote the rather poetic four-part series "Ethics in the Profession" for *The Nursing Times* (1909). They are "Ethics in Training,"[171] "Ethics in Hospital,"[172] "Ethics in Teaching,"[173] and "Ethics in Practice."[174] In defining ethics, she writes:

> The meaning of the word covers custom, usage, habit, and may refer to personal characteristic, or to the traditions of a community; hence, when talking of the ethics in the profession it means the customs and habits which the units of the profession are by degrees accumulating around the name and character of the trained nurse.[175]

Wood rightly points out that the traditions of the community and its practice experiences both further the tradition itself and generate new nursing ethical knowledge.

Regarding ethics teaching, she bids us consider "the ethics that may be derived from the subjects taught, the ethics of the taught, and the ethics of the teacher."[176] The "ethics of the subjects taught" refers to Mother Nature as teacher, and to a very Nightingalian perspective of putting patients in the condition for nature to work upon them. Here the student must discern and learn the laws of healing and mending the body, and the sadness of the problems of life, illness, and dying, as consequences of the violations of nature's laws. From this the nurse gains ethical knowledge—of the laws of health and illness, of mystery, of obedience, of the spirit of service, and of the need to become qualified. The "ethics of the taught" refers to how the student receives her nurse's training.

> Aware of her need of training in the arts that minister to the comfort of the sick, she watches the skill and listens to the words of the teacher, not only that she may gain dexterity, but that she may penetrate behind the act, into its spirit and reason, knowing that one day she must try her prentice hand on living flesh and quivering nerves. The ethics of the wards, gentleness, compassion, courage, selflessness, confront her here; it is no new lesson, it is only being taught by another teacher.[177]

Here, Wood tells us that as the student attends to the instructor, her learning is not simply that of *techne* but of character, as that newly learned *techne* (rational calculation) is to be employed on living, nervous flesh. This is the second derivation of ethics.

The third derivation of ethics is the teacher's own character as he or she looks within. "Fullness cannot come out of emptiness... what a man is, that he teaches." It is the work of the matron to place before the student "the dignity of the life of service, and show them the beautiful form of the spirit of service, the gentle compassion, the tender love..." [where] "the patients have been allowed to set the ethics of the hospital... Ethics in theory do not exist; they are severely practical, and are the external proof of the custom, habit, rectitude, and moral conscience of the individual."[178] Ethics is not an abstract, theoretical endeavor—it is the skilled hand on living flesh and quivering nerves. For Wood, "the masters and teachers of... ethics are the patients who from their beds of sickness... stretch out their hands... to those women who stand there... whose beautiful function is to render them service... of compassion."[179] It is, perhaps, all a bit heady, but an unusual and instructive insight from within the nursing tradition.

Given the extent of the journal literature and its richness, this is but an *amuse-bouche* that does not do justice to the banquet behind it, yet it is an invitation to that banquet.

Conclusion

Each of the themes above is ripe for further research and rife with policy implications. Many of the issues that they address have persisted from the start of modern nursing, for well over 150 years and have been refractory to resolution. The prescience of our early nursing leaders is breathtaking. For example, in 1928, an editorial raises the issue of *green spaces*: "It is not merely a question of recreation;

open spaces have a definite effect on the health of the city dweller."[180] Anywhere that there was an issue that touched upon health and well-being, there were nurses. Their ultimate resolution of all these issues would be, as nursing's early leaders insisted, in the *united* voice and action of nurses worldwide. It is time for nurses both to unite and for the millions of nurses worldwide to come together to tackle each one of the social and professional issues that these themes address. Minnie Goodnow's words are worth repeating:

> It is important also, in these days when all questions are becoming international ones, that nurses should know what is taking place on the other side of the world.[181]
> ... For many years [nurses] have gone out to the ends of the earth to help other countries develop good nursing... the world lies before nurses... shall we prepare for the challenge of humanity and then go to its help?[182]

If nursing had the strength of will and unity, coming together as one strong voice on these issues, then laws, social attitudes, and cultures would change, and these issues could be resolved. According to the 2019 WHO World Health Statistics Report,[183] there are approximately 20.7 million nurses and midwives in the world. That is strength enough to move any nation.

Some of these baker's dozen themes are discrete, but others have fuzzier boundaries and can merge. For example, the concern for children, and for illegitimate children in particular, overlaps with that of the young unmarried mother and the VD theme. There is no claim here that this typology of themes is definitive or exhaustive. The attempt here is to lay out themes that emerge from this research, to hint at the persistence of most of these concerns to the present, and to invite scholars to become immersed in the ethical riches of this essentially untouched body of literature. It would be difficult to examine these themes and not agree that nursing's ethical tradition is the bedrock of nursing's identity and is the core of pride of our profession. Broderick pulls all of these themes together when she speaks of nursing's concern for the whole of humanity. Listen to Albinia:

> The wakening of our profession throughout the civilized world to a deep sense of what each of us owe individually, not merely to our patient, to our hospital, or to our guild, not even to our country itself, but rather to the whole of humanity, is proceeding coevally with the wise and much needed development of training methods and of scientific knowledge, and the cultivation of a high professional ideal amongst us.[184]

Broderick, Dock, Burr, Fenwick, Snively, Robb, and all of the early leaders of modern nursing were adamant that nursing, as an educated, scientific, profession for women had something pivotal—and irenic—to offer to health care and to the needs of the humanity. They were and are correct.

Notes

1 Aeleah Soine, "The Relation of the Nurse to the Working World: Professionalization, Citizenship, and Class in Germany, Great Britain, and the United States before World War I," *Nursing History Review* 18, (2010): 51–80.

2 Portions of this chapter appear in Marsha Fowler, "The Nightingale Still Sings: Ten Ethical Themes in Early Nursing in the United Kingdom, 1888–1989," *OJIN*, May 2021. DOI: 10.3912/OJIN.Vol26No02PPT72

3 I am grateful for the Fulbright Research Award that supported this study. In addition, I am grateful to the Royal College of Nursing, London and its archivists for their assistance in this project.

4 See Chapter 9 on goods intrinsic to nursing.

5 John Dewey and James Tufts, *Ethics* (New York: Henry Holt and Company, 1908).

6 John Mackenzie, *A Manual of Ethics* (London: W.B. Clive, 1897).

7 American Nurses Association, "American Nurses' Association's First Position on Education for Nursing," *American Journal of Nursing* 65, no. 12 (Dec., 1965): 106–111.

8 Lynn Kirkwood, "Enough but Not Too Much: Nursing Education in English Language Canada (1874–2000)," in Christina Bates, Dianne Dodd, and Nicole Rousseau (eds.), *On All Frontiers: Four Centuries of Canadian Nursing* (Ottawa: Ottawa University Press, 2005), 190.

9 Ina J. Bramadat, "Nursing Education in Canada: Historical 'Progress'?" *Journal of Advanced Nursing* 14, no. 9 (Sept. 1989): 719–726; 720.

10 Ibid., 721.

11 Ibid., 721–722.

12 Barbara Fawkes, "A Year at Teachers College, Columbia University, New York," *The Nursing Times* (September 18, 1954), 10171019.

13 AEM, "Nursing as a Vocation," *The British Journal of Nursing* 45, no. 1183 (Dec. 31, 1921): 415.

14 E. Margaret Fox, "Vocation *versus* Profession," *The Nursing Times* X, no. 472 (May 16, 1914): 637.

15 Anon., "The Nurses' Social Union," *The Nursing Times* III, no. 90 (Jan. 19, 1907): 59.

16 Anon., Social Union, 59.

17 E.C. Pearce, *Nurse and Patient: An Ethical Consideration of Human Relations* (London: Faber & Faber, 1953), 78.

18 E. Margaret Fox, "What the Twentieth Century Nurse may Learn from the Nineteenth," *The British Journal of Nursing* (Dec. 9, 1910), 449.

19 Beatrice Edgell, *Ethical Problems: An Introduction to Ethics for Hospital Nurses and Social Workers* (London: Methuen & Company, 1929), 140–142.

20 A more contemporary, renewed Aristotelian virtue theory is found in the work of Alastair MacIntyre. This will be discussed in Chapter 9.

21 Ione Spaulding, "Professional Ideals," *The Nursing Times* (Oct. 21, 1955), 1196–1198. No Vol or Number available

22 Anon., "Ideal and Reality" (poem), *The Nursing Times* XV, no. 741 (June 15, 1919).

23 Miss F.J. Botting, "Ideals," *The Nursing Times* XV, no. 761 (Nov. 29, 1919): 1278.

24 "On Sœur Pierre's Paper," *The Nursing Times* XXIX, no. 1476 (Aug. 12, 1933): 763–764.

25 H.C.C. [Harriet C. Camp], "The Ethics of Nursing: Talks of a Superintendent with Her Graduating Class," *The Trained Nurse* 2, no. 5 (May 1889): 179.

26 Anon., "The Ethics and Etiquette of Nursing," *The Nursing Record & Hospital World* XVII, no. 444 (Oct. 3, 1896): 268–270.

27 Humphrey Rolleston, "Nurses Ancient and Modern," *The Nursing Times* XXVI, no. 1288 (Jan. 4, 1930): 7.

28 Anon., "The Ethics and Etiquette of Nursing," *The Nursing Record & Hospital World* (Oct. 3, 1896): 268.

29 Melia Kath, *Ethics for Nursing and Healthcare Practice* (Thousand Oaks, CA: Sage, 2013).

30 Editorial, "Professional Secrecy," *The Nursing Times* II, no. 42 (Feb. 17, 1906): 132.

31 Harold Kerr, "Ethics of Midwifery," *The Nursing Times* VIII, no. 371 (June 8, 1912): 622.

32 Editorial, "Professional Confidence," *The British Journal of Nursing* XLVI, no. 1190 (January 21, 1911): 41.

33 Editorial, "Professional Confidence," *The Nursing Times* (Jan. 12, 1918): 60.

34 Anon., "Sealed Lips," *The Nursing Times* XVIII, no. 879 (March 4, 1922): 202.

35 Barbara Fawkes, "Methods of Character Training," *The Nursing Times* (Aug. 14, 1954).

36 Fox, E. Margaret, *First Lines in Nursing* (London: Scientific Press, 1914), 4.

37 "naughty, adj. (and int.)," *OED Online*. June 2019. Oxford University Press. https://www.oed.com/view/Entry/125392?result=2&rskey=tnQxWV& (accessed July 6, 2019).

38 "empathy, n." *OED Online*. June 2019. Oxford University Press. https://www.oed.com/view/Entry/61284?redirectedFrom=empathy& (accessed July 4, 2019).

39 Goodnow was an American who, because of World War I, worked in France and England as well as the US.

40 Minnie Goodnow, *First-Year Nursing: A Text-Book for Pupils during Their First Year of Hospital Work*, 2nd ed. (Philadelphia & London: W.B. Saunders, 1916), 28.

41 Editorial, "Nursing...and Doctor's Opinions," *The Nursing Times* (January 11, 1957), 29.

42 Ibid., 29.

43 Ibid.

44 *Empathy* was not a term commonly used in this period and descriptions of *sympathy* more closely resemble what we today term *empathy*.

45 Wilhelmina J. Mollett, "Honour," *The Nursing Record* 1, no. 4 (April 26, 1888): 40–41.

46 Wilhelmina Jane Mollett, "Purity," *The Nursing Record* 1, no. 5 (May 3, 1888): 54–55.

47 Ibid., 55.

48 Wilhelmina Jane Mollett, "Courage," *The Nursing Record* 1, no. 7 (May 17, 1888): 76–78.

49 Ibid., 76.

50 Ibid., 77.

51 Charlotte A. Aikens, *Studies in Ethics for Nurses*, 2nd ed. (rev.) (Philadelphia: W.B. Saunders, 1923), 197.

52 Mollett, "Courage," 78.

53 Wilhelmina Jane Mollett, "Discipline," *The Nursing Record* 1, no. 9 (May 31, 1888): 99–101.

54 Ibid., 100.

55 Wilhelmina Jane Mollett, "Culture," *The Nursing Record* 1, no. 11 (June 14, 1888): 125–127, 125.

56 Ibid., 125.

57 "Empathy," Oxford English Dictionary Second Edition on CD-ROM (v. 4.0.0.3). Oxford, UK: Oxford University Press, 2009

58 Wilhelmina Jane Mollett, "Sympathy," *The Nursing Record* 1, no. 16 (July 19, 1888): 192–193.

59 Ibid., 193.

60 Ibid., 193.

61 Sara Fry, "The Role of Caring in a Theory of Nursing Ethics," *Hypatia* 4, no. 2 (1989): 87–103; 87.

62 M. Wiles. "The District Nurse and Etiquette," *The Nursing Times*, XXI, no. 1056 (July 25, 1925), 689–690.

63 Anon., "Recipe for a Good Nurse," *Nursing Times* 27, no. 1372 (Aug. 15, 1931): 899.

64 Anon., "Recipe for Making a Good Nurse," *Pacific Coast Journal of Nursing* XV, no. 5 (May 1919): 268.

65 May Just, "The Ideal Nurse: A Recipe," *The British Journal of Nursing* 102, no. 2225 (Jan. 1954): 8.

66 Anon., "Recipe for Making a Good Nurse," *Cassandra: Radical Feminist Nurses Newsjournal* 5, no. 2, (May 1987): 10

67 Fox, *First Lines*, I x.

68 I.M. Laycock, "A Scheme of Nurse Training," *The Nursing Times* (December 17, 1954): 1401.

69 Garside, R.F. "Assessment for Vocational Selection," *The Nursing Times* (March 14, 1958): 296–297.

70 E. Mira, "Character Tests for Nurses," *The Nursing Times* XXV, no. 1802 (Nov. 11, 1939): 1362–1363.

71 Editorial, "Careless Talk and...," *The Nursing Times* XLII, no. 14 (April 6, 1946): 259.

72 Editorial, "Wastage, Attrition and Discontinuation," *The Nursing Times* 61, no. 47 (Nov. 19, 1969): 1567.

73 Editorial, "Selecting Students," *The Nursing Times* (March 11, 1950): 247–248.

74 Royal College of Nursing, "Vocational Guidance and Selection Tests for the Nursing Profession," *The Nursing Times* XLII, no. 6 (Feb. 9, 1946): 296–297.

75 Terence Lee, "Predicting the Successful Nurse," *The Nursing Times* (April 29, 1960): 538–540.

76 Hillary Way, *Ethics for Nurses* (London: Macmillan, 1962). (UK: reprinted from *Nursing Times*.)

77 Anon., "Holiday in a Caravan," *The Nursing Times* XXI, no. 1042 (April 18, 1925): 354.

78 Mary Stollard, "A Holiday in Norway," *The Nursing Times* XXIV, no. 1211 (July 14, 1928): 855.

79 Two Nurses Over Forty, "The Joys of a Tent Holiday," *The Nursing Times* XXIV, no. 1216 (April 18, 1928): 998.

80 R.A. Cox-Davies, "The Eclipse—1927," *The Nursing Times*, XXIII, no. 1158 (July 9, 1927) 818.

81 Anon., "Shrive Tuesday Pancakes," *The Nursing Times* XXIII, no. 1140 (March 5, 1927): 263.

82 Lady Constance Howard, "Tasty Tid-bits and Dishes Dainty for Invalids and Convalescents," *The Nursing Record* 201, no. 8 (Feb. 4, 1892): 93.

83 B. Melville Nicholas, "Bird-Watching in Hospital," *The Nursing Times* XXXVI, no. 1860 (December 21, 1940): 1330.

84 Anon., "The Movement of Glaciers," *The Nursing Record & Hospital World* XII, no. 303 (Jan. 20, 1894): 53.

85 B. Melville Nicholas, "Before and After a Cuckoo Is Born," *The Nursing Times* XXX-VIII, no. 1933 (May 16, 1942): 329.

86 Clive Beech, "Honey," *The British Journal of Nursing* 102, no. 2234 (October 1954): 112.

87 Frank S. Stuart, "City of Golden Wax," *The British Journal of Nursing* 103, no. 2245 (Sept. 1955): 100.

88 Anon., "Life on Other Planets," *The Nursing Record and Hospital World* XIII, no. 347 (Nov. 24, 1894): 349.

89 Anon., "Poetry in Daily Life: I—Introduction," *The Nursing Times* XIV, no. 693 (Aug. 10, 1918): 832.

90 Maude Buckingham, "The Nurse 'Off-Duty'," *The Nursing Times* IX, no. 417 (April 26, 1913): 455.

91 Anon., "The 'Nursing Times' Lawn Tennis Competition, *The Nursing Times* XV, no. 735 (May 31, 1919): 536.

92 Jack Carrington, "Hints on Playing Table Tennis," *The Nursing Times* XXXVI, no. 1814 (Feb. 3, 1940): 124.

93 Editorial, "Our Needlework Competition," *The Nursing Times* IX, no. 439 (Sept. 27, 1913): 1067.
94 Anon., "A Fancy Work Competition," *The Nursing Times* III, no. 132 (Nov. 9, 1907): 995.
95 For this section, citations are only provided sufficient unto the task.
96 Anon., "The Modern Nursing Movement in France," *The British Journal of Nursing* XXXVIII, no. 988 (March 9, 1907): 179.
97 Minnie Goodnow, *Nursing History in Brief* (Philadelphia & London: W.B. Saunders, 1938), 18.
98 Goodnow, *Nursing History*, 311–312.
99 Anonymous, "Facts Trained Nurses Must Know," *The British Journal of Nursing* LII, no. 1349 (Feb. 7, 1914): 110.
100 Mona Grey, "World Health Organization, International Nurse," *The Nursing Times* 58 (Feb. 10, 1961): 178–179.
101 Barbara N. Fawkes, "Towards a 'European Nurse'," *The Nursing Times* 58 (Sept. 28, 1962): 1227.
102 "European Economic Community," *The Nursing Times* 58 (Sept. 28, 1962): 1228.
103 Soine, "The Relation of the Nurse to the Working World," 51–80.
104 Editorial, "Was it Worth While?" *The Nursing Times* 58 (June 9, 1961): 720.
105 *Suffragette*. Film (2015). https://www.imdb.com/title/tt3077214/
106 Editor, *British Journal of Nursing* XLII, no. 1097 (April 10, 1909): 291.
107 E.L.C. Eden, "The Nurses Social Union and its Objects," *The Nursing Times* 1, no. 24 (Oct. 14, 1905): 468.
108 Royal College of Nursing, "The Ward Sister as Citizen," *The Nursing Times* (Aug. 2, 1947): 534.
109 Albinia Broderick, "The Patriot Nurse," *The British Journal of Nursing* XLIII, no. 1114 (Aug. 7, 1909): 116. In *The Englishwoman.*
110 Editorial, "A Great Englishwoman," *The British Journal of Nursing* LXII, no. 1625 (May 24, 1919): 349.
111 Editorial, "The Trial of Edith Cavell," *The British Journal of Nursing* LXII, no. 1625 (May 24, 1919): 350.
112 A.E. Clark-Kennedy, "Edith Cavell: Pioneer and Patriot," *The Nursing Times* (Oct. 15, 1965): 1413–1415.
113 Anon., "Miss Cavell's Last Hours," *The Nursing Times* 13, no. 627 (May 5, 1917): 536.
114 Anon., "The Spirit of Edith Cavell," *The Nursing Times* 15, no. 734 (May 24, 1919): 505.
115 Editorial, "The Long Hours on Duty," *The Nursing Times* V, no. 196 (Jan. 30, 1909): 81.
116 Editorial, "Not a Nurses' Bill," *The Nursing Times* XXVII, no. 1348 (Feb. 28, 1931): 219.
117 Ernest C. Hadley, "The Present Transitional Period in the History of the Nursing Profession," *The Nursing Times* XXV, no. 1244 (March 3, 1929): 266–269.
118 Margaret Breay, "The Overstrain of Nurses," *The British Journal of Nursing* XLIX, no. 1282 (Oct. 26, 1912): 330.
119 Anon., "A Terrible Object Lesson," *The Nursing Record & Hospital World* XIX, no. 490 (Aug. 21, 1897): 143.
120 Ibid.
121 Anon., "Overwork," *The Nursing Times* 7, no. 298 (Jan. 14, 1911): 21.
122 Anon., "Overstrain of Nurses," *British Journal of Nursing* 50, no. 1293 (Jan. 11, 1913): 27.
123 Anon., "Overstrain of Nurses," *British Journal of Nursing* 61, no. 1613 (March 1, 1919): 134.
124 Editorial, "The Right of Life to Health," *The British Journal of Nursing* XLVI, no. 1188 (Jan. 7, 1911).
125 Anon., "Pay Hospitals for the Middle Classes," *The Nursing Times* 5, no. 211 (May 15, 1909): 397.

126 A. Broderick, "The Patriot Nurse," *British Journal of Nursing* 43, no. 1114, (1909): 116.

127 Miss Margaret Breay, "The Nursing of the Middle-Class Patient," *The Nursing Record & Hospital World* XXI, no. 536 (July 9, 1898): 26.

128 Editorial, "The Right of the Insured Sick to Skilled Nursing," *The British Journal of Nursing* XLIX, no. 1282 (Oct. 26, 1912): 329.

129 In the UK professional midwives need not be RNs.

130 Editorial, "Insured Sick," 329.

131 Anon., "Our Christmas Clothing Distribution," *The Nursing Times* IX, no. 448 (Nov. 22, 1913): 1323.

132 Editorial, "Tuberculosis and Poverty," *The Nursing Times* XXIX, no. 1466 (June 3, 1933).

133 Anon., "A 'Nightingale Probationer' in Poverty," *The Nursing Times* VII, no. 348 (Dec. 30, 1911): 1192.

134 Anon., "The Unmarried Mother—and Father," *The Nursing Times* XVI, no. 771 (Feb. 7, 1020): 168.

135 Dock, *Hygiene and Morality*, 135.

136 Lavinia Dock, "The Need of Education on Matters of Social Morality," *The British Journal of Nursing* LXII, no. 1125 (Oct. 23, 1909): 335–339.

137 Anon., "The Page Bill in New York," *British Journal of Nursing* 46, no. 1199 (March 25, 1911): 233.

138 Editorial, "London's Sick Babies," *The Nursing Times* XIV, no. 697 (Sept. 7, 1918): 91.

139 Anon., "The Unwanted Child," *The Nursing Times* (Aug. 31, 1912): 899.

140 Editorial, "Infant Protection," *The Nursing Times* (Jan. 25, 1957): 87.

141 M.L., "A Slum Baby," *The Nursing Times* (May 8, 1909): 385.

142 Anon., "Housing and Morality," *The British Journal of Nursing* LI, no. 1329 (Sept. 20, 1913): 230.

143 More than 100 years later, rising rates of child poverty were a concern at the meeting of the RCN congress in 2019.

144 John Raithby (ed.), *The Statutes of the Realm*. Complete set at Hathi Trust. Digital version of the 1963 reprint, by Dawsons of Pall Mall, London. https://catalog.hathitrust.org/Record/102430539?type%5B%5D=all&lookfor%5B%5D=statutes%20of%20the%20realm&ft=

145 Alan MacFarlane, *Illegitimacy and Illegitimates in English History* (2002). http://alan-macfarlane.com/TEXTS/bastardy.pdf

146 Anon., "Greater Care of the Illegitimate Child," *Nursing Times* 16, no. 782 (April 24, 1920): 488.

147 Anon., "Making His Name," *The Nursing Times* XXX, no. 1504 (Feb. 24, 1934): 168.

148 Anon., "Hardships of Illegitimate Children," *The Nursing Times* (Nov. 28, 1958): 1393.

149 Editorial, "Nurses and the Unmarried Mother," *The Nursing Times* XI, no. 524 (May 15, 1915): 575.

150 Editorial. "Nurses and the Unmarried Mother," *The Nursing Times*, XI, no. 524 (May 15, 1915), 575.

151 Anon., "Community of Knowledge," *The Midwife in The British Journal of Nursing* 77, no. 1932 (July 1929): 194.

152 A. Lombardini, "Our Great Adventure," *The Nursing Times* XV, no. 734 (May 24, 1919): 509–510.

153 Anon., "The Pure Milk Problem," *The British Journal of Nursing* XLVII, no. 1219 (Aug. 12, 1911): 125.

154 Editorial, "Clean Milk," *The British Journal of Nursing* XLII, no. 1106 (June 12, 1909): 465.

155 Anon., "Clean Milk," *The Nursing Times* XVIII, no. 913 (Oct. 28, 1922): 1048.

156 Anon., "Fire Tests with Flannelette," *The British Journal of Nursing* LXIII, no. 1125 (Oct. 23, 1909): 347.
157 Anon., "Waifs and Strays," *The Nursing Record* 10, no. 256 (Feb. 23, 1893): 99.
158 Editorial, "The Poor Law Child," *The British Journal of Nursing* XLIII, no. 1109 (July 9, 1909): n.p.
159 Royal College of Nursing, "The Rights of the Child," *The Nursing Times* (Aug. 19, 1955): 922.
160 Editorial, "Poor Things," *The Nursing Record & Hospital World* XXII, no. 581 (May 20, 1899): 390.
161 Brian Abel-Smith, *A History of the Nursing Profession* (London: Heinemann, 1960), 55.
162 Charlotte Aikens, "Hospital Ethics and Discipline," *Canadian Nurse* III, no. 4 (April 1907): 191–193.
163 Janet S. Ross and Kathleen J.W. Wilson, *Foundations of Nursing* (London: E. & S. Livingstone, 1956), 31.
164 Ibid., 26.
165 Ibid.
166 Ibid., 33–34.
167 Margaret Riddell, *Lectures to Nurses* (London: Faber & Faber [The Scientific Press], 1933).
168 Ross, Wilson, *Foundations*, 26–41.
169 E.C.N. Wilson, "The Practical Solution to Ethical Problems which Arise in the Course of Nursing Duties," *The Nursing Times* (Dec. 16, 1955): 1423–1424, and 1433–1434.
170 D.C. Baird, "Nursing—A World-Wide Social Activity," *The Nursing Times* (Dec. 23, 1955): 1449.
171 Catherine J. Wood, "Ethics in the Profession, I—Ethics in Training," *The Nursing Times* V, no. 195 (Jan. 23, 1909): 67–68.
172 Catherine J. Wood, "Ethics in the Profession, II—Ethics in Hospital," *The Nursing Times* V, no. 196 (Jan. 30, 1909): 87.
173 Catherine J. Wood, "Ethics in the Profession, III—Ethics in Teaching," *The Nursing Times* V, no. 197 (Feb. 6, 1909): 106–107.
174 Catherine J. Wood, "Ethics in the Profession, IV—Ethics in Practice," *The Nursing Times* V, no. 198 (Feb. 13, 1909): 126.
175 Catherine J. Wood, "Ethics in the Profession, I—Ethics in Training," *The Nursing Times* V, no. 195 (Jan. 23, 1909): 67.
176 Wood, "Ethics in the Profession, III—Ethics in Teaching," 106.
177 Ibid., 107.
178 Ibid., 107.
179 Wood, "Ethics in the Profession, II—Ethics in Hospital," 87.
180 Editorial, "Green Spaces," *The Nursing Times* XXIV, no. 1224 (Oct. 13, 1928): 1215.
181 Minnie Goodnow, *Nursing History in Brief* (Philadelphia & London: W.B. Saunders, 1938), 18.
182 Ibid., 311–312.
183 WHO World Health Workforce, 2019. https://www.who.int/hrh/nursing_midwifery/en/
184 Albinia Broderick, ICN photo title, *BJN* (Aug. 7, 1909): 116.

8

NURSING ETHICS BEFORE BIOETHICS

Prologue to the Future

Introduction

Buttons on the left. Buttons on the right. Women's clothing has buttons on the left, men's clothing has buttons on the right. Women's "boyfriend shirts" still button on the left, so aren't really "boyfriend" shirts. Zippers, too: slider on the left, slider on the right. Various reasons emerge including turning shoulder-forward for jousting, drawing a sword with the right hand, suckling a baby held in the left arm, women being dressed by a servant, and *sumptuary laws* that vainly attempted to restrict extravagance in dressing (buttons were an extravagance). Today, gender-neutral clothing opts for the men's side because—men still joust and draw swords? Then there is the issue of unisex shoes, *uni* meaning male. Women's feet are narrower overall in proportion to length, with a wider forefoot in relation to a significantly narrower heel. Women have wider hip structure causing a difference in foot strike (called the Q-angle), and a greater tendency to pronation. As women often weigh less than men, the midsole must be 15 percent less rigid so that a woman can bend the mid-shoe in walking or running. The height and length of the foot arch also differs. Today's unisex shoes are male normative. Can a woman wear men's clothing and shoes? Of course, but expect some chafing and blisters.

Nursing ethics and bioethics aren't exactly gendered. Then again, Isabel, Lavinia, Albinia, Mary, Charlotte, and Margaret over against Immanuel, René, Jeremy, Peter, Paul, John, John, and all the Johns—maybe they are. However, it is more likely that in attempting to walk in the shoes of bioethics, nursing has heel blisters because "that shoe don't fit." And it doesn't, but we need to see why by looking at nursing ethics before bioethics. We will look at themes and motifs such as nursing education as moral formation, student formation in the virtues, etiquette,

DOI: 10.4324/9781003262107-9

nursing as a calling, professional identity, the relational structure of nursing ethics and the duties generated by the different relationships. Though nursing ethics is not dilemma based, for those starving for dilemmas, we will look at dilemmas as case vignettes in Charlotte Aikens and Sister Rose Hélène Vaughan's dissertation.

Nursing Ethics before Bioethics

Nursing ethics developed over the span of approximately 150 years and is recorded in approximately 100 textbooks on nursing ethics and hundreds of articles, speeches, and other documents that are detailed in the first three chapters of this book. The corpus of that moral knowledge comes from several conjoined sources including the formal field of theological and philosophical ethics, the nursing moral tradition, narrative (oral and written), and practice its own unfolding literature. Here, we will survey the content of that knowledge. Patricia Benner, whose expertise in the domain of nursing practice as a source of ethics far exceeds my own, will address how practice generates moral knowledge in her chapter (see Chapter 9).

Nursing ethics prior to its colonization by bioethics bears little resemblance to bioethics. Early nursing ethics is nurse-centric, relationally based, addresses nurses' ethical comportment in all roles, is preventive in nature, incorporates nursing notions of *the good*, advances the social ethics of nursing, and sets forth ethical expectations for the profession as a whole. This first wave of nursing ethics is distinctive and differs significantly from contemporary bioethics in nursing, yet it remains largely unknown or dismissed, and glaringly under-researched. Nursing has lost sight of its living tradition of collective ethical wisdom and ethical identity, one that crafted an ethics that would and could sustain nursing practice today and could be further developed for nursing's future. It offers nurses a wise, nursing-focused, comprehensive, generous, and learned ethics that deserves to be reclaimed and renewed for today's nursing practice.

(My) Precipitating Research

In the process of deciding my dissertation topic (1980), and having been schooled in medical ethics (the emerging bioethics), the principles of biomedical ethics did not call to me. Bioethics did not attend to the issues of moral concern to nurses. I was, instead, attracted to the then current 1976 ANA *Code of Ethics for Nurses with Interpretive Statements* (*Code*), which had a depth, profundity, and nursing sensitivity that captivated me.[1] My dissertation topic became an examination of every iteration of the *Code* (and Lystra Gretter's 1893 Nightingale Pledge)[2] within its social context, to look at its progress and the social and ethical forces that shaped and informed it.[3] I subsequently became a member and then chair of the ANA Committee on Ethics, which allowed me to incorporate my research findings on nursing ethics into successive iterations of the ANA *Code of Ethics for Nurses with Interpretive Statements*.

The collateral findings of the dissertation were as important as the dissertation itself in the discovery of a breathtaking, fulsome literature in nursing ethics, written by nurses for nurses. It is an informed, insightful, extensive, embodied, situated ethics that is fully responsive to the values, obligations, and practice needs of nursing. This is, of course, what this book attempts to give away to nursing scholars in ethics in the hope of a more resonant nursing ethics to come.

Though we will focus on the US here, as a mandated part of the nursing curriculum, nursing ethics was not unique to the United States. Many of the member nations in the International Council of Nurses (ICN) also required curricular content in ethics. The *International Nursing Review*, 1926–1927, lists these nations as having curricular requirements for nursing ethics: Belgium, France, Greece, UK, Jugo-Slavia, Switzerland, Bulgaria, China, Germany, Sweden, Finland, and the US.[4] There does not seem to be, however, any national histories on the development of nursing ethics in these nations—which poses fertile ground for further research.

For the US and UK, to date, there has been no systematic analysis of this extensive body of pre-1965 nursing ethics literature, other than a preliminary descriptive incursion that identifies the works themselves, and examines the influence of the social context on the shape of this literature, and discovers some of the larger themes and motifs.[5,6,7,8,9] Further analysis of this literature is needed both comprehensively and topically; many of the topics (e.g., moral courage, sex trafficking, health disparities, gender disparities) in this heritage literature are also contemporary concerns. Some (actually many) of the concerns this literature addresses remain relevant today, 100-plus years later. The best starting point in examining this literature is with nursing leaders' understanding that nursing education was also moral formation.

Nursing Education as Moral Formation

Early modern nursing, from the founding of nursing schools in 1873 forward, viewed ethics education as essential, and held that the role of nursing education was both nursing preparation and moral formation, co-equally. It is not precisely that nursing students were considered morally unformed, though they were thought to be young, unexposed, ingenuous, and naive; rather, it was that students needed to be formed morally *as professionals and as nurses*. Nursing leaders believed that the educational environment must work, first, to shape the nursing student into a morally good nurse, imbued with notions of good in their nursing identity and practice and, second, to foster an understanding of what is right and wrong for the nurse to do not just in practice but as one who was possessed of a nursing identity. There was no separation of personal and professional identity; there was one inner identity—nurse—that suffused the totality of the person.

The incoming student, known as a probationer, was seen as a morally and educationally unformed girl who must be shaped into a morally good woman, professional/nurse, and citizen. Isabel Robb writes:

> the training school of a hospital may, therefore be regarded as a place not only for fitting women to properly undertake the care of the sick, but as an educational institution, where properly selected women are given such educational advantages that they can go forth equipped and ready to aid in the practical solution of social problems, which are to be mastered only by the help of intelligent womanly work.[10]

Nursing students would be equipped both for patient care and for addressing social problems. Their "educational advantage" specifically included "systematic" ethics education. Robb writes:

> Instruction in the science of ethics and the rules of etiquette should be commenced from the moment the pupil-nurse enters a hospital, and from the very beginning of her term of probation. It should go hand in hand with the training in the theory and practice of nursing, otherwise the pupil will fail to realize its proper degree of importance and thus much benefit will be lost to her. Such instruction should be practical and systematic, beginning with the moral laws and rules she will need first to put into practice, and progressively leading up to an appreciation of her greater and higher obligations to herself, to her profession and to humanity.[11]

In early nursing education, instruction in ethics began at the outset and saturated the entire curriculum including the practice components; it was not quarantined within a single course, though a course was also offered. It was taught by the head nurse of the school or hospital; that is, only by experienced, senior faculty, never by junior faculty. Early nursing education was a matter of development and support of moral character (character, virtues). Nursing required skill and that skill was technical, relational, and moral, all mixed together and baked; ethics was not frosting on the cake, ethics was baked into the cake itself.

Formation in the Virtues—Or the Moral Character of the Nurse

The ethics heritage literature, from the 1880s to 1965, discusses a wide range of virtues and excellences that are to be cultivated and modeled among nursing students and nurses, always situated within the context of nursing practice, the several nursing relationships (discussed below); and the community, bonds, and tradition of nursing. In both the US and UK, the term *character* or *moral character* usually stood in for *virtue*. In some instances, *attribute* would be used. Occasionally, the term *personality* was used, but generally, *personality* referred to the student's innate demeanor rather than moral character.

Across the literature, a large number of virtues and conjoined duties are discussed. Different terms may be used for the same virtue. They include truthfulness, rectitude, integrity, doing one's work decently and in order, avoiding impropriety, being a force for good, maintaining self-discipline and shunning personal laxity, unflinchingly standing firm on what one knows to be morally right, exercising moral pluck, voluntary observance of institutional rules and standards, and the exercise of self-discipline in ways that affirm personal moral and intellectual growth as well as both individuality and community; loving one's nursing work; being liberally (that is, broadly) educated, embracing an egalitarian respect for all regardless of social station or economic status; genuine compassion, empathy, kindness; and a love for humanity. These are attributes of moral character that could only be interiorized and understood as intrinsic to good nursing, within the immersive, lived, and tutored experience of nursing education and practice, and within the traditions of the community of nursing. It is, as noted in Chapter 7, a perspective based on Aristotle's virtue theory.

Specific virtues receive greater attention. Charlotte Aikens, in *Studies in Ethics for Nurses* (1923), writes that executive ability in the nurse requires "these two striking and important traits of character—moral courage and self-reliance. These two might be combined in the well-understood quality known as back-bone."[12] *Moral courage* is discussed in both the UK and US heritage literature from at least the 1880s, yet it finds its way into contemporary nursing ethics literature as if it were a new concept. In her 1925 work *Ethics: A Text-Book for Nurses*, Charlotte Talley includes a section for students on acquiring and practicing specific virtues in order to develop them. She advises several exercises including reflection on specific virtues, observing and examining instances of a particular virtue, keeping a notebook of these instances, and weekly self-examination.[13] Etiquette was understood to be an outward manifestation of inner moral character.

Etiquette

Nursing's ethics also attended to etiquette. The term *etiquette* is misleading and has unfortunately been misunderstood as simply good manners, often as tied to gender and class. The early nursing ethics literature has wrongly been dismissed as "primarily feminine etiquette" which is to misunderstand both this literature and *etiquette*.[14] The term *etiquette* is derived from the French where it referred to a ticket upon which was written a code of conduct for appearance at court, that is, a diplomatic protocol.

The application of the French word to a prescribed system of behaviour or ceremony at court is probably immediately after similar use of Spanish *etiqueta* (early 16th cent. in this sense), itself a loan from French in the sense 'label, note, notice'. The sense development apparently reflects the fact that the strict rules of protocol, hierarchy, and ceremony followed by the Spanish royal court in the 16th cent. were written in an official list.[15,16]

Originally designating the written note, in the sense-evolution (change in meaning over time) of the word, *etiquette* became a reference to the behavior itself. *Etiquette* similarly referred to "the order of procedure established by custom in the armed forces (esp. with reference to promotion and hierarchy), or in a legislative body, etc."[17] Thus, *etiquette* carries the meaning of formal behavioral protocol in which diplomacy is enabled, as well as that of military protocol. In the context of nursing, and hospital etiquette, *etiquette* does, indeed, have reference to *military discipline* and deals with the nurse-to-physician relationship, or nurse-to-nursing superiors, that is to *ward discipline*. As Anna Maxwell and Amy Pope note, "the etiquette of the army is, to a certain extent, repeated in the hospital. The reasons for its existence need not be discussed here; those who appreciate order and lack of friction will soon discover many for themselves."[18] The physician was the senior officer and the junior officers, nurses, were expected to stand in his presence and to obey his (lawful) orders, with discernment. Nurses were to wear the uniform with pride and neatness. Early nursing textbooks customarily characterized exemplary ward behavior as one of military discipline. For example, Minnie Goodnow (1912) writes,

> The organization and discipline of the hospital resembles that of the army. The so-called military discipline may be criticized or by some condemned, but it must continue to hold sway for the reason that in a hospital... *human life is at stake*.... The primary principle of military discipline is unquestioning obedience to superiors. This involves a formal etiquette. It embraces a strict code of honor, with punishment for its violation seemingly out of proportion to the offense. When an order has been given, it must be carried out with promptness and accuracy. If for any reason it cannot be done, that fact should be immediately reported to the proper authority with the reason assigned.[19]

Etiquette is not simply the superficial niceties of polite society. Rather, it refers to the protocols of ordered, disciplined, behavior of a quasi-military, hierarchically structured setting of the hospital. *Etiquette*, thus, refers to

> The canons of behaviour, such as courtesy, civility, and tact, that would allow diplomacy, negotiation, and relationships to proceed with a common relational understanding. Courtesy, civility, and tact were three attributes expected of the nurse that formed the interstices of relationships and communication, and even allowed for disagreement to be resolved.[20]

It is also etiquette that, in part, helps to set the moral tone (moral environment) of the practice setting. *Etiquette* demanded courtesy, tact, dignity, respect, cooperation, and more. Despite the foregoing etymology, some less capable authors of early nursing ethics texts were simply looking for a paragon of Victorian or *True Womanhood* and manners. In both the medical literature and nursing ethics literature, ethics and etiquette are knit together, often alliteratively as "manners and morals," "ethics and etiquette."

Nursing as a Vocation, Calling, Profession

From its early days, the American literature consistently and persistently refers to nursing as a profession, though it is what is called an eschatological affirmation; that is, it is "both here and now, and yet to come." Nursing aspired to become a full, and more importantly, recognized profession. The heyday of nursing literature defending nursing as a profession occurs in the 1940s and 1950s, with the defense of nursing as a profession in the *Tentative Code for Nurses* (1940) (material inappropriate to a code of ethics) and Genevieve and Roy Bixler's prominent article (1945) "The Professional Status of Nursing"[21] and its reprise, of the same title, in 1959.[22] Though it periodically becomes quiescent, the discussion of nursing as a profession has never ceased; the discussions consistently emphasize the now discredited trait characteristics approach of (a) the development of nursing's "distinctive body of knowledge" and (b) "autonomy" of nursing practice. Though leaders asserted that nursing was a profession—they simultaneously understood nursing as a calling or vocation as well. *Vocation* and *calling* mean the same thing, one from the Latin *vocare (to call)*, the other from the Anglo-Saxon (old English) *ceallian.*[23]

In a graduation address, Isabel Hampton (Robb) reminded the graduates of "the sacredness of their calling,"[24] which indicates that a calling is often thought of in religious terms, as in called by God, though that need not be. In essence, a calling is that to which one is drawn by virtue of one's predispositions, capacities, values, and perspectives, which may then be tutored and formed into the preparation and identity necessary for the exercise of one's calling. A calling intrinsically invokes one's passions and commitments, such as the well-being of others, social justice, walking with another who is suffering, birthing new life, presence at the end of life, and so on. The importance of a calling is that it can sustain one in the midst of difficulty. A calling is not about abilities; there are many things that one can do, and do well, but if it is not that to which one is called it becomes hard labor, grinding and wearisome. English psychologist Beatrice Edgell makes note of this for her British nursing audience (see Chapter 7). Nursing leaders consistently held notions of *profession and calling* together, but held together in tension. There are, however, two ways in which to understand *profession*—as an organized occupational practice requiring specific knowledge and skill, often represented by a guild, or, in an older sense of *what one professes*, e.g., I *profess* nursing, which more closely aligns its meaning with that of calling or vocation. Some authors incorporate both meanings of profession in their understanding.

There are two streams of discussion that follow: first, the nature of nursing education, and second, of just remuneration versus the exploitation of nursing labor. For example, Isabel Robb addresses both these concerns when she writes:

> In speaking of nursing as a profession for women, I have used the term advisedly. Some prefer the term vocation, or the Anglo-Saxon word, calling. The last, if made to bear the significance of a direct call from God to a consecrated service, would rather suggest, on first thought, a sisterhood with its religious restrictions; and surely profession means all that vocation does and more. The work of the clergy, the lawyer, and the physician is spoken of as a profession; the term implies more responsibility, more serious duty, a higher skill, and an employment needing education more thorough than that required in some vocations of life. Every day these qualities are more and more being demanded of the trained nurse by modern physicians and exacting laity...[25]

With reference to the gainfulness of a profession, she then states that:

> The trained nurse, then, is no longer to be regarded as a better trained, more useful, higher class of servant, but as one who has knowledge that is worthy of respect, consideration and due recompense—in a certain degree a member of a profession...[26]

More will be said, momentarily, about the attributes of the nurse, such as dedication, devotion, caring, and compassion, being such that they lend to a risk of exploitation. Exploitation, here, is preying upon nurses *because* of the values of the profession and the identity-based commitment of nurses to those values. Exploitation in the sense of just or unjust wages is often a bit different, and more directly related to institutional priorities and profit though ultimately is still predation. Robb, above, is alluding to four problems that, at the turn of the last century, nursing (in the home) faced: to distinguish itself from domestic service; to come to be regarded as a skilled profession; to retain the elements of calling; and to secure remuneration commensurate with nurses' education and skill and consistent with that of other professions.

Formation: What It Is and What It Is Not

Formation involved shaping the identity of a nursing student in a way that would foster the incorporation of the values, aims, ideals, goods, virtues, norms, knowledge, and skills of the profession as a part of one's identity. From the early days when the student is learning to *do* nursing, in the process of formation, the student *becomes* a nurse, so that personal and professional identity coalesce, are unified. Formation in nursing education is

> the method by which a person is prepared for a particular task or is made capable of functioning in a particular role. One forms, as well as educates,

priests, soldiers, nurses, and doctors in a process that moves beyond the knowledge content of those crafts to the moral content of the practices—the obligations entailed, the demands imposed—and thus to the moral formation of the practitioners.[27]

Early nursing engaged in *formation*, not *socialization*. Formation, as understood in nursing ethics, would in today's nursing education require an educational shift "from *socialization* and role-taking *to formation*,"[28] a shift that the Carnegie Foundation National Study of Nursing Education calls for.[29] *Socialization* involves learning to behave in certain ways, rather than the inner incorporation of those attributes and elements of identity that would in themselves give rise to the desired behaviors; *socialization* is external, *formation* is internal. Kathryn Halverson, et al. identify the attributes of professional identity:

> seven defining attributes for the concept of professional identity: internalized values and ideas, a sense of self that is derived and perceived from the nursing role, professional identity as a component of overall identity, engagement in duty and responsibility responsive to public interest and a concern for achieving social ends, perception of self that is influenced by the image of nursing, knowledge of what the role entails, and feelings of self-certainty in the role.[30]

Though this is a contemporary understanding it aligns with the understanding in the nursing ethics literature. This is the nurse who would not be, for example, disrespectful or lie to a patient because "that would be inconsistent with the very nature of nursing and who I am as a nurse." This is not a rational calculation (not "critical thinking") but rather a way of being-a-nurse that then guides practice in all the classes of relationship.

A Relational Motif for Ethics

Classes of Relationship

Early nursing ethics is relationally based. As has been noted elsewhere,[31] and in Chapter 4, the earliest American journal articles on nursing ethics (1889) begin by identifying seven classes of ethical relationship:

> For convenience sake, I will divide the duties of a nurse into seven classes: 1st. Those she owes to the family. 2nd. Those she owes to the doctor. 3rd. Those owing the family, friends, and servants of the patient. 4th. To herself. 5th. To her own friends. 6th. To her own hospital or school. 7th. To other nurses.[32]

The first relationship is, as always, to the patient. Given that approximately 80 percent of early nursing took place in the home, the patient and her or his family were the locus of concern; the patient was not simply the individual sick person. Over the decades, the number of classes of relationship would be reduced and reconfigured. The heritage literature follows a relational motif in articulating the duties that accrue to the nurse within each class of relationship. From the start, this gives nursing a structure within which to categorize and explicate nursing's ethical responsibilities, concerns, values, goods, and ideals. Many of the nursing ethics heritage books organize their chapters within this relational framework. A few of the books address only one relationship: nurse and patient. Let us move now to a few examples of ethical concerns within the assorted nurse relationships.

The Nurse–Patient Relationship as Compassionate, Whole-Person Care

The nursing ethics literature is sometimes written in first-person narrative, but always reflects the nursing experience of the author. In part, because this literature is not quite the rhetoric of today's academic journal articles with "theoretical frameworks," it tends to be dismissed. However, a more attuned reading of that literature is warranted in order to see the values, goods, and ideals that are embedded within it. For example, in her section "Seeing the Real Patient," Aikens writes:

> To see the real patient we must, in most cases, try to see him or imagine him in his natural environment; we must see him in relation to his family or relatives, or, lacking these, his associates, those with whom he mingles in everyday live.... We forget that in many cases an enforced stay, means loss of wages, frequently debt, worry from fear of losing a job, anxiety over family problems, perhaps overdue rent, perhaps hungry children, all these and more; yet in our shortsightedness, we see none of these things in the background as we move in and out among the patients. We need not only good judgment but we need a kind heart, and a mind that desires keenly to understand the whole man, we need to learn to see beyond the standing orders and general routine.[33]

The understanding of and exhortation to whole-person care, the notion of patient individuality, of kindness and compassion, and of a skilled understanding are all incorporated here. She concludes that section of her book with these words:

> A clear understanding of people is rarely reached until we have learned something of what constitutes pleasure to them and what their ambitions and disappointments have been. Would we be a little more patient, a little more kind, a little more attentive to their requests, would our service be a little less mechanical, if we could see back into their lives more clearly, see each patient in his own setting, surrounded by the people and things which make up his life? Is it part of our duty to try to see these things; to nurse the individual, not simply his disease? If so, how might we become proficient?[34]

It is a moral duty for the nurse to see the patient as person, as individual, in her or his totality, in giving kind, patient, and understanding care with imagination. This is care that is attuned to the individual's situation, context, and needs.

In her chapter "Tact and Imagination," Aikens has a section on the patient newly admitted to the hospital. She writes that, "Apart from standing [medical] orders... may each nurse not make out for herself a set of standing rules of ethics for new patients which might read somewhat as follows." Those rules of ethics include:

- Meet friends of the patient if possible and impress them with personal interest in the patient.
- Be sure to speak a few reassuring words of comfort and sympathy to patient as soon as possible after arrival.
- Find out when food was last taken. Give light nourishment if needed and permitted, and if meal is not near.
- Inquire sympathetically about length of illness. Inquire as to whether he feels comfortable at present.
- Find out if patient has dread of hospital, and is suffering from needless terrors, and try to remove dread.
- Never ignore the existence of new patient till something has to be done for him.
- Cultivate habit of showing helpful interest, and study how to be kind as needed in each case. Try to remember likes and dislikes when special points are mentioned.
- Remember that we are dealing with afflicted souls, hungry souls, as well as afflicted bodies.[35]

Here, Aikens is cultivating and inculcating (the term used in that period) the values and good central to nursing care such as concern, interest, reassurance, attention, sympathy, comfort, exploring needs, allaying fear, individuality, and compassion. These are her "standing rules of ethics for new patients."

Quoting physician Richard Cabot, Aikens writes:

Our profession, the profession to which you as nurses and we as physicians contribute what we can, brings us constantly into the closest contact with human souls. We are with our fellow creatures in their hours of storm and stress when what is deepest and truest in them comes to light. Such contact is sure to affect us in one of two ways. It can ennoble us or it can make us callous. There is no other alternative. Familiarity with the great spiritual experiences that attend birth, death, and bereavement, with the awful perplexity of choosing between one life and another, and the awful desolation of the sufferer who learns for the first time his malady is incurable, drives us all either to shut our ears to the poignant message of our work, hopeless of understanding its meaning, or else opens every sentence and every faculty to meet the world's revelations, with the faith that is the essence of religion.[36]

Nurse educators sought to prepare nurses who could face the poignant, joyous, terrorizing, and sorrowing moments in the lives of their patients with caring, skilled compassion—without becoming undone themselves.

Professional Secrets

The nurse–patient relationship is one of great intimacy. As Fox writes (see Chapter 7):

> In no other field of work... are you brought into such a succession of close and delicate intimacies with others. You are admitted where the patient's nearest and dearest relatives are excluded; you are told what is never breathed even in confidence to wife, mother, or son..."[37]

The nurse shares in intimate communication with the patient, but also observes what transpires in the home or in family and friend interactions. Thus, a concern for *professional secrets* is an early, pervasive, and enduring concern within the context of the nurse–patient relationship. I have written about this elsewhere[38] but, in brief, *professional secrets* are information that the nurse receives or observes, in the course of nursing practice, about the patient and family that is personal in nature, that the nurse must then decide whether or not to disclose to the physician. *Professional secrets* are broader and cannot be reduced to the contemporary discussions of *confidentiality* or *privacy*. Discussions of *professional secrets* are rooted in the nurse–patient relationship as one of trust and fidelity where the patient is the first object of nursing concern. Discussions of *confidentiality* and *privacy* are usually explicated within a framework of *patient rights,* and most frequently that actually means legal rights, not human rights. The term *medical secrets* was used in the nursing ethics textbooks that were written by physicians or clergy, which would set all secrets within the purview of the physician. Those ethics textbooks written by nurses used the term *professional secrets*; *professional* referred specifically to nursing, not medicine. Nurses recognized that not all of the secrets shared with them, or observed, should be shared with the physician. As nursing took place in the home, these secrets could pertain to anything or anyone in the household, whether family or not, and were not limited to the ill person or the illness. Nurses kept these secrets as professional secrets within nursing; the nurse made a judgment of what or what not to share with the physician. The early literature also speaks of nurses' *duty of conscience*; that is, the duty to form, hold, and act upon one's own moral judgments in patient care including issues of disclosure. Even then, there was a domain of autonomous nursing practice and discretion!

The language of human rights comes into nursing following World War II and draws upon Nuremberg and Helsinki documents, and Beecher's and related articles on human experimentation. It is at this point that nursing embraces the concepts of *privacy* and *confidentiality* as well as that of *patient rights*, though *privacy* and *confidentiality* are shallow concepts compared with *professional secrets*. In *The Nurse in Research: ANA Guidelines on Ethical Values* (1968), the section "The Protection of Human Rights" is divided into:

- Right of conservation of personal resources
- Right of freedom from arbitrary hurt
- Right of freedom from intrinsic risk of injury
- Rights of minors and incompetent persons[39]

Private duty nursing continues in the home until after World War II, at which point nursing moves into hospitals as *staff nursing*. A remnant of private duty nursing remained for a number of years when nurses were hired by the family to provide *special duty*, or "to special" the patient; that is, give private care in the hospital. Nurses who cared for patients in the home were in varying situations of wealthy, modest, and poorer homes. Though the poorest families would have visiting and not in-home nursing, the nurse might be situated in a home without heat, and with less nourishing meals, and requiring intense labor. Nurses could become exhausted and their health vulnerable. Care of self, under the larger category of duties to self, was not inconsequential.

Nurse-to-Self (Duties to Self)

Duties to self loom large (and uniformly) in the early nursing ethics textbooks. Self-care, as well as self-development, and personal flourishing are thick strands in nursing ethics, that do not appear in contemporary bioethics. Early nurse leaders and educators were adamant about duties nurses owed themselves. Clara Weeks (Shaw) prefaces her 1888 medical surgical nursing textbook with a chapter on the character and duties of the nurse. She states,

> Your duties may be classified as threefold: those which you owe to yourself, those due to the physician under whose direction you work, and such as relate immediately to the patient. Something is perhaps owing also to the school with which you are or have been connected.[40]

The *first* duties are those that the nurse owes to herself. Weeks specifically emphasizes "rest, food, and exercise." Emily Stoney, in her 1896 general textbook *Practical Points in Nursing for Private Practice*, writes:

> A nurse should improve her mind by reading the best books at her command, by going out and visiting friends, and by attending the theater twice a month; this will keep her in touch with outside affairs, and she will be able to converse intelligently with her patients.[41]

Duties to self are not simply those related to staying physically healthy; they include recreation, hobbies, friendships, reading, and more. In 1896, Harriet Camp's series of six relationship-based articles on ethics in *The Trained Nurse and Hospital Review*, two of the articles are devoted entirely to duties the nurse owes to self.[42]

Isabel Robb includes a wide range of concerns under duties to self: continuing education, self-development, maintenance of health, adequate rest and recreation, leisure hours profitably spent, reading, nutrition, friendships, spiritual development, habituation of various virtues, just compensation, savings for retirement, a daily hot bath in the evening for cleanliness and to aid sleep, vigorous brushing of the teeth, meals taken regularly, a "regular amount of well-ordered recreation," two weeks of vacation (required!), ongoing reading, and attending alumni association meetings.[43]

The range of activities that were recommended is extraordinary and extensive. Every ethics book contained at least one chapter on the duties of the nurse to herself, not simply in terms of health and physical well-being (though there was that), but also in terms of being involved in engaging interests, keeping the mind active in literature, poetry, theater—as well as reading nursing journals. Nurses were enjoined to travel to other countries to observe nursing there, but also to observe customs, landscapes, cuisines, and more. Nursing leaders and educators sought a person who was well-educated, well-rounded, and who had a well-balanced life. In 1930, Gladwin writes: "Because the body furnishes the only medium for self-expression and through it the mind and spirit, the real self, are revealed, her first duty to herself is to make her body as perfect an instrument as she possibly can."[44] Gladwin discusses the mind–body connection, and the advantage of striving for *perfect interrelated sanity* [health] *of body, mind, and spirit.*[45]

While it is noted that one must be healthy to give good nursing care (that is, health as an instrumental good), these injunctions to self-care and self-development, as well as professional development, were directed principally toward the well-being, happiness, and fullness of life of the nurse. Self-care, self-development, continued personal and professional learning, and personal flourishing are of paramount importance in nursing ethics, yet do not appear in the bioethics literature. It was, however, restored to the ANA *Code* from 2001, and further developed in the 2015 iteration of the *Code*.[46] It is interesting that the introduction of provision five, on duties to self, in the ANA *Code* was initially opposed, rather vigorously, then came to be welcomed.

Aikens' book contains chapters on health, recreation, and friendship.[47] However, she devotes a separate chapter to "Developing a Symmetrical Life," and writes that:

A fact that should never be forgotten is that, apart entirely from obtaining a nursing education and experience, every nurse while in training is developing a life.... so that she emerges from the training school a symmetrical well-balanced woman with a wholesome outlook on the world in general, and with right ideas as to the part she is to play in the world, is an important part of the training process.... Every nurse has a fourfold nature to be cultivated and developed. She has a physical, mental, spiritual, and social side to her make-up, all needing due care and cultivation, and the possibilities of becoming warped and stunted in growth, of becoming one-sided and narrow, are present in every nurse's life.[48]

For Aikens, "narrowness" imperils nursing care; it undermines the imagination and creativity requisite to excellence in nursing. Nursing requires a *symmetrical life* that today enters into discussions of work–life balance.

The early nursing journals, into the 1970s, are chockablock with travel diaries, book and poetry recommendations, reviews of works of fiction, essay contests, announcements for literary and theater events, recommendations for sports (suitable for young women), needlework and sewing patterns—and much, much, much more. This is a huge body of literature within the journals that is devoted to enhancing the personal life of the nurse. It is also an enthusiastic, warm, and lovely segment of the literature with a peek into the personal lives of nurses. The ethics textbooks written by nurses, and the nursing journals, all address ways in which the nurse can and must engage in activities that lead to a symmetrical life.

The Nurse-to-Nurse Relationship

There is not an abundance of material specifically on the nurse-to-nurse relationship. In part, the emphasis on discipline and all that it entails covers many of the expectations of nurse-to-nurse, to senior nurse, to nursing administration relationships. Early on, there is less explicit discussion of the nurse-to-nurse relationship as nurses predominantly worked in private duty in the home, and there was minimal contact with other nurses. However, when two nurses were needed in patient care, nursing school rivalries could come into play—and there were fierce school rivalries, each school having its own *registry* of graduates. Case referrals were made from these registries, and they determined which of their graduates would be called to a case. Robb (1912) writes:

> this obligation of loyalty must not only include the patient, the relatives and the physician, but must also be extended to fellow-nurses, not only of her own alumna, but also those belonging to other schools and other countries provided they are worthy of confidence.... Thus, when two graduates from different schools are associated in the care of a patient, each should regard it an as opportunity to broaden herself and perhaps learn new methods in her work. Their professional relations should be marked by mutual courtesy, respect and good-fellowship...[49]

Robb calls for "true harmony" and an "*esprit de corps*" among nurses.[50] A number of writers, in both the US and UK, speak of the "tone of a school" or the "tone of the hospital," both of which are discussions of the moral tone, or what today is called the *moral environment*, of education or practice. Aikens addresses the tone of a school in her chapter dedicated to the topic.[51] She begins the chapter by contrasting two hospitals. In one the halls are quiet; personnel address each other with respect, dignity, and formality; patient calls are responded to quickly and efficiently; discipline and etiquette are apparent; and "there is an air of alertness and consideration for the patients' needs, and of quiet dignity about the place that gives a feeling of confidence in the general management, and in the personnel of the nursing staff."[52] In the other hospital, there is chattering and shouting in the hallways, ample profanity and blasphemy, laughing and joking, a physician has his hand on a nurse's shoulder, a patient is catheterized and the screens are not pulled, flippant remarks are made about patients and they can be overheard. And more. The first setting displays a part of what Aikens means by a *good tone*. Aikens is describing and contrasting two actual training hospitals in which she had first-hand experience. But a bad tone of a school is more than a matter of a disturbing, noisy, negligent, profane, and frivolous, collective atmosphere. It also bears upon an individual nurse's responsibility.

> From the day a probationer arrives in a school she is helping to create the moral atmosphere in which she and other nurses are to live.... It may be asked, "What can one nurse do to improve conditions such as exist in the latter of the two training schools mentioned?"... She can refuse to belong to that class of people known as "the quiescent good."... Merely good intentions will not overcome bad practices nor improve conditions. Conditions grow worse, frequently, because good people do nothing. The "quiescent good" members of a school can often be roused to work for better moral standards, if one nurse musters courage to quietly protest against practices which are lowering the whole tone of the school.[53]

But there is still more to shaping the moral environment. Aikens discusses the treatment of probationer and junior students.

> One of the tests of character which comes to every nurse, comes in the attitude or manner which she assumes toward probationers and juniors.... It is essential for the highest good of the school that every nurse radiate that spirit of helpfulness and kindness which should permeate every institution for the care of the sick. There are numerous little methods which a kind-hearted thoughtful nurse may use who has not forgotten the bewilderment and depression of the first few weeks of her probation period, that will do much to lessen that horrible feeling of loneliness and timidity which a probationer feels, in a strange place, where she is on trial, and under close observation.[54]

Aikens discusses, as well, the relationship between nurses (students) and principals, and nurses with physicians—and the necessity of keeping relationships with physicians professional and not seeing a physician outside the hospital.

Beyond the schools and training hospitals, nursing leaders called for cordial relations generally among nurses, and within professional associations, a unity of purpose and concert of efforts. But friendships among nurses was a tetchy issue.

Enduring Taboo—Lesbian Presence in Nursing

Bullough and colleagues write that "it was not until after World War II that a career and marriage became possible for larger numbers of women."[55] Based on the Bullough three-volume biographical collection, approximately 76 percent of the early nursing leaders were and remained unmarried. Because of social conventions and legal disabilities imposed upon married women, women at the turn of the century would have strong reasons not to marry and a distaste for its constraints. By social convention, women who married would cease to be active in nursing and, depending on social stature, might instead become a "patron" of nursing. It is likely that a significant number of these leaders devoted their lives to nursing simply out of a love of nursing and thus remained single. It is also likely that a significant proportion of those women were lesbian, and entering nursing would give them both a professional life of greater freedom than enjoyed by women generally, and cover for being lesbian. Within nursing, there were homosocial communities, female networks, and strong and enduring female friendships, as well as economic friendships. Some of these communities and some of these friendships were lesbian, some mixed, and some heterosexual. It is fair to say that single women built modern nursing and that some, perhaps many, of those women were lesbian.

Lesbians were widely stigmatized in society, and there were homonegative attitudes in nursing. There is no great breadth of research on lesbian contributions to early nursing, or the ways in which they might have been oppressed or disadvantaged, or accepted.[56,57,58,59] This is difficult research to conduct from today's distance. The commonly effusive, sometimes overdrawn, intimate, loving style of letters between women of the late 1800s and early 1900s, or even in their personal diaries, does not lend itself easily to definitive analysis beyond that of close friendship. The early ethics literature contains a few indirect lesbophobic statements casting it as a danger to nursing students, as if lesbianism were a communicable virus. In a discussion of friendship in nursing in her ethics textbook, Aikens writes, "It is hard to keep one's affections always within safe limits, yet it is just as well to know that friendship has its dangers, and to guard against these dangers when possible."[60] Isabel Robb, too, warns nurses about friendships: "Sentimental, intense personal friendships between nurses are a mistake, and are rarely productive of good. In some instances, they must be regarded as forms of perverted affection; they are always unhealthy…"[61] By 1942, Phyllis Goodall writes in (her unfortunate book) *Ethics: The Inner Realities*:

> In dormitory life or in any other way of life, avoid crushes for they will rob you of all healthy, natural desire to mingle with groups of people and within your life they will harbor evils and miseries that jealousy can bring. When carried too far, they will turn your emotions from their natural bent and cause you to have an unnatural and unhappy attitude toward men… the best rule in friendship is to be fond of many and familiar with none.[62]

There is a fear within the early nursing literature that requiring young women to reside in shared living quarters (dormitories) could cause them to become lesbian; the best way to avoid this was to restrict friendships and familiarity. There are undoubtedly other sources yet to be uncovered, but as a taboo topic there may not be beyond these three.

While a UK, and not a US, journal, there is one brief and curious article in the *Nursing Record* in 1888 that is of interest. Its title is "Are Women Clubbable?" It has reference to the private gentlemen's clubs of London, and probably universities, military, working men's and sports clubs, and more. They were initially places for wealthy and aristocratic "gentlemen," but became accessible to professionals. They provided a range of amenities such as dining and parlors for reading or socializing, card rooms, and many held public debates. James Boswell quoted Doctor Johnson as first using the term "clubable," in the late eighteenth century, to mean— of men—agreeable, companionable, and sociable.[63] Women were not admitted to these clubs and were not thought to be *clubbable*. Initially, women were excluded from these clubs, or when included could attend but not speak.

> These clubs strongly excluded women, since women were supposed to be incapable of serious or thoughtful discussion—as Pope had put it in his *On the Characters of Women*: No thought advances but her Eddy Brain// Whisks it about, and down it goes again.[64]

Exclusion was also based on the fact that these gentlemen's clubs could devolve into rowdiness based on the amount of port that was consumed.

The *Nursing Record* article has specific reference to lesbian clubs, and from what I can ascertain is the earliest and only reference to lesbians in nursing journals of the period and is, thus, of some historical importance. It begins with a reference to Grecian vases depicting Sappho of Lesbos (the eventual derivation of the term *lesbian*). In English, the first extant appearance of the term *lesbian* as either a noun or an adjective, and without reference to Sappho or her Greek island, occurs in 1732. However, the use of the category or adjective lesbian did not become common until the late 1800s.[65] Laws pertaining to homosexuality generally applied only to gay men, not lesbian women, in part because lesbian sex was not regarded as sex.[66] The article is not sexualized and not about lesbians per se, but rather the clubs that they had formed that might provide a model for nurses' participation in women's clubs. It is brief and is transcribed in full here:

There is an interesting article in the *Women's World* for this month upon Sappho by Miss E. Jane Harrison, and among other things she writes:—"These Lesbian women had their clubs, in which they developed to the full that particular form of social enjoyment which comes to women from the society of women—only an enjoyment that supplements, nowise supplants, their enjoyment of the society of men. These Lesbian clubs and societies met not for the discussion of domestic machinery—a thing permissible and even laudable, yet scarcely stimulating—but for the keen and emulous culture of the arts. This social instinct between women and women has for centuries been well-nigh dead. How should they care to meet and talk when they had nothing, or but two things, to talk of?—two for the middle classes—economy and husbands; two for the upper—fashion and scandal; interesting for five minutes, bearable for ten, wearisome exceedingly (saving the last) for fifteen. But the true social instinct among women is reviving, is possible now to ask a dozen women to meet without the melancholy conviction that one-half will bore and the other be bored. Well, who knows? They *were* in Sappho's days. One thing is certain—a woman who does not know the joy of meeting a chosen few of her college friends—her own elect—at a well-appointed feast (Sappho herself loved 'things delicate') has a fine sensation yet to try. It is a joy that man, with his keener and healthier *flair* for pleasure, has ever been careful to secure, this privilege to keep some social unions for his own sex alone, and most reasonably. Between man and woman there is and must ever be that mysterious and all-pervading thing—that barrier, or rather the most intimate bond, of diversity which we label sex. The very magnetism that draws has the power also to paralyse; the very charm that inspires speech can in a moment confound its freedom. Strife between a man and a woman, even in words, is a graceless and, save for the lightest parrying, should be an impossible thing; between man and woman there is no 'give and take'; each must give all, and though friendship is possible, *camaraderie* stands forever forbidden by a thousand beautiful conventions from within, not from without. So for *camaraderie*, for all absolute relaxation of social strain, for all keen unflinching conflict of wits, we will do as the Lesbian women did—have our women's clubs." The experiment to ascertain whether women are clubbable now-a-days is going to be tried, at any rate. The Somerville Club, which is only for ladies, was formally opened on April 10th. The members of the ladies committee received daffodils tied with yellow ribbon, and in a short space of time all the rooms were so crowded that it became almost impossible to move. They were very bright and pretty, with draperies of Madras muslin, the paint and paper being stone color and a greyish blue. In the evening, there was a meeting, at which Mrs. Symes Thompson took the chair and Mrs. Scharlieb gave an opening address on "Some advantages of Club Life for Women."... Among the lectures will be one on "Browning as a Teacher of the Nineteenth Century." Debates are also to be opened by Miss Hagemann on "Corporal Punishment,"... "The Place of Women in Practical Politics." Nursing so far has not attracted the club's attention, but it will doubtless not be long before it does so. Anyway, the movement is one more sign of women uniting to help themselves, and we wish it all success.[67]

This piece is noteworthy in that it is the only reference I have found in the early nursing journals to lesbians. It does not condemn lesbians, or sexualize them, but rather enviously focuses on their women's clubs, places of learned camaraderie and debates, something its author believes would benefit nurses.

It is difficult to interpret literature of the late 1800s and early 1900s when attempting to research lesbian contributions to nursing. The common, often overblown, rhetoric of intimacy between women (or sisters and cousins) is subject to misinterpretation; the nomenclature of *lesbian* was unsettled; and homosocial communities, female networks, and long-term female friendships, as well as economic (co-residential) friendships existing into the mid-1900s were confounding. One of the functions of social ethics is "housekeeping"; that is, to look within to see if a group lives what it affirms. Nursing cares for LGBTQ+ patients, and patients of all races and ethnicities, and affirms respectful, dignified, care for all—while, dissonantly, lesbians within nursing are still hidden among us. Nursing is now in a period of intensive self-examination for unacknowledged racism, and yet nursing has remained quietly heteronormative and homonegative. There is more housekeeping to be done.

The Nurse-to-Physician Relationship

The relationship with the physician, including concerns for medical incompetence or negligence, sexual harassment, and verbal abuse, are substantial but tend to be addressed rather cryptically. Vaughan takes note of these instances in her dissertation (see Chapter 3). From the start, there is a concern for incompetent physicians, but even more, for a terrible tension for the nurse who must be loyal even to an incompetent physician, yet whose priority and first allegiance is to the patient. Robb (1900) takes great pains to explain that the nurse is not qualified to judge a physician's ability or to question his treatments, neither may she ever criticize the physician to the patient or family. At some point, however, Robb had to give a nod to reality, and she writes:

If a nurse has made up her mind that a physician is incapable, she can always find some means of refusing to take charge of the nursing of his patients, but once having put herself under him, let her remain loyal and carry out his orders to the letter. Nor is it honorable in the nurse ever to cast discredit in any way upon the physician...[68]

When the issue is not expressly physician incompetence, but abuse, she writes:

> But if truth must be told, rare instances occur in which the physician is unworthy of the respect both of the nurse and patient, ... she [the nurse] is not expected to put up with unjust or rude behavior... she is fully justified in leaving the case as soon as an efficient substitute has been found to take her place.[69]

For Robb, any question about the competence or appropriateness of medical care must come from the patient or the family, not the nurse. Gladwin is perhaps one of the more direct commentators on medical malpractice and the nurse. In 1930, she writes:

> The question of the inefficiency or malpractice of a physician may arise. There are, unfortunately, unworthy men in the medical profession, just as there are nurses without conscience or honor.... No rule can be given to serve as a safe guide on all occasions.... The atmosphere is sometimes cleared when the nurse remembers that she owes her first allegiance to her patients. No nurse should sow seeds of doubt regarding the physician's work in the mind of the sick one but it may be her duty to lead the family to think of a consultation. She should not yield to her first impulse to throw up the case, but should remember that the patient who has fallen into the hands of a quack or a dishonest, inefficient practitioner needs her much more than more fortunate ones,... nurses have helped physicians to save many lives and occasionally a nurse has saved a life in spite of a physician.[70]

In the more capable ethics literature, a subtle distinction is made: nurses are to be *devoted* to the patient but *loyal* to the physician. *Devotion* supersedes *loyalty*.

By the 1930s, a linguistic shift had begun. Rather than call attention to the physician by specific mention in nursing documents, the *nurse-to-physician* relationship begins a shift, first to *nurse-to-the-medical profession,* then to *nurse-to-other health professionals.* The 1926 ANA *Suggested Code,*[71] an unadopted precursor code of ethics, contains these classes of relationship: nurse to patient, nurse to medical profession, nurse to allied professions, nurse to nurse, and nurse to her profession (includes legislation, i.e., society). The 1940 *Tentative Code for the Nursing Profession,*[72] another precursor but unadopted code, continues the relational motif with these classes of relationship: to the profession, to the patient, to the medical profession, to other nurses, to the employer, to the public, to others (as human beings), and to herself. (The classes of relationships will continue to reconfigure.) In both iterations of the *Code,* the emphasis is on the *medical profession,* and there is only passing mention of the individual *physician.* However, the relevant passage is telling in the way it is stated:

> Loyalty to the physician demands the nurse conscientiously follow his instructions, and that she build up the confidence of the patient in him. At the same time, she will exercise reason and intelligence in carrying out orders. She is to

avoid criticism of him to anyone but himself, and, if necessary, to the proper administrative authorities, in the institution or agency, where both may be working, or to the local medical professional society.[73]

Note that the nurse is being directed to speak with the physician initially (principle of fair warning) and then to report a physician as necessary and if the institution is unresponsive to go outside to the professional medical association. The nurse works up the ladder in reporting but does not allow it to dead-end in the hospital. Still, that ladder is all within medicine's house. The *Code* continues:

> Because a nurse is conscientious in carrying out a physician's directions for the proper care of his patient and conforms to the rules and policies of the institution or agency in which she is serving, it need not follow that she necessarily conforms to the physician's ideas of society or other policy. Nor does it mean that she approves of all the policies and practices of the institution or agency, in which she is serving, or of the professional organization of which the physician may be a member.[74]

The nurse need not embrace the institution's, or physician's, or medical profession's social or political ideology! In general, nursing had not. Nursing had its own notion of the good society, or more specifically a society in which conditions and structures foster health and well-being. The disparity between nursing's view of the good society and that of medicine will become apparent in the arguments over the creation of Medicare in the 1960s. The president of the American Medical Association (AMA) led the charge to oppose Medicare, a proposed publicly supported health insurance, initially for those over the age of 65.[75] The AMA vigorously opposed Medicare, and the *Journal of the American Medical Association* ran screeds against this "danger of socialized medicine." The AMA sent a letter to the ANA asking for support in opposing Medicare legislation. The ANA pointedly did not join the AMA; nurses were generally in favor of publicly supported health insurance. Medicare became law in 1965.[76] Nursing's position on Medicare shows that nursing had its own mind on social issues. Long given to social reform, nurses mingled among the people as district/visiting nurses, public health nurses, school nurses, settlement house nurses, seeing first-hand the social conditions that affected health, caused disease and illness, or fostered preventive health care. These experiences informed nursing's relationship, not just to physicians and medicine, but to society.

The Nurse-to-Society Relationship (Social Ethics)

While I much admire physician Edmund Pellegrino and his exquisite writings on the physician–patient relationship and physician virtues, he misunderstands *etiquette*, and he misunderstands nursing. In 1964, in the *American Journal of Nursing*, he writes that *etiquette* affirms the *dignity* of the physician's calling. *Etiquette* is about discipline and good order, not dignity. It is also about the moral tone of ward relationships. Pellegrino criticizes the ANA *Code* (1960 iteration) and writes that "the truly ethical core of the codes of both professions [medicine and nursing] derives from the dignity and rights of the patient as a person."[77] He objects that the majority (9 of 17 provisions) of the *Code* is about

> The dignity and prerogatives of the profession, rather than with the rights and duties flowing from the human nature of the patient. For example, being a good citizen, participating in nursing organizations, in legislation, in establishing terms of employment are good ends in themselves but they are independent of the direct duties owed to the patient.[78]

Pellegrino was one of the shepherds of the emerging bioethics, a physician, who revered the Hippocratic tradition and affirmed the American Medical Association codes of ethics. Here he is trying to bend nursing ethics to his medical ethics. Nursing is nursing, not junior medicine, and there is an incommensurability of the ethics of the two professions. The medical codes focused on the preservation of the status, income, and prerogatives of the physician as well as the physician–patient relationship.[79] Nursing ethics does not descend from the Hippocratic corpus, nor the medical tradition, and is not bound by its norms. Nursing and women's history, and the philosophy that informed nursing leaders, necessitated that it be socially and civically engaged. The successive iterations of the ANA *Code* have a consistent insistence that nurses be civically engaged *for the health of society*. Pellegrino's view of the proper content of a code is medically normative and oriented to the individual patient, in addition to glossing over the self-serving components of the AMA codes. His imposition of a medical ethical perspective on nursing ethics stands in contrast to Densford's position that nursing needs persons of *social sensitivity*.

> Much like personal sympathy, it goes beyond the immediate situation, impelling action in the promotion of desirable conditions. The socially sensitive student, for example, is concerned not only to recognize symptoms and give treatment but to investigate and use her influence for correcting the social conditions which give rise to the condition. Dr. Hilda Taba cites an example of a child suffering from malnutrition. The socially sensitive nurse is one who not only wishes to care for the child and treat it well but who is concerned also to see that the conditions which originally led to malnutrition are corrected.[80]

Nursing has, until recent years, been possessed of a reformist bias, and has engaged in "unladylike commotion" that Lavinia Dock called for—and got her arrested at least thrice. Densford calls upon nursing to do just that:

> Did Socrates, Jesus, Savonarola, Galileo, Lincoln, and Florence Nightingale adapt themselves to the society of their day? Did they fit in? Were they so well

adjusted that they caused no trouble for the people or institutions with which they came into contact?... Obviously not, since Socrates and Jesus were condemned to death, Savonarola was mobbed [hanged and burned at the stake], Galileo came close to losing his life, Lincoln was assassinated, and Florence Nightingale had to struggle against the conservatism and lack of vision of her contemporaries... we glorify them for opposing evil institutions and for creating new and better ones.[81]

Discussions of nurses' relationship to society pervade the early literature and are usually discussed under the topics of *citizenship*, *democratic ideals* or *democracy*, and *love for humanity*. Throughout, and consistent with the philosophy of Pragmatism, there is a commitment to *democracy* that flavors the writings, and indeed Densford's book has a chapter called "Living Democratically." While space does not permit us to explore it, Densford's book also contains a prescient section on "racial inequality" and another on "social equality."

By the 1940s and 1950s (after Nuremberg), the literature begins to include discussions of *human rights*. From early days, there is a concern for those who live in poverty who require nursing care, for the social construction of poverty and illness, and for health disparities.[82,83,84] Aikens writes:

> The established order of things sometimes has to be upset before much progress can be made. There are conditions that are not right in regard to nursing which should be worked at till better conditions are assured. In the private nursing field especially, nurses are most unequally distributed—patients who sadly need their skill are unable to secure it; nurses who seriously need work are held back from accepting calls to nurses where their help is sorely needed.[85]

Aikens calls for nurses to have a *pioneering spirit* and to pioneer nursing service beyond the established order of things.[86] In an extremely popular textbook on nursing history (1944), Elizabeth Jamieson and Mary Sewell make an astonishingly direct and loaded statement. They write:

> As we scan the great mural depicting the story of mankind, there may be discerned the long and devious course of the evolution of nursing, throughout which the woman's skill in caring for the unfortunate has served always as an instrument of social progress... today's professional nurses are recognised as the utilisation of woman's special gifts in raising the level of the social order through the medium of nursing. At times, her work has been smothered by great forces of hatred and intolerance, the fruits of her labors apparently lost. Yet we see, always, a surging forward in spite of temporary retardation and decline.[87]
>
> In a world of apparent crass materialism, glorifying the destructive forces of war as a means to desired ends, there is observable also, side by side with building of tanks, submarines, and airplanes, the development of an idealism which conceives the possibility of a world affording equality of races, economic

security, and peace... In an age in which society is assuming new responsibility in relation to the underprivileged, the aged, the sick, and even the delinquent, emphasis is changing from mere alleviation of suffering to a scientific viewpoint which demands the searching out of causes of poverty, disease, and crime....At the same time governments are proposing to secure food, shelter, and health for their peoples, according to need and regardless of ability to pay. More and more it is being recognized that only by creating a sense of relationship and understanding among all the various groups of society may there be brought about any permanent amelioration of the condition of the unfortunate.[88]

Jameson and Swell note that nursing works toward social progress; has been resisted, obstructed, and undermined by medicine; they express concern for the socially constructed determinants of health and illness and the social safety net; express contempt for the military–industrial complex, and express a utopian hope for social unity in the amelioration of "the condition of the unfortunate." Even after the Progressive Era has ended, nursing retains progressive concerns for the welfare and well-being of the populace and its health.

This passage is typical of the persistent theme of social criticism and social change across the 150 years of nursing ethics literature. Nursing and nurses are interested in the plight of "the unfortunate," and *social justice* in relation to social structures, so are involved in social programs, social activism, and social legislation. These obligations and concerns go well beyond a concern for health disparities focused on specific diseases or access to/cost of health care within the health-care system, which is central to bioethics' concerns for *distributive justice* in relation to the health-care industry.

Had nursing's origins been different, would nursing ethics have had a more constrained concern for social structures? Granted, the contemporary social activism of nursing is not as broadly engaged today or as activistic as it was in nursing's earlier days; however, there remains a steady stream of assertive feminist critique and feminist ethics within nursing, and the current ANA and ICN codes of ethics consistently require social engagement from all nurses in all roles.

There is an anonymous piece in the 1902 *AJN* that celebrates "The Nurse as a Factor in Political Reform." It is important in that it points to the fact that nurses were broadly engaged with politics and society for the betterment of society, not simply the betterment of health. The author writes:

After the downfall of Tammany [corrupt political machine], the public press commented to some extent upon the work of the "Settlements" [Settlement Houses] as a factor in bringing about this great victory, and special mention was made of the fact that the women of the "Nursing Settlement" on Henry Street had been largely influential in rousing the women of upper New York to a knowledge of the terrible conditions that existed in the slum districts under Tammany rule.

This circumstance is of interest to the profession at large, for the reason that nurses, for the first time to our knowledge, are given recognition as political reformers, a place which we believe in the future they will fill with great honor.

The fact that the Mayor of Boston has nominated a woman to be Overseer of the Poor is another great step in political reform, and we believe that this position could be filled to especial advantage by trained nurses, both in our large cities and our smaller towns, and even in the country districts.

We would like to see a trained nurse appointed as one of the assistants to the Health Officer in every large city where so much of the work of this department is done in connection with women and children. A successful trained nurse, as she comes towards middle life, is a woman of exceptionally well-balanced judgment, her sympathies are keen, her judgment is cool, and her familiarity with many phases of society make it impossible for her to be influenced by the sentimental picturesqueness of poverty. She sees the world more from a man's stand-point, but deals with its problems with that finer delicacy of touch which it is generally conceded women possess.[89]

The relational structure of nursing ethics, and as it endures in the contemporary ANA *Code of Ethics for Nurses with Interpretive Statements*, provides a basis for reclaiming and renewing nursing ethics for today, without the constraints and limitations for nursing practice of bioethical dilemma and conflict ethics.

Ethical Dilemmas and Conflicts in Early Nursing Ethics

While nursing ethics was neither conflict nor dilemma focused, it was not oblivious to conflicts or dilemmas. However, abstract, *a priori*, philosophical rules and principles, divorced from any context, were not understood to be helpful. Nursing ethics relied on furthering the moral values and character of nurses within the context of relationships to prevent or forestall dilemmas or conflicts. Where they did occur, nurses had been taught and trained/mentored in the clinical apprenticeship and apprenticeship for moral comportment to bring the values and good of nursing to bear upon the situation, to refrain from bending like a willow in the wind, and to show *pluck* (or *backbone* or *moral courage*); that is, to stand by the values nursing affirmed, and their own conscience, and to refuse any compromise that would harm the patient or the moral integrity of the nurse. Ethical dilemmas and conflicts are not entirely absent from the nursing ethics literature, but they are anything but the core focus.

However, for those who hunger and thirst for dilemmas and conflicts, there are case examples here and there, but the two chief sources of dilemma material are the works of Charlotte Aikens[90] and Sister Rose Hélène Vaughan.[91] The cases or dilemmas are dated, but the ethical issues underlying them are common today. That is to say, that while settings change (home care to hospital care), nursing practice changes (e.g., nurses give injections), diseases change (Spanish flu to Covid), the underlying ethical issues are relatively stable.

There are approximately 100 examples in Chapter 25 of Aikens' book, drawn from day-to-day nursing. In terms of Andrew Jameton's largely ignored three-fold categorization of clinical ethical concerns, Aikens' examples include both *ethical uncertainty* as well as *ethical dilemmas* (*moral distress* being the third of Jameton's categories).[92] Aikens advances a nursing-specific ethics. Every chapter of her text-book is followed by short essay questions for nursing students, questions that are as relevant today as they were in 1916 when they were published. Hers are questions of nursing ethics, questions in which medically normative bioethics has little interest, such as:

- What is an ideal? Of what value is it in life?
- Explain what you mean by the term "duty."
- Show that in performing one's duty one may have a curious mix of motives.
- What is conscience? What effect does it have on the life and work of a nurse?
- Describe the nurse you have met who came nearest to your ideal.
- How may a nurse help in securing or maintaining the right moral atmosphere in a hospital?
- What should a nurse do when a male patient, of whose character she knows practically nothing, begins to flatter her and assert his undying devotion to her?
- What ethical principle does a nurse violate when she gives to others information which has come to her because of her work as a nurse?
- Should the accepting from patients of small favors or other gifts be permitted among nurses in a hospital?
- Show how the principle of honesty enters into the taking of temperatures and the keeping of records.
- What course should a nurse pursue who discovers that she has given a wrong dose of a medication to a patient?
- What do you understand by the term "professional relations" [boundaries]?
- Are we ever placed in situations where it is impossible to do right, if we honestly want to do right? Give illustrations to prove that this is or is not so.
- Show how the quality of imagination in the nurse may affect the comfort of her patients.
- How may poise of soul be cultivated?
- What is meant by the term "vocation?" In what sense does it differ from "occupation?"[93]

Aikens' is a textbook meant for students, so these questions are intended for ethical reflection in the process of nursing identity formation. Note that these questions are largely those of moral uncertainty that are addressed within Aikens' chapter. And, hey, there is one question on *moral distress*. The questions of principles that Aikens raises are addressed in two chapters under the more general rubric of "Old Fashioned Virtues." These are not principles of biomedical ethics, in the Beauchamp and Childress understanding; rather, they are the consequence of a morally formed character, virtues, and ethics enacted in the context of patient care, hospital relations, and personal life. Aikens also incorporates approximately 100 ethics cases or vignettes in her book. Here are some examples with my "translation" to contemporary nursing:

> A doctor asks a nurse who has just returned from a case of scarlet fever to assist him at an operation the following morning. He insists that there is no danger. The nurse fears that she might carry infection. What should she do when the doctor says he will assume all responsibility? [Think about the Covid-19 pandemic.]
>
> A nurse is called to an obstetrical patient on the second day after the birth of the child. The baby's eyes are infected. The patient, privately to the nurse, blames the doctor... The doctor privately tells the nurse that the husband is to blame, and that he had previously had gonorrhea and thought himself cured. What should the nurse do when questioned by the patient as to how the infection occurred...? [Think about the nurse's double-bind, truth-telling, paternalism, and gender...]
>
> A nurse is called to nurse a child critically ill with pneumonia. The family wish her to apply onion poultices to the feet, and to rub a certain ointment on the chest. The treatments will probably not do any harm. What should the nurse do about it? [Think about cultural practices and cultural sensitivity.]
>
> A [student] nurse who has an unusual memory is able to pass written examinations taking a full 100%, in many, and a high grade in all. Her practical work is very inferior. She seems to lack judgment and tact and is not always truthful. What should the [school] principal do in regard to this case? What point should be considered? [Think about a nurse-educator's and a school's responsibilities.]
>
> A visiting nurse is engaged by a family to assist at a birth and to visit the patient afterward. The doctor's manner when he arrives shows very plainly that he does not wish the nurse to assist him in any way. She offers to prepare a disinfectant solution for his hands, and asks whether he wishes anything sterilized, etc. He gruffly declines all such suggestions and does not even wash his hands before making an examination to determine the progress of labor. What should the nurse do in such a case during the labor? If a septic condition follows the birth in such a case, and the nurse knows the doctor is careless or incompetent, what are her duties in this matter? [Think about a nurse's response to physician incompetence, negligence, carelessness or wrong-doing.][94]

Aikens' textbook is a remarkable work that has continuing relevance and is to be commended for study among those interested in nursing ethics and bioethics now, over 125 years later. The caveat here is that the reflection or essay questions she poses reflect the book's emphasis on moral character, nursing and moral identity, and that identity in practice—not cases and dilemmas which appear at the end of the book. The book, overall, reflects Aikens' own lived experience and intimate knowledge of nursing practice.

Rose Hélène Vaughan's 1935 master's "dissertation" (introduced in Chapter 3) also addresses cases or dilemmas in nursing ethics. She did so at the behest of the Roman Catholic priest (Dom Thomas Verner Moore) who served as the dissertation director for her master's degree in nursing. Moore, a philosophical theologian, was in the process of writing a book on ethics for nurses and wanted cases for his book. Moore's book is a standard treatise on Catholic medical-ethical concerns (abortion, sterilization, euthanasia, etc.) and displays little or no familiarity with nursing, understanding of nursing, or knowledge of nursing ethics. When Vaughan provides him with ethical "incidents" in nursing practice, he includes them in his book but does not actually address them. Thus, Vaughan's dissertation would serve dual purposes. These circumstances explain why Vaughan focused on dilemma-ethics and why her dissertation is unlike the prevailing nursing ethics literature. Still, it is an interesting source for ethical incidents encountered by nursing students, or ethical questions that they raise and not incidents per se. The population from which the incidents or questions are drawn is that of nursing students in Catholic schools of nursing, so that some of the questions raised are peculiar to the specific population and their age group. So, there are incidents identified in choosing to sleep instead of going to Mass, questions about dating or physical contact with one's date, questions about drinking, smoking, informing parents, and the like.

As noted previously, Vaughan creates 33 categories, and some subcategories, in the typology of her incidents. The categories are very dependent upon the Roman Catholic tradition of moral philosophy. Far and away, the most common of her incidents are within the nurse-to-physician relationship, followed by those in the nurse-to-nurse relationships; she termed these "problems of cooperation."[95] Over the 33 categories, there is a broad range of concerns, and a mix of youthfulness, inexperience, and experience, such as these:

- Are we allowed to give a narcotic to a patient that is very sick which might tend to shorten life?
- While getting ready to make formulas for the babies I realized that I had not sterilized the medicine glass. Thinking "Oh, well, what's the difference?" I was about to use it unsterilized. My conscience began to trouble me. I boiled the glass.
- Why is it unethical for a nurse to go out with her male patients?
- A graduate nurse was caring for a patient who died. The interne and the nurse treated the body very disrespectfully and acted as though it were a dummy of some sort. I wondered how they would feel if the person were one of their own relatives in the hands of another nurse or doctor.
- I don't know if this seems to be only in my imagination or if it really exists, but when a physician is examining a female patient and you are sure he is taking liberties outside of his profession, is there any way the nurse can tactfully prevent it?

- A patient insists on making unwelcome advances to his nurse. The nurse does everything in her power to stop these without making herself and her patient conspicuous. What should she do? Leave the case or threaten the patient?
- Nurses are often criticized for having close friendship between themselves—is there any harm in this affair?
- When a patient is not improving rapidly as might be expected, the question is often asked of the nurse, "Whether it would be advisable to change physicians". This is rather a delicate subject and one she is often confronted with.
- We have a patient on our floor who is proving herself a regular nuisance. She thinks she is much sicker than she really is and puts on her light when she wants nothing at all. We are very busy on our hall and such acts are very irritating. It is difficult to practice control, but I suppose to show her our anger would do no real good.
- Is it considered permissible to remove the appendices of two eight-year-old orphan girls who manifested no symptoms merely as an illustration at an anesthetist convention?
- Should a nurse undertake a task and persist in carrying it out even though she realizes herself incapable of doing so?
- Interne and nurse going into a vacant room and closing the door.
- What can a student nurse do in the situation of being forced into the profession by her parents?
- Probably the most difficult problem a nurse has to face is that of being tactful. Each patient has a different outlook and disposition and must be treated accordingly. I never realized before how really important self-control and confidence are. I learn more about it every day and am beginning to have a different idea of life in general.[96]

Perhaps my favorite of Vaughan's collected incidents is this: "Now that beer is legal, is it alright for a nurse to accept a glass of Pabst Blue Ribbon Beer just as she would Fannie Mae chocolate?"[97]

Despite these "incidents," the early ethics literature differs from contemporary nursing ethics literature in that it is not problem-oriented; it is virtue-oriented, relationally oriented, and *calling*- or *vocation*-oriented, and these form the strands within which problems might be discussed and addressed. There is no rationalist philosophical ethics that is brought to bear. Note that virtue ethics does not lead to breakdown or dilemma-based ethics; it leads to relationally based ethics, an aim of which is to avert ethical problems or conflict by maintaining relationships; it is a preventive ethics.

As nursing moved away from nursing ethics and into bioethics, there was, however, one persistent, nagging, vestige that should have signaled the existence of a prior, nursing-focused ethics: *The ANA Code of Ethics for Nurses with Interpretive Statements (Code)*.[98]

The *Code of Ethics* for Nurses as Anomalous

In an era of nursing bioethics, the *Code* is a glaring anomaly. With origins in the late 1800s, and successive revisions for over a century, and a new revision beginning, the *Code* represents the "old magik" that resides in nursing ethics before there was a bioethics. Despite efforts in the 1984 *Code* revision to incorporate more of bioethics, its inclusion was limited largely to bits and bobs of language, but did include some concepts such as privacy, confidentiality, self-determination, and informed consent, concepts derived from historical events, historical contexts, and the law. Recall (in Chapter 5), that these concepts in bioethics surface after the Nuremberg documents, after the Beecher[99] and Pappworth[100] articles, after the period when physicians had lost public trust and stature, and after life-prolongation medical interventions raised questions of futility. Nursing had its own, more nuanced, and more nursing-relevant predecessor concepts in the nursing ethics literature (as in the *professional secrets* mentioned above) that were reflected in the ANA *Code* and were refractory to conversion to bioethics. The ANA *Code* remains within the nursing ethics tradition that generated it.

The ANA *Code* continues and advances an enduring nursing ethics with its renewal approximately every ten years. Lystra Gretter's Nightingale Pledge was an oath, patterned after the Hippocratic Oath, and parts of it could not be understood without reference to the Hippocratic Oath. It was not, however, a code of ethics. There were two predecessor codes, the *Suggested Code* of 1926 and the *Tentative Code* of 1940. The first adopted code was the *Code for Professional Nurses*, approved by the ANA House of Delegates in 1950. It contained 17 enumerated provisions. Over the decades the number of provisions would vary and would become more conceptual and less directly prescriptive.[101] Eventually, the *Code* would be published with Interpretive Statements. The Interpretive Statements provide some explanatory material but, more importantly, provide guidelines for the application of the provisions in different settings or under different conditions. The Interpretive Statements are now regarded as a part of the *Code* itself.[102,103]

The *Code* is neither derivative nor representative of bioethics. Its contents retains a relational structure and explicates the duties of nurses within each of the relationships. It incorporates an enduring concern for a broad social ethics and for nurses' duties toward themselves; and addresses issues, values, and ideals central to nursing ethics that do not appear in the general bioethics literature, and sometimes, not even in the nursing bioethics literature. When our committee presented, to the ANA House of Delegates, the draft revision that would become the 2001 *Code*, several nurses took to the mic, in tears, asking that the *Code* not be changed because "I love this Code." They explained how it had helped them in practice. They could not conceive that it could continue to be revised to become responsive to nursing practice as it developed and changed. The *Code* deserves that love as it is a code by nurses, for nurses, and addresses nursing with a deep intimacy and abiding familiarity born of generations of nursing experience, practice, and tradition.

It should, in itself, point us back to our heritage of nursing ethics and prompt us to reclaim that ethics for a new day.

Conclusion

Nursing needs to delve deeply into its 150 years of early ethics literature in order to come to an authentic expression of nursing ethics that is not simply a medical or bioethics with buttons on the blazer moved to the other side, while keeping the same cut. In 1984, a great friend of nursing, Andrew Jameton, wrote that "Nursing is the morally central health profession. Philosophies of nursing, not medicine, should determine the image of health care and its future directions."[104] He is correct. Solid work in nursing's ethical heritage will in fact demonstrate that nursing ethics is and can be superior to all others in its service to the ethical needs of nurses and nursing. Nurses have well over 100 years of nursing ethics, before bioethics, an ethics that is virtue- and practice-based, wise, thoughtful, extensive, and informed. Yet, it has lain fallow and forgotten for the past 150 years as bioethics usurped and colonized nursing ethics. The nursing ethics literature from the 1800s to the 1960s, and the successive revisions of the *Code* beckon us to gather the harvest bounty that is offered toward an authentic expression of nursing ethics.

Notes

1 American Nurses Association, *The Code for Nurses with Interpretive Statements* (Kansas City, MO: ANA, 1976).
2 L. Gretter, *The Florence Nightingale Pledge* (Detroit, MI: Farrand Training School for Nurses, Harper Hospital, 1893). Personal photograph of the original autograph manuscript.
3 Marsha D. Fowler, *Nursing's Ethics, 1893–1983: The Ideal of Service, the Reality of History.* Dissertation (Los Angeles: University of Southern California, 1984).
4 International Council of Nurses, *International Nursing Review, 1926–1927,* volumes 1–2. (Geneva: ICN), 1–349. https://babel.hathitrust.org/cgi/pt?id=uc1.b3506464& view=1up&seq=5
5 Fowler, *"Nursing's Ethics, 1893–1983."*
6 M.D.M. Fowler (2016), "Heritage Ethics: Toward a Thicker Account of Nursing Ethics," *Nursing Ethics* 23, no. 1 (2016): 7–21.
7 M.D. Fowler, "Nursing's Code of Ethics, Social Ethics, and Social Policy." *Nurses at the Table: Nursing, Ethics, and Health Policy,* Special report, *Hastings Center Report* 46, no. 5 (2016): S9–S12.
8 M.D. Fowler, "Why the History of Nursing Ethics Matters," *Nursing Ethics* 24, no. 3 (2017): 292–304.
9 M.D. Fowler, "The Influence of the Social Location of Nurses-as-Women on the Development of Nursing Ethics," in H. Kohlen and J. McCarthy (eds.), *Nursing Ethics: Feminist Perspectives* (London: Springer, 2020).
10 Isabel Robb, *Nursing Ethics: For Hospital and Private Use* (New York: Koeckert, 1900), 47.
11 Ibid., 16.
12 C.A. Aikens, *Studies in Ethics for Nurses,* 2nd ed. rev. (Philadelphia: W.B. Saunders, 1923), 197.
13 C. Talley, *Ethics: A Textbook for Nurses* (New York: G.P. Putnam, 1925), 122–126.

14 Sara Fry, "The Role of Caring in a Theory of Nursing Ethics," *Hypatia*, 4, no. 2 (1989): 87–103; 87.

15 "etiquette, n." OED Online, June 2022, Oxford University Press (accessed July 30, 2022). https://www.oed.com/view/Entry/64853?redirectedFrom=etiquette&

16 M. Wiles, "The district nurse and etiquette," *The Nursing Times* XXI, no. 1056 (July 25, 1925): 689–690.

17 "etiquette, n." 1c. OED Online, June 2022, Oxford University Press (accessed July 30, 2022). https://www.oed.com/view/Entry/64853?redirectedFrom=etiquette&

18 Anna Maxwell Pope and Amy Pope, *Practical Nursing: A Text-book for Nurses* (New York: G.P. Putnam, 1914), 15.

19 Minnie Goodnow, *First Year Nursing* (Philadelphia: W.B. Saunders, 1912), 19–20.

20 Marsha D. Fowler, "Ethics and Etiquette," *Journal of Christian Nursing* 37, no. 1 (Jan./March, 2020): 13.

21 Genevieve K. Bixler and Roy W. Bixler, "The Professional Status of Nursing," *American Journal of Nursing* 45, no. 9 (1945): 730–735.

22 Genevieve K. Bixler and Roy W. Bixler, "The Professional Status of Nursing," *American Journal of Nursing* 59, no. 8 (1959): 1142–1146.

23 "call, v." OED Online, March 2023, Oxford University Press (accessed April 15, 2023) https://www.oed.com/view/Entry/26411?rskey=zySLqg&result=1

24 Ethel Johns and Blanche Pfefferkorn, The Johns Hopkins Hospital School of Nursing, 1889–1949 (Baltimore, MD: The Johns Hopkins Press, 1954), 82–83.

25 Robb, *Nursing Ethics*, 32–33.

26 Ibid., 37.

27 Patricia Benner, Molly Sutphen, Victoria Leonard-Kahn, and Lisa Day, "Formation and Everyday Ethical Comportment," *American Journal of Critical Care* 17, no. 5 (September 2008): 473–476.

28 Ibid., 474.

29 P. Benner, M. Sutphen, V. Leonard Kahn, and L. Day, *Educating Nurses: Teaching and Learning a Complex Practice of Care* (San Francisco and Stanford, CA: Jossey-Bass and Carnegie Foundation for the Advancement of Teaching, 2009).

30 Kathryn Halverson, Deborah Tregunno, and Ivana Vidjen, "Professional Identity Formation: A Concept Analysis," *Quality Advancement in Nursing Education – Avancées en Formation Infirmière* 8, no. 4, Art. 7 (2022): 1–16. https://qane-afi.casn.ca/cgi/viewcontent.cgi?article=1328&context=journal

31 Fowler, "Why the History of Nursing Ethics Matters."

32 HCC [Camp, Harriet C.], "The Ethics of Nursing: Talks of a Superintendent with Her Graduating Class," *The Trained Nurse* 2, no. 5 (1889): 179.

33 Charlotte Albina Aikens, *Studies in Ethics for Nurses* (Philadelphia: W.B. Saunders, 1916), 99.

34 Ibid., 100.

35 Ibid., 103.

36 Ibid., 138.

37 E. Margaret Fox, "The Ethics of Nursing and the Care of the Nurse's Own Health," in *First Lines in Nursing* (London: Scientific Press, 1914), 1–10.

38 Fowler, "Why the History of Nursing Ethics Matters."

39 ANA Committee on Research and Studies, "The Nurse in Research: ANA Guidelines on Ethical Values," *Nursing Research* 17, no. 2 (March–April, 1968): 104–107.

40 Clara Weeks (Shaw), *A Text-Book of Nursing* (New York: D. Appleton and Company, 1888), 15.

41 E.A.M. Stoney, *Practical Points in Nursing for Private Practice* (Philadelphia: W.B. Saunders, 1896), 18.

42 H.C.C. "The Ethics of Nursing: Talks of a Superintendent with Her Graduating Class," *The Trained Nurse* 2, no. 5 (May 1889): 179. The author's name is not given in the

article. She was a female superintendent of a school of nursing in Brooklyn, NY, Harriet C. Camp.

43 Isabel Adams Hampton Robb, *Nursing Ethics: For Hospital and Private Use* (New York: E.C. Koeckert, 1900).

44 M.E. Gladwin, *Ethics: Talks to Nurses* (Philadelphia: W.B. Saunders, 1930), 73–74.

45 Ibid., 74.

46 M.D.M. Fowler, *Guide to the Code of Ethics for Nurses: Development, Interpretation and Application,* 2nd ed. (Silver Spring: American Nurses Association, 2015).

47 Aikens, *Studies in Ethics for Nurses* (1916).

48 Ibid., 163.

49 Robb, *Ethics,* 258–259.

50 Ibid., 144.

51 Aikens, *Studies,* 143–151.

52 Ibid., 143.

53 Ibid., 144–145.

54 Ibid., 146–147.

55 Vern Bullough, Lilli Sentz, and Alice Stein, *American Nursing: A Biographical Dictionary,* Vol. 2 (New York: Garland Publishing, 1992), xiv.

56 Blanche Wiesen Cook, "Female Support Networks and Political Activism: Lillian Wald, Crystal Eastman, Emma Goldman," in Nancy F. Cott (ed.), *Social and Moral Reform,* vol. 17/1 (Berlin, Boston: K.G. Saur, 1994), 302–334. DOI: 10.1515/9783110971101.302

57 Susan M. Poslusny, "Feminist Friendship: Isabel Hampton Robb, Lavinia Lloyd Dock and Mary Adelaide Nutting," *Image: Journal of Nursing Scholarship* 21, no. 2 (1989): 64–68.

58 Mary Ann Bradford Burnam, *Lavinia Lloyd Dock: An Activist in Nursing and Social Reform.* PhD dissertation, (Columbus, OH: The Ohio State University, 1998).

59 Carole A. Estabrooks, "Lavinia Lloyd Dock: The Henry Street Years," *Nursing History Review* 3 (1995): 143–172.

60 Aikens, *Studies in Ethics for Nurses* (1923), 209.

61 Robb, *Ethics,* 140.

62 Phyllis A. Goodall, *Ethics: The Inner Realities* (Philadelphia, PA: F.A. Davis, 1942), 175–176, 187.

63 "clubbable, adj." *OED Online,* March 2023, Oxford University Press (accessed March 27, 2023). https://www.oed.com/view/Entry/34790?redirectedFrom=clubbable

64 David Doughan and Peter Gordon, *Women, Clubs and Associations in Britain* (London: Routledge, 2006), 9.

65 "lesbian, n. and adj." OED Online, March 2023, Oxford University Press (accessed April 10, 2023). https://www.oed.com/view/Entry/107453?redirectedFrom=lesbian&

66 Enze Han and Joseph O'Mahoney, *British Colonialism and the Criminalization of Homosexuality: Queens, Crime and Empire* (London: Routledge, 2018).

67 Anon., "Are Women Clubbable?" *The Nursing Record* 1, no. 3 (April 19, 1888), 33.

68 Robb, *Ethics,* 251.

69 Ibid., 257.

70 Gladwin, *Ethics,* 105–106.

71 American Nurses Association, "A Suggested Code: A Code of Ethics Presented for the Consideration of the American Nurses' Association," *American Journal of Nursing* XXVL, no. 8 (August 1926): 599–601.

72 American Nurses Association, "A Tentative Code: For the Nursing Profession," *American Journal of Nursing* 40, no. 9 (September 1940): 977–980.

73 Ibid., 979.

74 Ibid.

75 Wilbur Cohen, "Reflections on the Enactment of Medicare and Medicaid," *Healthcare Financing Review,* Annual supplement (1985): 3–11.

76 M.D. Fowler, *Nursing's Ethics, 1893–1983: The Ideal of Service, the Reality of History.* Dissertation (Los Angeles: University of Southern California, 1984).
77 Edmund D. Pellegrino, "Ethical Implications in Changing Practice," *American Journal of Nursing* 64, no. 9 (September 1964): 110–112, 111.
78 Ibid., 111.
79 Fowler, *Nursing's Ethics*, 224–226.
80 Katharine J. Densford and Millard S. Everett, *Ethics for Modern Nurses: Professional Adjustments I* (Philadelphia: W.B. Saunders, 1946), 22–23.
81 Ibid., 30.
82 Marsha D.M. Fowler, *Guide to Nursing's Social Policy Statement: Understanding the Essence of the Profession from Social Contract to Social Covenant* (Silver Spring, MD: American Nurses Association, 2015), 189–191.
83 Fowler, "Nursing's Code of Ethics, Social Ethics, and Social Policy."
84 Marsha D. Fowler, "The Influence of the Social Location of Nurses-as-Women on the Development of Nursing Ethics," in Helen Kohlen and Joan McCarthy (eds.), *Nursing Ethics: Feminist Perspectives* (London: Springer, 2020).
85 Aikens, *Studies in Ethics for Nurses* (1923), 230, 250.
86 Ibid., 262.
87 Elizabeth Jamieson and Mary Sewell, *Trends in Nursing History*, 2nd ed. (Philadelphia: W.B. Saunders, 1944), 622–624.
88 Ibid.
89 Anon., "Editorial Comment: The Nurse as a Factor in Political Reform," *American Journal of Nursing* 2, no. 4 (January 1902): 301.
90 Aikens, *Studies in Ethics for Nurses* (1916).
91 Rose Hélène Vaughan, *The Actual Incidence of Moral Problems in Nursing: A Preliminary Study in Empirical Ethics*, Dissertation (Washington, DC: Catholic University Press, 1935).
92 Andrew Jameton, *Nursing Practice: The Ethical Issues* (Upper Saddle River, NJ: Prentice Hall, 1984).
93 Aikens, *Studies in Ethics for Nurses* (1916).
94 Ibid., 295, 300–301, 282, 288.
95 Vaughan, *Incidence*, 21–22.
96 Ibid., 45–90.
97 Ibid., 47.
98 American Nurses Association, *The Code of Ethics for Nurses with Interpretive Statements* (Silver Spring, MD: ANA, 2015).
99 Henry K. Beecher, "Ethics and Clinical Research," *New England Journal of Medicine* 274, no. 24 (June 1966): 1456–1460.
100 Maurice Henry Pappworth, "Human Guinea Pigs: A Warning," *Twentieth Century Magazine* (1962): 66–75. See also: Maurice Henry Pappworth, *Human Guinea Pigs: Experimentation on Man* (London: Routledge & Kegan Paul, 1967). See also: M. Pappworth, "'Human Guinea Pigs' – a History," *British Medical Journal* 301 (December 1990): 1456–1460.
101 Marsha Fowler, "A Chronicle of the Evolution of the Code for Nurses," in G. White (ed.), *Ethical Dilemmas in Contemporary Nursing Practice* (Washington, DC: American Nurses' Publishing, 1992), 149–154.
102 Fowler, *Nursing's Ethics.*
103 Marsha Fowler, "Nursing's Ethics," in A. Davis and M. Aroskar (eds.), *Ethical Dilemmas and Nursing Practice*, 4th ed. (Norwalk, CT: Appleton & Lange, 1997), 16–33.
104 Jameton, *Nursing Practice*, xvi.

9

STUDYING EXPERT ETHICAL COMPORTMENT AND PRESERVING THE ETHICS OF CARE AND RESPONSIBILITY EMBEDDED IN EXPERT NURSING PRACTICE

Patricia Benner

The starting points of this chapter are, first, to get beyond three social imaginaries that impede interdependence and caring for one another; a Cartesian and Kantian social imagination of moral thought and agency;[1] and a technological self-understanding with a primacy of autonomy and problem solving. The second focus in on an *ethics of care and responsibility* from the Christian and virtue ethics traditions as they show up in expert nursing practice.[2]

The key taken-for-granted *social imaginary* in the late modern era is to imagine that human beings' most basic way of being-in-the-world is as separate, private, subjective, and idiosyncratic individuals, standing over an objective world (as if a disembodied mind is separate from all other minds). On this Cartesian view,[3,4,5] the mind is separate from the body, and the body and mind stand apart from one another and "outside of" and separately from the world. For the first point, Charles Taylor points to three main social imaginaries of late modernity all of which understand the self as apart from their skillful and perceptive embodied engagement in the world.[6] Taylor notes that the late modern person is not enfleshed, the person is excarnate,[7] leaving out the nature of embodied intelligence, perception, and skilled know-how. This *representational view* of the mind posits that schema, thoughts, and concepts (representations) lodged in the mind,[8,9] separated from body and world, determine what and how objects in the world are perceived.[10,11] This Cartesian view is refuted by current learning sciences, and philosophy. Morality, steeped in a Cartesian view of the mind, is refuted here by nurses' skilled embodied know-how and insights revealed in nurses' narratives about caring for patients and families. For the second point, these narratives demonstrate *a relational ethics of care* that demonstrate skills of *attentiveness*, *involvement*, and *responsiveness* that allow these nurses to recognize and care for embodied and dependent patients (see

DOI: 10.4324/9781003262107-10

the section, below, "Following the Body's Lead, A Caring Ethic of Recognition, and Knowing the Other").[12,13,14,15,16,17,18]

Immanuel Kant's view of morality, moral agency, and actions centers on the person's will, uninfluenced by emotion. These particular aspects of Kant's moral theory have influenced ethical discourse in the West, in general, and *biomedical ethics*, in particular. The pervasive Cartesian understanding of the way persons exist in the world, i.e., as private separate disembodied minds, along with Kant's vision of morality centered on the individual governed by emotion-free will alone are both part of our common late modern social imaginary enmeshed with a technological understanding of the self-social imaginary.[19,20,21,22] Our current era of late modernity is governed and shaped by the pervasive taken-for-granted technological self-understanding that modern persons are rational, autonomous problem solvers, who, in a Cartesian fashion, stand over against problems, taking control, and exercising autonomy to master the situation.[23,24,25]

These three briefly presented social imaginaries that shape our self-understandings and ways of being-in-the-world, along with the social imagination that our most basic self-understanding is that of engaging with others in transactions and exchanges of "mutual benefit" (see Taylor, *Modern Social Imaginaries*), hide our embodied interdependence, and our member-participant selves who are finite, embodied, and necessarily interdependent and dependent.[26] These self-understandings cause *practices of care and responsibility* to be marginalized and overlooked in public institutions, discourse, and social practices. The Cartesian, Kantian, and technological views of moral agency of the self misrepresent and misunderstand our interdependent, dependent, and embodied existence, and guide much of our moral and ethical discourse. They are false self-understandings that hinder caregiving and care-receiving practices as finite, embodied, vulnerable, and dependent member-participants of society, families, and communities.

As embodied, finite member-participants, we are first and foremost socially constituted, embodied, and interdependent. As human beings we *live* our embodied, finite human ways of being in the world, and as *a life manifestation* it is natural to respond to a vulnerable person in need with care; we have to have a *reason* not to care, according to Løgstrup.[27] Kari Martinsen, a Norwegian nurse philosopher, following Løgstrup and her own theory of caring, also holds that care is a *life manifestation* and a natural human response to meeting a vulnerable embodied other.[28] They define this natural response of care in response to another's vulnerability, a *life manifestation*, a pre-cultural part of being born into an already created world where care is possible.

We are formed, according to the pervasive modern social imaginary as separate autonomous, individuals—separate agents—who have mastery over the frailties of finitude, embodiment, and interdependence—imagining that, as autonomous agents, we primarily engage in mutually beneficial exchanges with others. But this social imagination of how we exist in the world comes at unsustainable and extremely high costs, personally, socially, and societally. Fortunately, skills, capacities, *virtues* of *attentiveness*, and *responsiveness* of *care and responsibility* are rich and abundant in the ethical comportment of most civil, decent persons who respond to persons who are injured or in need of care along with the expert nurses we studied, who are positioned and knowledgeable about providing care to ill and vulnerable persons. The *ethics of care and responsibility* is marginalized, and not well supported by the staffing and work design patterns in health-care institutions. Yet, expert nurses sustain them in their practice, staying true to the nursing mandate to provide care to the ill and vulnerable. These caring practices are illustrated below by expert nurses who responded to nonverbal patients by *following the body's lead*, and to the importance of *knowing the patient* in nursing practice.

Narratives and observations of nursing practice demonstrate nurses' *attentiveness* and *responsiveness* to patients' embodied strengths, concerns, vulnerabilities, and embodied intentionality. This *ethical comportment of care and responsibility* exemplifies *attunement* to particular embodied patients, and an ethical comportment of responsive, responsible care.[29]

This chapter argues that practice communities and their shared narratives of exemplary practice based on *everyday ethical comportment* form practice traditions steeped in notions of good internal to the practice that act as moral sources for practice. *Ethical comportment* is defined as the skilled know-how of embodying and enacting notions of good in particular clinical nursing practice situations.

In contrast to *ethical comportment*, *biomedical ethics*, a principle-based, procedural-based decision-making ethics,[30] is a narrower approach to ethics, using the application of formal principles to ensure rights and justice in situations where ethical conflicts, dilemmas, or puzzles exist. The formal moral principles used in biomedical ethics are based upon what is the right thing to *do*, rather than on what are good ways to *be*, in order to provide excellent care in particular situations. Biomedical quandary and procedural ethics depend on everyday skillful ethical comportment and practical moral reasoning formed by the members of the health-care practice community to exercise a biomedical principle-based, decision-making approach to ethics. Quandary and procedural ethics focus on breakdowns in everyday ethical comportment, and on the adjudication of rights in situations of moral dilemmas, injustice, or infringement on patients' rights. Biomedical ethics focuses on what is the right thing *to do* rather than on ways *to be* and *do good*. The moral goals of defining rights and seeking justice defines obligations and duties, rather than the nature of a good life and good practice.

To examine notions of the good life, what is worth being and preserving, one must study everyday expert ethical comportment and narratives of actual practice embedded in communities of practice.[31] Principle-based procedural approaches to ethics focusing on adjudicating rights and principles cannot stand alone as a moral discourse or practice, because they cannot provide a positive statement of the good, and yet they depend on an everyday ethical comportment and practical knowledge of what constitutes good practice in particular situations. As Benner, Tanner, and Chesla (2009) note:

> Skillful comportment is more complicated than any theoretical account. For example, a theoretical discourse about rights and justice is deprived for two reasons. First, the formal theory cannot point out all the skilled know-how… encountered in practice, and second, a formal procedural ethics cannot account for the qualitative distinctions and complexities in living it out.[32]

Charles Taylor's work on (a) the nature of practical reasoning, exemplified in nursing by science-using clinical reasoning, (b) the notion of *strong evaluations* as opposed to simple preferences, and (c) the role of story in capturing ethical comportment and qualitative distinctions in socially organized practices all enrich the ethical discourse in health care. These ethical themes in Taylor's work will appear throughout this chapter.[33,34]

The Nature of Clinical Reasoning, a Science-Using Form of Practical Reasoning

Taylor contrasts reasoning that occurs across time through changes in the patient's clinical condition with "snapshot" or static reasoning that provides "yes" or "no" answers at particular points in time.[35] Scientific reasoning breaks the situation down into non-overlapping elements and explicates all the relevant criteria for making an absolute judgment at a particular point in time. Unlike scientific reasoning, clinical and ethical *reasoning in transitions* is comparable to a "moving picture" rather than a presentation of separate slides in a PowerPoint presentation. Clinical reasoning across time allows gains and losses in understanding across time to be considered along with a range of possible intervention consequences and futures. The good practitioner must be *attuned* to the clinical situation in order to skillfully intervene in ways that are true to the patient's clinical needs, concerns, and changing clinical condition. Ethical comportment requires good science and caring practices and their situated skillful use in particular practice situations.

Moral Choices as "Strong Evaluations"

Charles Taylor's notion of *strong evaluations* (in *Sources of the Self*) is of strong choices rather than simple choices or decision-making because the choice matters as to how the person understands what he stands for and how and what he wants to be. Strong evaluations are linked to how the person wants to live her or his life. For example, nurses make strong evaluations as opposed to simple consumer choices, or strictly "cause and effect choices." Nurses' strong evaluations are based on qualitative distinctions, for example between alleviating patient suffering or the possibility of increasing it. They attend to these qualitative distinctions in their nursing care through *attentiveness* and skills of *involvement* with the patient and demonstrating *relational ethical comportment with particular patients and families*. Such strong qualitative distinctions are distinctions of moral worth. For example, one can only make strong evaluations about qualitative distinctions in actual clinical situations of ethical comportment in relation to specific moral concerns such as dominating control versus liberating care in actual relationships with patients with particular concerns.

The Role of Story in Capturing Ethical Comportment and Qualitative Distinctions in Socially Organized Practices

As Taylor (in *The Language Animal*) states in his chapter "How Narrative Makes Meaning":

> I want to defend the idea that stories give us an understanding of life, people, and what happens to them which is peculiar (i.e., distinct from what other forms, like works of science and philosophy, can give us) and also unsubstitutable (i.e., what they show us can't be translated without remainder into other media).
>
> What can we communicate about people and life in a story? A story often consists in a diachronic [evolving in time] account of how some state or condition (usually the terminal [or concluding] phase) came to be. This can illuminate things in various ways. It often gives us an idea of "how things came to be," in the sense of explaining why, or giving causes. It can also offer insight into what this terminal phase is like: we can perhaps now appreciate more its fragility or permanence, or value or drawbacks, and the like. The story can also give us a more vivid sense of the alternative course not taken, and so how chancy, either lucky or unlucky, the outcome was. And it can also open out alternatives in a wider sense, it can lay out a gamut of different ways of being human.... Now everybody would probably grant my first assertion above, that narrative constitutes a way of offering insight into causes, characters, values, alternative ways of being, and the like. But many would baulk at the second affirmation, that this form is unsubstitutable. Of course, it may be in some cases, but the thesis here is to the effect that valid insight in the above matters can be given in story which cannot be transposed to the medium of science, atemporal generalization, and the like.[36]

The expert nursing narratives presented in this chapter are accessible to other nurses who share similar nursing practices of advocating for the most effective and astute care of patients, often with shared perceptual acuity in understanding the clinical condition of the patient, and/or understanding of their role as the compassionate stranger, or one who bears witness and offers presence or solace to someone who is suffering or facing death, and more. Clinical narratives offer insights that are neither adequately described or understood, nor explained without the particular unfolding engaged story of meeting and coming to understand another's human plight and/or clinical condition. Narratives can disclose *knowing how and when* (reasoning across time, and situated thinking-in-action) in contrast to objectified, detached lists of *knowing that and about*. A narrative is often accessible and understandable because it is an account of clinical reasoning through transitions in the patient's condition or concern. Løgstrup (in *The Ethical Demand*) calls such an account *the Particular Universal*, and I have called them *paradigm cases* because they gather up meanings in a particular clinical situation that enable the meanings and clinical know-how to be recognized in particular clinical situations. And I agree with Løgstrup that nurses' clinical narratives of their practice are singular universals that have comparative and disclosive powers. Nurses' clinical narratives about their practice cannot be reduced to generalizations, covering laws, or mandates, much less to checklists for things to notice or do. Each must be understood as an unfolding story moving through transitions in the patient's condition and the nurse's understanding of that person's concerns and experience of illness and suffering, as well as their changing clinical condition.[37]

Distinctions between Virtue and Care Ethics

A key contrast between *virtue ethics* and *care ethics* lies in the *way* virtues or *notions of the good* are taken up in the two traditions. The Greek virtue tradition focuses on the inner character of the actor, whereas the Judeo-Christian tradition focuses on relationships, interactions that are relational; for example, how virtues are expressed and enacted in specific relationships and interactions, particularly unequal relationships that go beyond mutual exchange of mutually beneficial good, where the relational members have different and unequal vulnerabilities and strengths.

In studies of excellent nursing practice, my colleagues and I have described relational and skillful attunement characterized by the virtues of *openness* and *responsiveness*. In this chapter, I use narrative examples of *following the body's lead* when patients are nonverbal. An excellent relational caring practice focuses on meeting the other with recognition, acknowledgment, and respect that seeks to allow the other to be who they are, fostering support, growth, and/or self-acceptance or self-understanding.[38,39,40,41,42]

Pellegrino describes the idea of virtue for medical education as:

(1) excellence in traits of character, (2) a trait oriented to ends and purposes (that is to say, teleologically), (3) an excellence of reason not emotion, (4) centered on a practical judgment [*phronesis*], and (5) learned by practice.[43]

Pellegrino's points 2, 4, and 5 also hold true in care ethics. However, distinct contrasts with care ethics can be made between points 1 and 3. Possession of excellent individual traits is desirable in care ethics. However, a care ethics shifts the focus away from the individual's fixed possession of inner character traits, to relational qualities that emerge within the context of relationship. These are relational qualities such as attunement, recognition, and understanding and responding to the other in a caring relationship, attending to vulnerabilities, supporting strengths, dependency needs, embodied intentionality, empowerment, open communication, and so on. Care ethics focuses on the *other's* concerns and needs in the relationship. Focusing on one's "inner character" can create an excessive focus on one's self and own traits and skills. This focus on self fosters self-involvement that interferes with getting to know the other person, their interests, strengths, fears, and concerns in the other's own terms. The relational virtues that include skills of openness and responsiveness are required for a respectful meeting of the other. But they do not just sit as inner, permanent traits uninfluenced by meeting the other:

> One's capacity for responding to those in a caring relationship depends on openness [and responsiveness]. Though the expert caregiver must develop expert attunement to the other, no technique, personal attribute, or skill can guarantee that the other will respond. On the other hand, the response may be far greater than what the caregiver would predict, based upon what he or she offers. Because solicitude itself, is shaped by finitude and thrownness [from Heidegger, how a person is "thrown" into the present or future in relation to their past, characteristic of human being's sense of temporality... existence in time], being *in* a particular relationship precludes choosing clairvoyantly what to offer or what the offering will mean to the other. Such a dynamic and co-constituting relationship is better understood in practice [by the engaged caregiver] and in narrative than in formal theories and laws.[44]

There is an even greater contrast to point 3 of the virtue tradition—the emphasis on reason not emotion in the virtue tradition. How emotional openness, responsiveness, and attunement foster rationality will be further explored later. Care ethics uncovers and demonstrates the relationship between emotion and rationality.[45]

Here, a care ethic departs from a traditional Greek Virtue ethics and also departs from a Kantian will-based, emotion-free, moral decision-making and instead explores the relationships between emotion and rationality. In a care ethic and in all human beings, all the time, emotional access and attunement, and emotion-based perceptual grasp make rationality possible.[46] A care ethic necessarily emphasizes particularity and relationship, both of which require emotional connection, skills of involvement, attunement, and responsiveness. Links between emotion and rationality must not be misconstrued here as *emotivism* or a disruption of reason implied by irrational or unattuned emotional responses typically and falsely attributed to the risks of *all* emotional states in the virtue tradition's separation of emotion from rationality. An Aristotelian vision of emotion governed by reason is a step in the right direction because it comes closer to capturing the way that one's emotional responses are developed in the acquiring of a practice or a habitus.[47]

A normative virtue ethics, when blind to cultural differences in persons' ways of being in the world, can create false normative expectations incongruous with another's cultural values and ways of being-in-the-world. Openness and responsiveness require that the notions of good of all concerned, be explored and uncovered before assuming that one's own cultural values are shared by others. Similarly, a focus on one's traits, talents, and inner character, when it becomes primary, produces a form of *moralism* that also blocks meeting the other in his or her own terms, because of an inward focus on one's own character or virtue. The health-care provider–patient relationship is for the sake of the patient's growth and well-being and coming to understand and know the other person's concerns, and interests are essential to an authentic caring relationship.

Cynicism and disillusionment over power and profit motives and current health care might tempt us to settle for benign benevolence for the sake of improving society. But displacing one's primary concerns for the other, to ensure self-development or improving the society, does not ensure benevolence in the larger society and diminishes a coherent understanding of authentic care of the other in particular situations.

Care ethics and Aristotelian *phronesis* (practical wisdom) share a vision for responding to the particular:

> Responding to the general situation occurs when one follows ethical maxims and gives the standard acceptable response. When an individual becomes a master of his culture's practices or a professional practice within it, he or she no longer tries to do what *one* normally does, but rather responds out of a fund of experience in the culture and in the specialized practice. This requires having enough experience to give up following the rules and maxims dictating what *anyone* should do, and, instead, acting upon the intuition that results from a life in which talent and sensibility have allowed learning from the experience of satisfaction and regret in similar situations. Authentic caring in this sense is common to Paulian *agape* and Aristotelian *phronesis*.[48]

Recovering the primacy of the good over the right in many particular instances, as recommended by Pellegrino and Thomasma,[49] requires a common understanding of what it is to have a practice.

The aim of this comparison of distinctions between virtue and care ethics is to revive understanding of health care as *a caring practice carried out by practitioners of trustworthy character* who are engaged in *care ethics*. The goal is not to replace rights and principle-based ethics because health care also requires respectful treatment of rights for creating equity in the care of strangers. Ensuring patient rights will continue to be necessary in cases of extreme breakdown. However, repair of injustice and loss of patients' rights require insights into good ways to be, and respond in particular unjust situations drawing on notions of good from both the virtue and care traditions:

> Learning to be a good nurse requires mastering the science, technology and theory required to practice, but also the caring practices and helping skills to be a good

nurse who engages in ethical and clinical reasoning. This practice-based approach to ethics holds that moral agency is both agent-centered and practice-centered. Biomedical Ethics... rely on the moral grounding of the ethical comportment of excellent practitioners functioning in practice communities.[50]

Notions of good in ethical comportment in specific situations are lodged in a practice as noted by Joseph Dunne:

> A practice is not just a surface on which one can display instant virtuosity. It grounds one in a tradition that has been formed through an elaborate development and that exists at any junction only in the dispositions (slowly and perhaps painfully acquired) of its recognized practitioners.[51]

Experience refers to the turning around, the adding of nuance, the amending or changing of preconceived notions or perceptions of the situation.[52]

A study of expert nursing practice uncovered a commonly occurring dialogue and conflicts between clinical nursing care, clinical reasoning and judgments, and the generalizations drawn from formal research studies of patient populations.[53] This research sought to give public language to situated thinking-in-action, everyday ethical concerns, and practices by expert nurses working in a community of practicing nurses.[54,55,56,57,58]

One of the goals of this chapter is to illustrate some of the practical gaps between formal procedural ethical theory, biomedical ethics, and the three social imaginaries of the relationships with others laid out at the beginning of the chapter. To accomplish these aims, narrative examples, focusing on commonly occurring expert recognition and caring practices of the nurses whose nursing practice we studied through observations and narrative accounts, are presented here.[59,60,61] These nurses' experienced-based narratives[62] illustrate practical reasoning, skilled know-how, and notions of the good internal to excellent nursing practice. Research observations along with informal interview questions about observations were a second source of research data.[63]

Ethical comportment—in contrast with ethical decision-making, confronting and resolving ethical conflicts, dilemmas, and practice breakdowns—focuses on the actions and embodied intentionality of nurses in actual nursing practice. Ethical comportment goes beyond ethical decision-making, seeking to uncover ways of relating to and caring for patients in particular patient-care situations.

Knowledge embedded in expert nursing practice includes skilled know-how, voice, posture, attentiveness, noticing, and perceptual and recognition skills, as well as skilled responsive readings of the situation, constituting nurses' everyday ethical comportment, an experience-based instantiation of socially organized practice. Ethical comportment encompasses more than prescriptive or formal theories that medical bioethics typically describes or explains.

This view of the everyday ethical comportment and knowledge embedded in practice demonstrates a dialogical relationship between theory and narrative accounts of actual clinical nursing practice. For example, nurses at different skill levels were found to have different levels of perceptual recognition ability, and thus different levels of moral agency and imagination at different levels of skill acquisition, from Novice to Expert levels in the Dreyfus Model of Skill Acquisition.[64]

The writings of Hubert Dreyfus,[65,66] Alasdair MacIntyre,[67] Charles Taylor,[68] and Joseph Dunne[69] explain and describe practice as socially organized and embedded, self-improving, and with notions of good internal to it. Sara Ruddick's (1995)[70] understanding of mothering as a practice with socially embedded knowledge and skill, with a sense of responsibility for the impact of one's knowledge and judgments on those involved in the relationship, also provides strong arguments for considering practice as a moral source and guide to engaging in excellent practice. All these authors have guided the author's approach to a socially organized practice that has notions of the good internal to it, and is self-improving as a moral source.

Sullivan and Rosin define practical reasoning of which clinical and moral reasoning are examples in contrast to scientific or critical reasoning:[71,72]

Practical reason, once central to education… has been all but eclipsed in the focus on utility on the one side and on abstract analytical thinking on the other…. Practical reasoning is concerned with the formation of a particular kind of person—one who is disposed toward questioning and criticizing for the sake of a more informed and responsible engagement. Such persons use critique in order to act more responsibly as it is the common search to realize valuable purposes and ideals that guides their reasoning. Practical reason grounds the academy's great achievement—critical rationality—in human purposes that are wider and deeper than criticism…. In the end, practical reason values embodied responsibility as the resourceful blending of critical intelligence with moral commitment.[73]

This perspective on practice as socially embedded and organized with notions of good internal to well-prepared and experientially taught practitioners is a sharp contrast to a rational-technical view of practice that attempts to remove practitioner judgment through applying the latest scientific research and technology, artificial intelligence alternatives to clinicians' clinical reasoning in particular situations, or application of ethical principles and rules to guide moral conduct.[74]

In this view, practice is a moral source in its own right. Borgmann (2003)[75] holds that practice has far more complexity than theory or science can capture. In philosophy, this is called the "limits of formalism."[76] Theory is not sustainable without an ongoing robust self-improving practice maintained by well-prepared highly skilled practitioners.[77] Theory, however, both constitutes and is constituted by practice-based ethical comportment, skills, and notions of excellence supported by the practitioners.[78,79,80] Theory without practice has no examples that can instantiate theory, create a dialogue between theory and practice, possibly correcting both, and thus theory is vacuous without practice as a basis for understanding what the derivative, generalized, and reduced accounts of the world presented in theory. In addition to seeking to "put theory into practice," nurse educators need to create a dialogue between practice and theory as both sources for correcting and modifying the other, as a way to enrich and enlarge theory by innovative practices and yet unarticulated aspects of the situated thinking-in-action and caring practices of expert nurses in actual nursing practice.

The beginning practitioner, due to lack of experience, must rely on rules and principles but, as experience-based proficiency develops, can perceive a given situation in terms of past whole concrete cases.[81] This practice-based, (practicalist) view corrects for a radical separation of the knower and the known characteristic of a Platonic and Cartesian view of theory.[82]

For the past 41 years, I and my colleagues have been studying the practice of nurses, listening to their stories of their practice, and the visions of excellent practice that sustains them.[83] In narratives of learning, the point is to convey experiential learning, to describe situations that taught the practitioner something new, or altered her or his clinical understanding, or self-understanding as a practitioner.[84] In a narrative of objectification and distance, the storyteller is more of an observer than an engaged participant, and typically tells the story as a strictly cause and effect account.[85]

Following in the footsteps of early Greek philosophers such as Plato and Socrates, US health care has focused on technical rationality to create certainty and limit variations in health-care delivery. But technical-rational technicality, while useful, is not sufficient for sound clinical reasoning and clinical judgments.[86,87] Practical rationality has all but been ignored by managerial practices in the health-care industry.[88,89] For example, hospitals use guidelines and checklists to manage practice, but seldom seek to find out what frontline knowledge workers such as nurses and physicians are learning directly from frontline expert clinicians' practice.[90,91]

Rational-technical thinking, with its quest for certainty based upon generalizations from population statistics,[92] is inadequate because it leaves out clinical reasoning and judgment required for particular patients across time and in particular contexts:

Her [e.g., clinical experts'] adeptness then, lies neither in a knowledge of the general as such, nor in an entirely unprincipled dealing with particular. Rather, it lies precisely in the mediation between general and particular in the ability to bring both into illuminating connection with each other. This requires perceptiveness in her reading of situations as much as flexibility in her mode of "possessing" and "applying" the general knowledge.[93]

Judgment is more than the possession of general knowledge; it is the ability to instantiate this knowledge with relevance and appropriateness or sensitivity to context such as available clinical experts, particular clinical events and timing, and so on. In each fresh actuation, there is an element of creative insight through which it makes itself equal to the demands of a new situation. Because of this element of "excess," beyond what has already been formulated, which the expert clinician proves herself recurrently capable of, the clinical expert generating clinical judgments lies partly in the tacit dimension.[94,95]

Clinical reasoning and judgments in nursing and medicine are laden with patient particularities (e.g., age, co-morbidities, patient sensitivities, concerns, and more) and contextual issues, such as timing, technical and personnel resources, and availability of relevant experts. Invariable rational technicality that ignores judgment about particular patients, contexts, and changes across time is dangerous to patient safety and quality of care. These same arguments apply to the invariant application of rules, guidelines and biomedical ethical principles applied to ethical comportment and ethical concerns related to particular patients.

Nursing is typically described in terms of "knowing that and about" formal decontextualized rational-technical accounts of nursing knowledge that do not describe, nor account for "knowing how, when, and why" or situated thinking in action and clinically reasoning across time about changes in the patient's clinical condition and responses to therapies. Narrow rational technicality cannot account for judgments made through clinical reasoning across time for acutely ill patients with particular co-morbidities, sensitivities, and varying levels of tolerance for technologies and treatments. Population statistics, and generalized scientific guidelines are used to limit errors in clinical judgments by clinicians. Yet these attempts to ignore context, variance and particularities of specific patients to eliminate the judgment of clinicians are dangerous to the extent that they ignore context and patient and situation particularity.

A patient cared for by a group of nurses, whose practice was in our research study, was badly injured in a motor vehicle accident and was hospitalized for over three months with multiple fractures and injuries. All the nurses on the unit on all shifts learned how to position him with the least amount of pain. He was finally able to leave the hospital, walking! The nurses felt disappointed that they did not get a chance to say goodbye and wish him well. A few weeks later, he came back to see the nurses, saying:

> I had to come back and tell you how your care has changed my life. I am an accountant, and I believed that life was about exchanges, that you got only what you offered the other. You get what you give. But I had nothing to offer you, in my brokenness, and helplessness, and you cared for me, with no expectations of any return on my part. Nurses on all shifts learned how to position me with the least amount of pain. I no longer believe that life is mere exchange and that you get what you earn. You showed me that life is more than equal exchanges.

Charles Taylor (2003)[96] points out that our current modern and postmodern social imaginary and self-understanding of imagined relationship with others is one of mutually beneficial exchanges, as discussed at the beginning of the chapter. The expert nurse's narrative examples of care above demonstrate that caregiving requires more than relatively equal mutually beneficial exchanges. Nursing practice requires that nurses meet particular others who are vulnerable and require authentic care with compassion and solidarity. Society could not function without the care of nurses, teachers, parents, social workers, and myriad other caregivers to those requiring support and nurture.

The notions of caring practices and concern for the well-being of others is central to the notions of good embedded in nursing as a practice. Nursing, loving generous parenting, teaching, or childcare cannot operate on "mutually beneficial" exchange mentality. The essential caring practices embedded in society offer an antidote to our frayed sense of connection and relatedness to one another.

Breakdowns and pathologies of caring are written about extensively in psychological and nursing literature on caregiving.[97,98] *Sentimentalism*, one of the pathologies of caring, means that the caregiver elaborates the suffering of others, turning the patient or family emotions back on oneself, as if it were the caregiver's own world and self that are at risk.[99] The skills of connection and care require that caregiver—care-recipient relationships are free from sentimentalism, i.e., patient/family emotions focused back on the caregiver rather than the patient and situation at hand.

Unwanted illness and loss often, and understandably, bring protests of anger and disappointment, "not me, not here, not now," that can somehow through compassion and care get transformed into openness and hope, "yes, me, yes now, and how?"[100] I have witnessed this transformation often, in the most ordinary comforts and gifts, of hope, fortitude, connection, and the patient's ability to receive care when most would rather be more independent than possible, except for short interludes. As a nurse, I learned that I could be with those whose world was threatened, offer whatever I could, based upon my concern for the well-being of the patient and family and my skilled knowledge and frontline placement in health care. Offerings of care require tact and attunement to patients so that families can receive and accept care without undue anxiety and threat. As a nurse, a compassionate stranger, I return home to a relatively intact world without excessive personal suffering.

Moralism, like sentimentalism, involves a similar distortion in caring relationships.[101] For example, you realize that you do not have the required skills, virtues, and moral fiber to offer compassionate care for someone and you seek help. As a result of falling short of skill and strength of character, one works on changing attitudes, character, and skills in order to offer empathic, compassionate care. However, after correcting one's own character development, attention should shift back to the one(s) cared for. To stay focused on one's own character involves an incurvature of emotion on the self, diluting the needs of the other. Avoiding moralism[102] requires avoiding focusing on oneself while focusing on the other, responding to the other as "other," but not wholly "other."[103,104]

Much of my research and teaching career has been focused on the development of expertise in nursing practice. One of the robust findings of our studies of nurses' skill acquisition and practice is that without effective skills of involvement that include *openness, responsiveness, attentiveness, curiosity*, and *genuine caring practices* directed towards the one cared for, one cannot develop expertise or mastery.[105] If the nurse is detached, objectifying, and distant, she or he will be cut off from learning from experience, while being effectively cut off and protected from learning about the other's concerns, suffering, vulnerabilities, and needs. Over-involvement and sentimentalism also prevent expertise in nursing care.

The following narrative accounts of practice[106,107] come from *Advanced Beginners*, newly graduated nurses, *Competent* nurses, intermediate nurses who have two years of work experience and have enough clinical experiences to recognize recurring patterns in patients' clinical condition, and *Expert* nurses, those who have at least five years of work experience and are recognized by peers and supervisors as expert clinicians. Each group was assessed through observation and interviews grouped according to the Dreyfus Model of Skill Acquisition.[108,109]

These nurses' practical knowledge was described by direct observation and informal bedside and small group narrative accounts of actual examples of these nurses' practice. The sample consists of 130 nurses in intensive care units in eight different hospitals in three different regions of the United States. All nurses were interviewed in small groups three times. In the small-group interviews, nurses gave narrative accounts of their clinical practice. The members of each group were asked to do active listening, question the storyteller for any needed clarification, and offer similar or contrasting incidents.

In addition to Advanced Beginners to Expert nurses in the Dreyfus Model of Skill Acquisition,[110] we also studied nurses with five or more years of experience but who were not selected as preceptors or considered experts by their peers.[111] Their narratives were fragmented due to lack of clear memories of patients or situations, and provided primarily an objectified, outside-in account with little description of their concerns or responses in the situation. Jane Rubin characterized their description of clinical reasoning to be limited to "cause and effect" thinking.[112] These nurses had not effectively learned to take up the practice of nursing and had limited narrative memory, and almost no qualitative distinctions or distinctions concerning patients' moral worth and vulnerabilities. Recognition practices (i.e., recognition of changes in patients and recognition of patient concerns, characteristics, and bodily tendencies) were a pervasive theme in the expert nurses' narratives. Nurse participants characterized these practices as *knowing a patient* or *following the body's lead*.

Following the Body's Lead, a Caring Ethic of Recognition, and Knowing the Other

Moral agency, from Kant on, has been connected to one's ability to make autonomous choices, guided by will, not emotion. We discovered in studies of critical care nursing practice that practicing nurses neither limit nor exclusively link moral agency with the ability of the patient or nurse to make will-based autonomous choices.[113,114,115,116,117] This is particularly evident in expert nurses' care of premature infants, babies, young children, and in expert nurses' approaches to caring for adult patients with various levels of prolonged coma. Expert nurses, in caring for nonverbal patients, frequently talked about the importance of *following the body's lead*.[118] They followed the patient's *body's lead* by figuring out what the infant needed, by how active, agitated, or quiet infants and nonverbal adults were by levels of their embodied activity.

This form of moral agency called *following the body's lead* is a skillful recognition of the infant, child, or semi-conscious, nonverbal patient, associated with "bodily intentionality," described by the nurses as bodily characteristics, *leanings*, *tendencies*, and *action states*. Of course, these subtle recognition practices lack explicit clarity, the level of clarity possible for fully conscious deliberate choices made by alert, verbal, well-functioning adults. Silent patients cannot rely on Kant's notion of rational will, but expert nurses engage in emotionally attuned and *fuzzy recognition* of imprecise, vague, or ambiguous responses of nonverbal patients and ambiguous practical moral situations. Expert nurses judge how restful or comfortable the patients are by studying the ways their body responds to their care. For these nurses, it is unimaginable to care for these nonverbal, young, or often semi-conscious patients without responding, and recognizing their *expressions of embodied intentionality* to guide the timing of their nursing care, use of technology, and so on.

For these expert nurses, caring for nonverbal patients requires that they recognize, notice, and respond to whatever patients communicate by their embodied actions through an ethic of *attentiveness*, *curiosity*, and *responsiveness* to the *embodied evidence* of the infant's, child's, or adult's needs and levels of comfort and suffering. Expert nurses refine recognition practices and responses to the embodied "preferences" and tendencies of their patients. This form of practical knowledge (*phronesis* or practical wisdom) and clinical reasoning demonstrates *knowing how and when* and situated thinking across transitions rather than *knowing that and about*.[119] Knowing that and about accounts are objectified, elemental accounts of knowledge and skills leaving out situated-thinking-in-action, relational qualities, communication, transitions, timing—all contextual aspects and more.

For nonverbal adult or infant patients, nurses tried to avoid misusing technology in order to avoid harming patients, while seeking to do good and act responsibly toward patients. The following nurse illustrates this notion of avoiding harm:

> I think she was between 700 and 800 grams. And she was clearly declaring herself ready [to be weaned from the ventilator] and I was sure that was what would happen. So I went directly to the attending [physician] with the blood gasses [showing oxygen saturation] and I said, "1 think she's trying to tell us something. I don't see how you can keep ventilating this kid." Except that I knew

that he didn't usually do things like this and that something was just wrong. And I needed to be satisfied why this small gestational-age baby couldn't be extubated. In my own mind, I needed to be satisfied. And so, I did push it one more time, risk wrath and all this stuff [from the physician], because I wasn't settled with it.

This nurse's knowledge of the infant's embodied capacities prompts her to take a stand for good practice, a stand that she knows that the physician would take if he had not thought that this baby was at a younger gestational age than was the case. She finally clears up the confusion and the infant is successfully extubated. She concludes with an ethical maxim: "Like I say, if you're not helping, you're doing harm with ventilating. It's a little thing but if that kid wasn't extubated that day, then there's always chances of things going wrong and all this trauma." Her attentiveness and care guide her to an ethic of "safe use of technology." She advocates for the infant's particular needs and avoids blindly following inappropriate physician orders. The nurse's underlying question seems to be, "What if I usurp the patient's own best capacities for healing?" To count as caring, the nurse's practice must serve the patient's own growth, recovery, concerns, and embodied intentionality. As noted earlier, Sullivan and Rosin (2008)[120] call attention to how practical reasoning, unlike critical or scientific reasoning (a rational-technical approach), is always concerned with ensuring that one's reasoning, actions, and decisions are made with a sense of responsibility as to how the patient will be impacted. For silent patients, intentionality can only show up as embodied intentionality, through reading and understanding patients' bodily responses.

Intensive care nursery nurses repeatedly describe their observations of particular embodied tendencies of babies. These expert nurses attribute the distinct ways that infants declare themselves in ways that guide what they do for the infants. One might argue that the babies have moral worth and embodied forms of agency, without making stronger claims for member-participant or autonomous will-based agency. It is possible to think that this is 'pure projection' by the nurses, but the nurses' descriptions of the babies' characteristics are definitive, realistic, and recognizable by other expert caregivers. Such recognition expertise is not infallible. However, the nursing care of premature infants depends on its general reliability to guide interventions and inquiry. These expert nurses relate to infants in their care as human beings with needs and capacities for embodied expressiveness. Through the nurses' experience-based knowledge, the infants are accorded common humanity with their recognizable embodied intentionality. Nurses perceive particular infants as growing stronger and more organized in their behaviors. Moral worth, based on autonomous choice, is supplanted by the nurses' expert recognition of the particular infant's embodied intentionality. Moral agency, based on autonomous choice, cannot apply to the nonverbal infant or other silent patients, but through the nurses' relationship, observational skills, and attentiveness, nonverbal patients are recognized by making themselves known to these expert nurses, through embodied tendencies, capacities, evidence of comfort, and discomfort responses. Because these nurses form an understanding and connection with particular infants, they do not take an oppositional "all-or-none" position, "either autonomous or incapable of being understood" that would overlook embodied intentionality exemplified by infants and silent patients with needs and capacities for embodied expressiveness. Through the nurses' experience-based knowledge, the infants are accorded member-participant status in our common humanity with their embodied actions and expressions of feeling states. Moral worth, based on autonomous choice, is supplanted by the nurses' expert recognition of the particular infant's embodied intentionality evidenced by bodily tendencies, responses to the environment and levels of emotional and bodily responses.

Expert nurses note that their skillful practice of following the body's lead becomes more astute over time with experience. This careful experience-based practical reasoning from experiential learning about particular patients' embodied tendencies and capacities demonstrate these expert nurses' clinical grasp and perceptual acuity and their ability to tailor their care accordingly. As the nurses acknowledge, they are sometimes mistaken; this experience-based attunement is more than mere projections. For example, in the following interview the nurse describes how she painstakingly learned to feed a critically ill premature infant:

Nurse 1: This kid just started throwing up a lot whenever we tried to feed him, so it was just trying different things. First off, feeding him more slowly, burping him better, which didn't really seem to matter. Feeding him more slowly, trying to catch him at a time before he started crying really hard, and having a bottle at the bedside ready to go as soon as he indicated that he was hungry just so he wouldn't get worked up, because then he seemed more likely to throw up.... He liked a certain nipple best, a certain speed. He liked the formula warmed to the exact right degree and just the whole combination of things that helped him eat better.

Nurse 2: That is amazing, they have little individual personalities even when they're young. We had a baby who wouldn't eat anything warmed. Everything had to be cold. We had to write this down for everyone.

Nursing practice dictates a response-based ethic that depends on knowing and according shared recognition of particular infants and patients. An ethic of care and responsiveness requires experiential learning about particular infants, families, and communities. This relational, experiential knowledge can only be shared with particularized descriptive narratives and direct observations of practice:

Researcher: You were all talking a little bit about *knowing* a kid. I don't know if you could each talk a little bit about what is it to know a kid? Especially, a 600-gram kid. Do you "know" a 600-gram kid?

Nurse 1: Absolutely, if you don't you're dead. (Laughter)

Researcher: This is a question that I thought about. What about getting attached to a kid, too? I wondered in the early period when you first were in ICN and working with these really young kids who, from my point of view, seem kind of undifferentiated. Did you get attached to kids then, or did it take a while before you really felt like these little ones have personalities and are different?

Nurse 2: I think it took a little while to really get attached to the very small ones. It's as they get a little bit older. When they're two days old they don't really have any personality and they do all look alike. They're not quite human. They've got really translucent skin and they are red and squirmy. But after they get older, a little bit older, when they're a month old or so and they're sort of into the chronic stage that they start developing their idiosyncrasies and you know whether they're going to tolerate suctioning well or twit out for half an hour. Things like that. Whether feeding them makes them feel better or feel worse.

Nurse 1: Yeah, what comfort measures work and what don't. Do they like to be bundled? Do they like to suck their fingers or does that make them have bradycardia. That sort of thing. You learn about each kid. I think you learn it really quickly though. I can go in and take a chronic preemie that I don't know and by the end of the 12 hours, I know exactly what works.

Nurse 2: Yeah, because you know what to try.

Nurse 1: Yeah. What's the most likely thing to learn and you go down the list until you find something that does [comfort].

Nurse 2: It took a while; it took years probably to get to that point. That I could get in there, try all my little tricks, figure out what works and what doesn't, and get the kid squared away. Although sometimes they don't [get squared away], and sometimes nothing works.

These nurses describe skilled ethical comportment based on focused attentiveness, responsiveness, and comforting measures, learned from working with many premature infants. This is similar to the attentiveness and skill reported earlier that enabled the nurse to recognize when the child was ready to be weaned from artificial ventilation. The nurses are quick to point out that their knowledge does not reduce the "other" to total recognition—one nurse reminds the other nurses in the small group interview that sometimes "nothing works." This practice of knowing the patient includes verbal patients and families, but is particularly striking when discussed in relation to the nonverbal infant or adult:

Nurse: I got to know her in a semi-sedated level and paralyzed, on a level you get to know a lot of patients in ICU. You still feel like you know them, but I got to really know her family very well, her mother, her husband, her father, and her brothers...

Researcher: You talked about that you can know a patient when they are sedated, just talk about what you mean by that for the sedated patient.

Nurse: It's something, I think, that's hard to describe, but I feel like I get to know them differently than when they're normal, I'm sure. But there's some sense of who this person is. It's like when you touch them, or when you say something to them, what happens on their monitors. Or maybe just to see what the effect of what you're doing shows up in what's happening to the patient, how they look, even when they're paralyzed just whether their features look a little different, something… if they seem to be comfortable when you are there. You get to know them through talking to their family about how they are. They give you all these stories. When I contacted nurses that had taken care of her when she was a pediatric patient because she had a lot of episodes down on Peds to find out how they'd handled the parents and what she was like. I don't know, you just get to really know them. I felt like I really knew her. I felt like she was a little baby, almost, like an eight-year-old or a ten-year-old, that needed a lot of special attention and that she probably throws tantrums if she doesn't get her way. And that gets in the way of how she's going to recover because she couldn't afford to do that.

Knowing each particular patient is central to fostering patient recovery. These expert nurses consider the patient to be someone who can be known as a human being, even though she is not fully conscious. Recognition practices and understanding nonverbal patients are imprecise moral arts. Sometimes, the person is misunderstood. However, the lack of certainty or even misunderstandings do not diminish the importance of attentive responsiveness and the attempt to recognize and understand nonverbal patients.

To be accorded human status, persons require some measure of recognition and understanding. This is the nemesis of the romantic quest to define oneself outside of societal forces or community, opinion, or responses of others (see Taylor, *Sources of the Self*). Without recognition from others, one ceases to exist socially.[121] Recognition and social understanding are essential to constituting others and allowing others to be known and to be socially recognized. The nursing discourse of knowing a patient[122] points up the distinctions between mere explanation based on criteria or principles, and the moral art of understanding made possible through engaged reasoning and action in specific relationships and situations.

The Dialogue between Explanation and Understanding: A Moral Art

The moral art of understanding and attentiveness is illustrated in a narrative by nurse Linda Sawyer,[123] in which she begins working with Ellen, a woman with diabetes. Ellen's disease had been explained by medical science, but the problems of living with her disease had not been understood, nor well-managed, nor were physicians' and nurses' attentiveness and ethical responsiveness sufficient to understand the embodied illness experience of rapid steep ascents and descents of blood sugars for this patient with brittle diabetes. Explanations for the disease and symptoms were well-defined, but the patient's daily lived experience of extremely labile high and low blood were neither understood nor considered in the medical treatment plan. Understanding of her daily experience was overlooked in the medical focus on explanation.

Nurse Linda Sawyer: The joy of Home Health Nursing for me is the ability to spend more time with a patient in order to make an impact on the person's health status and quality of life. Ellen was diagnosed with juvenile diabetes at age 5 and soon after that also developed a seizure disorder. I first met Ellen when she was being seen by our agency for stasis ulcers of her heels... On this admission, I became the case manager. She was 38 years old and described as intellectually slow. She lived with a very loving family who were knowledgeable about her condition. She and her family belonged to a very supportive church. On this admission, Ellen had a stasis ulcer of her left heel and cellulitis of her foot with an open wound the length of the bottom of her foot. Ellen had frequent grand mal seizures and was on two anticonvulsant medications, and also had frequent hypoglycemic reactions. The family, patient, and physicians described these problems as "to be expected" and "that's Ellen."

I always have difficulty accepting that things couldn't be better and see part of my role as one of a detective. Ellen's mother told me that Ellen always had several episodes of hypoglycemia a week, often causing her to be admitted to the hospital or go to the emergency room. Often her mother would get phone calls at work from various emergency rooms telling her that Ellen had been riding the bus or shopping and had become unconscious.

Her mother could recognize hypoglycemia at night from subtle changes in her breathing. Ellen was not doing blood glucose monitoring, and I taught her and her mother to check her blood sugar level four times a day. Her record showed wide ranges from 40 to above 400 even in the same day. I discussed this with her physician, who then referred Ellen to a diabetic specialist. The specialist worked out a sliding scale of short- and long-acting insulin to decrease hypoglycemia at night. Her mother and I then did some fine-tuning of the regimen to stabilize Ellen at home [adjusting the dosages in response to the patient's responses].

Meanwhile, diabetic complications were increasing. [In the narrative, the nurse gives a detailed list of the complications and her responses to them. Her goal was to make adjustments that would give Ellen as much independence and control as possible ...]

I'm lucky in my job that I can continue to see Ellen long-term since she has an unstable condition, and the health care plan understands that my care keeps her from being hospitalized or requiring more expensive care. Ellen has not been admitted to the hospital in over three years and has only been to the emergency room twice. Her mother says that Ellen has never been so stable with her diabetes and seizures, and how relieved they are to not go through constant emergencies. Ellen jokes with me on our visits and says, "Give me a chance, Linda. Just give me a chance." A chance is what I try to give Ellen every day—a chance to be able to walk on her two feet for as long as possible, a chance to live with her chronic illness.

Even the shortened narrative[124] reveals moral engagement and practical reasoning. Explanation had become a way of coping with the troubling problems in Ellen's life: "It was to be expected; after all, these are the typical complications of diabetes." But scientific explanation and disengaged observation could not ensure that Ellen, her family, or her health-care practitioners understood how to engage in the daily treatments and recognize and respond to changes, patterns, diabetic crises and suffering. Self-care and care from others require an engaged relationship of practical reasoning (*phronesis*, practical wisdom) and understanding. Skilled ethical comportment is shaped by attentiveness and responsiveness and the ability to recognize changing patterns of responses of the patient to treatment and illness. Of course, it would be far better for Ellen to be able to recognize the changing patterns, and this increased independence is Linda Sawyer's goal in teaching Ellen and her mother blood glucose monitoring. Here, day-to-day practice must inform the quest to make the patient as "independent as possible" rather than the impossible goal of complete patient autonomy.

It is especially difficult to recognize a changed pattern when one is living with the change slowly over time. In this case, Linda Sawyer's distance and professional knowledge helped her to recognize a problem had arisen and to react appropriately. She noticed that Ellen's blood sugar patterns had changed, and she began to do detective work rather than dismiss the problem as unresolvable. This process of recognition and response requires the practitioner to know the particular patient and establish a relationship characterized by attentiveness and a skilled engagement. Knowing a patient makes attunement and responsiveness possible.

The Role of Emotional Responses in Learning Ethical Comportment

Engaged reasoning and ethical responsiveness can only be experientially learned. Unlike Kant (2002),[125] Taylor links emotional responses with ethical understanding:

> What I know is also grounded in certain feelings. It is just that I understand these feelings to incorporate a deeper, more adequate sense of our moral predicament. If feeling is an affective awareness of situation, I see these feelings as reflecting my moral situation as it truly is; the imports they attribute truly apply.[126]

Sentience, Taylor claims, is central in recognizing *distinctions of worth* and whether one has a good understanding or grasp in a situation. Emotional response, recognition, and ethical comportment are inextricably linked.[127] In her book, *From Detached Concern to Empathy* (2011), Jody Halpern points out that empathy requires a form of emotional reasoning rather than objectified detached thoughts about what the concepts and mental content of another's person's separate mind might be, a Cartesian and Kantian view of rationality, emotion, and empathy.[128] Her argument is that, unlike a Cartesian understanding of a *representational mind*, human beings have direct emotional and perceptual access to the world through their emotional responses to the situation.[129] The Cartesian view of the representational mind and *mediated epistemology* through images, ideas, concepts, and schema stored in the private mind, proposed by Descartes has been soundly disputed. Valenced emotions are essential for perception, and emotional responses allow for fuzzy recognition such as noticing family resemblances and similarities and dissimilarities in whole situations.[130,131] There is no strictly will-based emotion-free perception.[132,133]

The Dreyfus and Dreyfus (1988)[134] Model of Skill Acquisition demonstrates how expert practice and situated skilled know-how depend on learning gaining an increasingly differentiated meaningful world, i.e., developing a *sense of salience* where some things just stand out in clinical situations as more or less important, without having to figure them out. A sense of salience requires experiential learning of judgment, perception, and distinctions of worth and goods in particular persons and situations.

The role of emotion in experiential learning is tied to perceptual grasp and noticing similarities and contrasts between past whole concrete cases. The clinician learns experientially about better and poorer outcomes in particular patient/family concerns. Learning from similarities, distinctions, and contrasts between various real clinical situations with all their variations help to create an informed and attuned perceptual grasp of an emotionally imbued meaningful world of dangers, possibilities, concerns, risks, and contingencies in one's everyday immersion in the world.

Perception and noticing depend on emotional responses to immersion in the world.[135] For example, initially, Advanced Beginners[136,137] may be flooded with anxiety and fear of making a mistake and may attempt to dampen their fearful anxiety-laden emotional responses. But already at the Competent stage, a sense of discomfort or dread may cause the nurse to re-examine his or her interpretation of the situation. At the Competent stage, anxiety is more intelligent and the competent nurse is more situationally attuned to a discordant lack of a good perceptual grasp in a clinical situation that does not unfold as expected. At the Proficient stage, attunement increases to the point that emotional responses signal the nurse to notice changing relevance because increasingly a loss of a good perceptual grasp of the situation is felt by the nurse.[138] With expertise, emotional responses, the skill of noticing and seeing, are associated actions that are increasingly tied together.

Taylor's view of agency as relational, i.e., co-constituted, and emotionally attuned and related to distinctions of worth and meanings, guided our understanding of the nurses' changing forms of agency illustrated in the narratives:

> Agents are beings for whom things matter, who are the subjects of significance. This is what gives them a point of view in the world. What distinguishes persons from other agents is not strategic power, that is the capacity to deal with the same matter of concern more effectively. What springs to view is that persons have qualitatively different concerns.... The centre is no longer the power to plan, but rather the openness to certain matters of significance.[139]

Openness and responsiveness to matters of significance allow the experienced practitioner to develop a sense of salience that facilitates perceptual grasp, leading to early warnings of significant changes in patients.[140]

Engaged reasoning makes visible different capacities and vulnerabilities than can be noticed by disengaged reasoning. Both skillful engaged reasoning and critical reflection are needed for an ethic of care, so that distortion, self-deception, and patterns of oppression do not cloud one's perceptions. However, disengaged rational-technical reasoning alone is not sufficient for informed, caring practices including skills of involvement with particular patients that improve clinical reasoning and judgment.

Nurses' understanding of the clinical situations when moving from competence to proficiency increases their ability to respond to matters of significance—often in the form of the ability to change perspectives on situations based on emotional responsiveness to the unfolding clinical situation. Proficient nurses' stories describe changing preconceptions, plans, and predictions in response to a particular situation.[141] Emotional responses are also linked to being open or closed to the situation's demands. Nurses use maxims that point to experientially gained wisdom that help them to stay open to the situation. For example, one nurse states, "Take care of these patients and get fooled a million times." Staying open to being possibly fooled curbs tunnel vision, confirmation bias, and projection. Being aware of biases and controlling for biases such as hidden racism and other biases such as confirmation biases[142] that can creep into our clinical reasoning and judgments are an ongoing practice challenge and necessary scrutiny.

Another nurse talks about the ethics of vigilance, watching to make sure that excessive or no longer needed treatments or tests deleterious to the patient are erroneously continued:

> Nurse 1: It's even minor stuff... "Why are you going to exsanguinate this kid when is sitting up watching TV eating?" (Continue unnecessary blood tests)... It's just little stuff like that. And when they [new nurses] get a little more experienced, they and their assessment skills get better, they can notice that maybe they're wheezing a little bit or that they're a little cold. They're a little blue or something. But it's like cleaning up.

Attentiveness and *noticing* are qualitatively different caring practices. Attentiveness is required for catching the multiple details that can be missed in nursing care. Attentiveness is based on a deliberate set of habits and practices. Noticing is less deliberate than attentiveness and is dependent on expert engagement and a *sense of salience* (i.e., having some things just stand out as more or less important). As noted earlier, a sense of salience (meaningfulness) guides recognition of the unusual or unexpected events. Noticing and recognizing the other is essential to an ethic of responsiveness and giving the other moral worth.

Conclusion

Being in the situation with the best scientific, theoretical knowledge, and educational mentoring and situated coaching[143] for noticing qualitative distinctions enhance experiential learning and the development of clinical expertise and expert ethical comportment. Both experiential learning and expert ethical comportment require noticing what does and does not work in specific situations, with the goal of improving a clinical situation and not making it worse, and the goal of improving future practice. The notions of good represented by norms and moral principles cannot be extended and enriched without a concomitant focus on particular clinical situations, with their context, timing, and concerns of patients and families, relational possibilities and so on instead of mindlessly applying generalized rules or guidelines without considering these contextual variations.

A practice offers new possibilities, creative thinking, and discovery, allowing for improving, developing, and enriching both practice and theories about practice. Caregivers, close others, and health-care workers extend the moral agency of patients through noticing and attending to their vulnerabilities and recognizing embodied intentionality of silent patients. A theoretical moral system that only recognizes autonomous, fully deliberate conscious, emotion-free decision-making as the only form of moral agency misses this rich moral source of agency afforded to silent patients by expert attentive and responsive caregivers, along with the agency and clinical impact that occurs with fuzzy recognition of subtle changes in patients' clinical condition that allow for lifesaving early warnings. Expert recognition practices for silent patients extend the moral possibilities of caregiving and decrease inherent vulnerabilities of silent patients. Abstract principles are necessary for orienting and alerting the learner to the appropriate regions of concern and for clarifying the public discourse on choices but, without attentiveness to the patient by caregivers, abstract principles cannot ensure that clinicians will recognize when moral norms or values are present or salient. Explanation cannot ensure understanding that will engender an ethical response in particular situations as noted in Linda Sawyer's narrative above.

One can only talk about what one sees and notices, and this removes narrative accounts from purely subjective accounts. Stories can depict and reflect actual real experiences. The storyteller reports thoughts, feelings, and experiential knowledge that portray meanings inherent in the story. Stories of skillful ethical comportment by expert clinicians can be a source for experiential learning for others and a moral source for situated thinking-in-action and ethical comportment.

In the United States, health-care systems are driven by the need for efficiency, efficacy, safety, and pressures for cost cutting and increasing profits. The focus on speed and efficiency often crowds out attentiveness afforded by engaged reasoning and attentiveness. The drive for speed and efficiency short-changes quality improvement strategies of listening and understanding the knowledge and discoveries of frontline knowledge-workers such as nurses and physicians. Telling and hearing stories is rare, or non-existent in busy short-staffed health-care systems. Telling stories of experiential learning in practice can improve the development of local practical knowledge and the shared expertise of communities of clinicians. Stories help identify moral infractions, concerns, and notions of good in ways that are covered over in formal decontextualized accounts of "knowing that and about" to characterize nursing practice. Likewise, formal ethical theories often cover over moral concerns and distinctions that frequently occur in actual practice situations. Objectified institutional reports of costs, patient outcomes, and patient complications, by focusing on outcomes alone, ignore the means, i.e., the caring practices, that make good outcomes possible.

Narratives of practice when told to others give voice to moral conflicts, concerns, exemplary ethical comportment, clarifying notions of good central to excellent practice. Ethical analyses of moral dilemmas, practice breakdowns, and conflict offer most when the moral concerns of all participants are heard and understood and when no one imagines that they can account for excellent practice without narrative examples. Analysis of ethical breakdowns aimed at adjudicating disputes and determining rights comprise only a small portion of our ethical concerns and experiences. To examine distinctions of worth, relational ethics of care, and rival interpretations of competing goods in particular clinical situations, narratives of particular practice situations are essential.[144] Studying and describing skills of involvement, attentiveness, openness, curiosity, responsiveness, and responsibility embedded in everyday nursing practice uncover moral sources instantiated and embedded in nursing practice, and are essential for understanding everyday ethical comportment of nurses. Like practices of knowledge development in high reliability organizations, we need to study the knowledge and experience of frontline expert practitioners through observation and storytelling.[145]

Generalized statistical knowledge and "knowing that and about" without also examining "knowing how and when" and situated thinking-in-action render expert practice in particular situations invisible:[146]

The question is whether we can as a society see the web of care that constitutes socially embedded practical knowledge (demonstrated here by expert nursing practice), the knowledge that is associated with preserving human worlds, and come to value this skillful, courageous comportment. All of the caring practices such as nursing, mothering, fathering, education, child care, care of the aged, social welfare, care of the earth may be potential saving practices, even as they are threatened and marginalized by a society that creates myths about ever-expanding possibilities to manage and control all aspects of life. Explanation and detached ways of knowing cannot replace the situated action and possibilities created by being with particular concrete others. Without the careful skillful care required for rearing children, educating [and caring for] the young and old, caring for our earth, our technological breakthroughs are meaningless. Indeed, we will not have the necessary safety nets for the breakthroughs since each breakthrough brings with it a potential fallout requiring new networks of care.[147]

Notes

1 Charles Taylor, *Modern Social Imaginaries* (Durham, NC: Duke University Press, 2003).
2 All the research data used in this article were originally published in the following two book chapters: P. Benner, "Finding the Good behind the Right: A Dialogue between Nursing and Bioethics," in F.G. Miller, J.C. Fletcher, and J.M. Humber (eds.), *The Nature and Prospect of Bioethics, Interdisciplinary Perspectives* (Totowa, NJ: Humana Press 2003); and P. Benner, "A Dialogue between Virtue Ethics and Care Ethics," *Theoretical Medicine*, 23 (1997): 1–15. (Reprinted in the book in honor of Edmund Pellegrino, *The Moral Philosophy of Edmund Pellegrino*, D. Thomasma (ed.) (Dordrecht: Kluwer).)
3 René Descartes (1628), "Rules for the Direction of the Understanding," in E.S. Haldane and G.R.T. Ross (eds.), *The Philosophical Works of Descartes*, two volumes reprint (Cambridge: Cambridge University Press, 2022).
4 Patricia Benner, "Overcoming Descartes' Representational View of the Mind in Nursing Pedagogies, Curricula and Testing," *Journal of Nursing Philosophy* 23, no. 4, Special Issue: The Role of Philosophy in the Nursing World (Oct. 2022).
5 Patricia Benner, "Teaching and Learning Clinical Reasoning: Maximizing Human Intelligence, Expert Clinical Reasoning, Scientific Knowledge, and Decision-Making Supports," in Martin Lipscomb (ed.), *Nursing Philosophy* (London: Routledge, 2024).
6 Charles Taylor, *A Secular Age* (Cambridge, MA: Harvard University Press, 2007), 164–209.
7 Ibid., 17.
8 Herbert L. Dreyfus and Charles Taylor, *Retrieving Realism* (Cambridge, MA: Harvard University Press, 2015).
9 Charles Taylor, *The Language Animal: The Full Shape of Human Linguistic Capacity* (Cambridge, UK: Cambridge University Press, 2016).
10 Dreyfus and Taylor, *Retrieving Realism*.
11 Taylor, *The Language Animal*.
12 Mica R. Endsley, "Expertise in Situation Awareness," in K. Anders Ericsson, Robert L. Hoffman, Aaron Kozbelt, and A. Mark Williams (eds.), *Cambridge Handbook of Expertise and Expert Performance*, 2nd ed. (Cambridge, UK: Cambridge University Press, 2018), 714–741.
13 Elizabeth Ennen, "Phenomenological Coping Skills and the Striatal Memory System," *Phenomenology and the Cognitive Sciences* 2 (2003): 299–325.
14 Shaun Gallagher and Dan Zahavi, *The Phenomenological Mind*, 3rd ed. (London: Routledge, 2021).
15 Shaun Gallagher, *How the Body Shapes the Mind* (London: Clarendon, 2005).

16 Alva Noë, *Out of Our Heads* (New York: Hill & Wang, 2010).
17 Hubert L. Dreyfus, "Misrepresenting Human Intelligence," *Thought* 61, no. 243 (December 1986), 430–441.
18 Immanuel Kant, Three Critiques, three-volume set: *Vol. 1: Critique of Pure Reason*; *Vol. 2: Critique of Practical Reason*; *Vol. 3: Critique of Judgment*, UK edition (London: Hackett Classics, 2002).
19 Martin Heidegger, *Being and Time*, trans. John Macquarrie and Edward Robinson (New York: Harper & Row, 1962).
20 Hubert L. Dreyfus, *Being in the World: Commentary on Division I, Being and Time* (Cambridge, MA: MIT University Press, 1991).
21 Patricia Benner, "The Roles of Embodiment, Emotion and Lifeworld in Nursing Practice," *Journal of Nursing Philosophy* 1, no. 1 (2000): 1–15.
22 Ashley Moyse, *Resourcing Hope for Aging and Dying in a Broken World* (New York: Anthem Press, 2022).
23 Heidegger, *Being and Time*.
24 Charles Taylor, *Modern Social Imaginaries* (Durham, NC: Duke University Press 2003).
25 Ashley Moyse, *Resourcing Hope for Ageing and Dying in a Broken World* (New York: Anthem Press, 2022).
26 Patricia Benner and Judith Wrubel, *The Primacy of Caring* (Englewood Cliffs, NJ: Prentice-Hall, 1989).
27 Knud E. Løgstrup, *The Ethical Demand* (Notre Dame, IN: University of Notre Dame Press, 1997).
28 Kari Martinsen, *Care and Vulnerability*, trans. Linn Elise Kjerlan (Oslo: Akribe Publishers, 2006).
29 Benner and Wrubel, *Primacy of Caring*.
30 Tom Beauchamp and James Childress, *Principles of Biomedical Ethics*, 8th ed. (Cambridge, MA: Harvard University Press, 2019).
31 Patricia Benner, Christine Tanner, and Catherine Chesla, *Expertise in Nursing Practice: Caring, Clinical Judgment, and Ethics*, 2nd ed. (New York: Springer, 2009).
32 Ibid., 329,
33 Charles Taylor, "Explanation and Practical Reasoning," in *Philosophical Arguments* (Cambridge MA: Harvard University Press, 1995), 51–53.
34 Charles Taylor, *Sources of the Self* (New York: Cambridge University Press, 1989).
35 Charles Taylor, "Explanation and Practical Reasoning," 51–53.
36 Charles Taylor, *The Language Animal* (Cambridge, MA: Harvard Belknap, 2016), 281–282, 292.
37 Patricia E. Benner, Patricia Lee Hooper-Kyriakidis, and Daphne Stannard, *Clinical Wisdom and Interventions in Acute and Critical Care: A Thinking-in-Action Approach*, 2nd ed. (New York: Springer Publishing, 2011).
38 Ibid.
39 Benner et al., *Expertise in Nursing Practice*.
40 C.A. Tanner, P. Benner, C. Chelsea, and D.R. Gordon, "The Phenomenology of Knowing a Patient," *Image* 25, no. 4 (1993): 273–280.
41 Ibid.
42 P. Benner, "Finding the Good Behind the Right: A Dialogue between Nursing and Bioethics," in F.G. Miller, J.C. Fletcher, J.M. Humber (eds.), *The Nature and Prospect of Bioethics: Interdisciplinary Perspectives* (Totowa, NJ: Humana Press, 2003).
43 Edmund D. Pellegrino and David C. Thomasma, *A Philosophical Basis of Medical Practice* (New York: Oxford University Press, 1981).
44 Patricia Benner, "The Quest for Control and the Possibilities of Care," in *Heidegger, Coping and Cognitive Science: Essays in Honor of Hubert L. Dreyfus*, Mark Wrathall and Jeff Malpas (eds.) (Cambridge, MA: MIT. Press, 2000), 293–309, 296.

45 P. Benner, "The Roles of Embodiment, Emotion and Lifeworld in Nursing Practice," *Journal of Nursing Philosophy* 1, no. 1 (2000): 1–15.

46 Antonio Damasio, *Descartes' Error: Emotion, Reason and the Human Brain* (New York: Penguin Press, 2003).

47 P. Bourdieu, *The Logic of Practice*, R. Nice trans. (Stanford, CA: Stanford University Press, 1980/1990).

48 H.L. Dreyfus, S.E. Dreyfus, and P. Benner, "Implications of the Phenomenology of Skillful Ethical Comportment," in Benner et al. (eds.), *Expertise in Nursing Practice*, 326–327.

49 David C. Thomasma, *The Influence of Edmund D. Pellegrino's Philosophy of Medicine* (Dordrecht: Springer Dordrecht, 1997). DOI: 10.1007/978–94-017–3364–9

50 P. Benner, "The Role of Experience, Narrative, and Community in Skilled Ethical Comportment," *Advances in Nursing Science*, 14, no. 2 (1991): 1–23.

51 J. Dunne, *Back to the Rough Ground: "Phronesis" and "Techne" in Modern Philosophy and in Aristotle* (Notre Dame, IN: Notre Dame University Press, 1992), 378–380.

52 Hans-George Gadamer, *Truth and Method*, trans. rev. J. Weinsheimer and D. Marshall (New York: Bloomsbury Press, 1975).

53 P. Benner and J. Wrubel, "Skilled Clinical Knowledge: The Value of Perceptual Awareness," *Nurse Educator* 7, no. 3 (1982), 11–17.

54 Benner et al., *Expertise in Nursing Practice*.

55 Benner et al., *Clinical Wisdom*.

56 Benner, "Finding the Good behind the Right," 113, 140.

57 Benner, "The Roles of Embodiment," 1–15

58 Tanner et al., "Knowing a Patient."

59 Benner et al., *Expertise in Nursing Practice*.

60 Benner et al., *Clinical Wisdom*.

61 P. Benner, "A Dialogue between Virtue Ethics and Care Ethics," *Theoretical Medicine*, 23: 1–15. (Reprinted in the book in honor of Edmund Pellegrino, *The Moral Philosophy of Edmund Pellegrino*, D. Thomasma (ed.) (Dordrecht: Kluwer, 1997).)

62 C. Geertz, "Deep Play: Notes on the Balinese Cockfight," in P. Rabinow and W. Sullivan (eds.), *Interpretive Social Science: A Second Look* (Berkeley, CA: University of California Press, 1987).

63 Benner et al., *Expertise in Nursing Practice*.

64 Ibid.

65 H.L. Dreyfus, and C. Taylor, *Retrieving Realism* (Cambridge, MA: Harvard University Press, 2015).

66 H.L. Dreyfus, and S.E. Dreyfus, with Thom Anthanasiou, *Mind Over Machine: The Power of Human Intuition and Expertise in the Era of the Computer* (New York: The Free Press, 1986).

67 Alasdair MacIntyre, *After Virtue: A Study in Moral Theory* (London: University of Notre Dame Press, 1981).

68 C. Taylor, *The Language Animal, the Full Shape of Human Linguistic Capacity* (Cambridge, MA: The Belknap Press, Harvard University, 2016).

69 J. Dunne, *Back to the Rough Ground*.

70 S. Ruddick, *Maternal Thinking: Toward a Politics of Peace* (Boston, MA: Beacon Press, 1995).

71 W. Sullivan and M.S. Rosin, *A New Agenda for Higher Education, Shaping the Mind for Practice* (Carnegie Foundation for the Advancement of Teaching, and San Francisco: Jossey-Bass, 2008).

72 Jane Rubin, "Impediments to the Development of Clinical Knowledge and Ethical Judgment in Critical Care Nursing," in Benner et al. (eds.), *Expertise in Nursing Practice*, 171–198.

73 Sullivan and Rosin, *New Agenda*, xvi.

74 J. Dunne, "An Intricate Fabric: Understanding the Rationality of Practice," *Pedagogy, Culture and Society* 13, no. 2 (2009): 367–389.

75 Albert Borgman, *Power Failure* (Grand Rapids, MI: Brazos Press, 2003).

76 H.L. Dreyfus, *What Computers Still Can't Do: A Critique of Artificial Intelligence* (Cambridge, MA: MIT Press, 1992).

77 Borgman, *Power Failure*.

78 MacIntyre, *After Virtue*.

79 Joseph Dunne, "An Intricate Fabric: Understanding the Rationality of Practice," *Pedagogy, Culture and Society* 13, no. 2 (2005): 367–389.

80 Benner, "The Roles of Embodiment."

81 P. Benner, "Novice to Mastery: Situated Thinking, Action, and Wisdom," in Elaine Silva Mangiante, Kathy Peno, and Jane Northup (eds.), *Teaching and Learning for Adult Skill Acquisition: Applying the Dreyfus and Dreyfus Model in Different Fields* (Information Age Publishing, 2021).

82 Benner, "Teaching and Learning Clinical Reasoning."

83 Benner et al., *Clinical Wisdom*.

84 P. Benner, "The Role of Narrative Experience and Community in Expert Ethical Comportment," *Advances in Nursing Science* 14, no. 2 (1991): 1–21.

85 Rubin, "Impediments."

86 Benner et al., *Clinical Wisdom*.

87 Robert J. Wears and Katherine M. Sutcliffe, *Still Not Safe: Patient Safety and the Middle-Managing of American Medicine* (New York: Oxford University Press, 2020).

88 Ibid.

89 Benner et al., *Clinical Wisdom*.

90 Wears and Sutcliffe, *Still Not Safe*.

91 Karl Weick and Kathleen Sutcliff, *Managing the Unexpected: Resilient Performance in an Age of Uncertainty* (San Francisco: Jossey-Bass, 2007).

92 Joseph Dunne, "An Intricate Fabric: Understanding the Rationality of Practice," *Pedagogy, Culture and Society* 13, no. 2 (2005): 367–389.

93 See note 1.

94 J. Dunne, "An Intricate Fabric," 376.

95 Michael Polanyi, *The Tacit Dimension* (London: Routledge & Kegan Paul, 1967).

96 Charles Taylor, *Modern Social Imaginaries* (Public Planet Books, 2003).

97 Mary V. Wrenn and William Waller, "Pathology of Care: The Concept of Care from an Economic Philosophy Perspective," *Oeconomia, History, Methodology, Philosophy* 8, no. 2, (2018): 157–185. DOI: 10.4000/oeconomia.3195

98 Warner Mendenhall, "Co-dependency Definitions and Dynamics," *Alcoholism Treatment Quarterly* 6, no. 1 (1989): 3–17. DOI: 10.1300/J020V06N01_02 To link to this article: https://doi.org/10.1300/J020V06N01 02)

99 Knud Løgstrup, *The Ethical Demand* (London: University of Notre Dame Press, 1997).

100 Benner and Wrubel, *Primacy of Caring*.

101 Løgstrup, *Ethical Demand*.

102 Ibid.

103 Emmanuel Levinas, *Totality and Infinity* (Pittsburgh, PA: Duquesne University Press, 1961).

104 Emmanuel Levinas, *Humanism of the Other* (Chicago: University of Illinois Press, 1972).

105 Rubin, "Impediments."

106 Benner et al., *Clinical Wisdom*.

107 Benner et al., *Expertise in Nursing Practice*.

108 Benner, "Novice to Mastery."

109 Benner et al., *Expertise*.

110 Benner, "Novice to Mastery."

111 Rubin, "Impediments."

112 Ibid.

113 Benner et al., *Clinical Wisdom.*

114 Benner et al., *Expertise in Nursing Practice.*

115 Benner et al., "Knowing a Patient."

116 Benner, "Finding the Good."

117 Patricia Benner, "A Dialogue between Virtue Ethics and Care Ethics," *Theoretical Medicine*, 23 (1997): 1–15. Also in D.C. Thomasma. (eds.), *The Influence of Edmund D. Pellegrino's Philosophy of Medicine* (Dordrecht: Springer Publishing, 1997).

118 Benner, "Dialogue."

119 Benner et al., *Clinical Wisdom.*

120 William Sullivan and Matthew Rosin, *A New Agenda for Higher Education: Shaping a Life of the Mind for Practice*, 1st ed. (San Francisco: Jossey-Bass, 2008).

121 Charles Taylor, *Sources of the Self: The Making of Modern Identity* (Cambridge, UK: Cambridge University Press, 1989).

122 Tanner et al., "The Phenomenology of Knowing a Patient."

123 Benner, "Finding the Good."

124 Published in its entirety in Benner, "Finding the Good."

125 Kant, Three Critiques.

126 Taylor, *Sources of the Self*, 248.

127 Ibid.

128 Halpern, *From Detached Concern to Empathy*, 2011.

129 Benner, "Teaching and Learning Clinical Reasoning."

130 Ludwig Wittgenstein, *On Certainty*, trans. G.E.M. Ancombe and G.H. von Wright (New York: Harper Torch Books, 1972).

131 Noë, *Out of Our Heads.*

132 Taylor, *The Language Animal.*

133 Dreyfus and Taylor, *Retrieving Realism.*

134 Hubert Dreyfus and Stuart Dreyfus, *Mind over Machine: The Role of Intuition in an Age of the Computer* (New York: New York Free Press, 1988).

135 Taylor, *The Language Animal.*

136 Dreyfus and Dreyfus, *Mind over Machine.*

137 Benner et al., *Expertise in Nursing Practice.*

138 Hubert L. Dreyfus, "On Expertise and Embodiment: Insights from Maurice Merleau-Ponty and Samuel Todes," in Jörgen Sandberg, Linda Rouleau, Ann Langley, and Haridimos Tsoukas (eds.), *Skillful Performance Enacting Capabilities, Knowledge, Competence, and Expertise in Organizations* (New York: Oxford University Press, 2017), 149.

139 Charles Taylor, "Explanation and Practical Reason," in M. Nussbaum and A. Sen (eds.), *The Quality of Life* (Oxford: Clarendon Press, 1993), 208–231, 209.

140 Benner et al., *Clinical Wisdom.*

141 Benner, "Novice to Mastery."

142 Charles P. Friedman, Guido G. Gatti, Timothy M. Franz, Gwendolyn Murphy, Frederic Wolf, Paul Heckerling, Pau Fine, Thomas Miller, and Arthur Elstein, "Do Physicians Know When Their Diagnoses Are Correct? Implications for Decision Support and Error Reduction," *Journal of General Internal Medicine* 20 (2005): 334–339.

143 Benner, et al., *Clinical Wisdom.*

144 Ibid.

145 Friedman et al., "Do Physicians Know when Their Diagnoses?"

146 Benner et al., *Clinical Wisdom.*

147 Benner, "The Quest for Control," 309.

10

A CLOSET FULL OF ETHICS FOR SEASONAL WEAR

Living in Southern California, I discovered that it was not possible to buy a coat suitable for a Siberian winter when I needed one. My closets are full and are in serious need of a clear-out. I have casual clothes, work clothes, dress clothes, gym clothes, camping and hiking clothes, cycling clothes, academic regalia, church vestments, Southern California winter clothes (called sweaters), Northern California winter clothes (puffy jackets), winter clothes for the Siberia project (ummm, with animal fur), and more. The clothes serve different climates, weather, and purposes, so are not mixed-and-matched to wear together. Some are clothes that I need only occasionally, but have to keep for when their specific purposes arise. So it is with this book. There are bits and pieces of ethics clothing in the closet that one rarely finds worn in nursing circles that should, nonetheless, be pulled out of the closet for different seasons and purposes. This chapter is a closet chapter. Chapter 4 introduced nursing ethics as a social ethics. Social ethics is about the positive agenda of building a good society, as well as the negative agenda of identifying and changing the harmful aspects of society. It is about substantially more than social justice alone: it is about a vision of and for good persons in a good society, but of course including social justice as well. This chapter extends the discussion of social ethics in nursing, in contrast to the nominal use of the term *social ethics* in bioethics. More specifically, this chapter introduces the discipline of social ethics and its three basic functions that rely upon *moral suasion*. Social ethics emerges from the context of Pragmatism, and Progressivism in which *associationalism* furthers the political action of unenfranchised women and nurses in society. The chapter then looks at the three periods of the historical social ethics movement and the role of religious social ethics in US society. The chapter discusses the enduring links of social ethics to nursing ethics, as well as its links to the formative period of bioethics. Social ethics, as it engages in social criticism and seeks social change, is

DOI: 10.4324/9781003262107-11

intrinsically activist and political, and a form of advocacy. The chapter includes a brief examination of the pivotal Hart–Devlin debate, which received considerable attention in the fields of ethics and law, but relatively none in bioethics. The Hart–Devlin debate is important both to social ethics and nursing ethics as it addresses the question of the legislation of morality, important to considerations of legislation regarding, for example, homosexuality, reproductive rights, book bans, pornography, child marriage, and more. Thus, the Hart–Devlin debate is important to nursing, whether in the expectation of informed voting by individual nurses, or in the engagement of nursing's political action committees. While there are remnants of social ethics still active in nursing, much of that tradition was lost with the movement of nursing into colleges and universities, and hospitals. It is, however, a rich heritage that offers abundant wisdom—experiential, practical, and theoretical— if we would simply take it out of the closet in its season.

Social Ethics: What It Is Not

One of the key relationships of nursing ethics has always been nurse or nursing-to-society, though that relationship has languished following nursing's move into the university. It has since been recovered in part in the ANA *Code of Ethics for Nurses with Interpretive Statements*, 2001,[1] and amplified in the 2015[2] revision and will be again in the 2025 revision now underway. Chapter 4 discusses early nursing's social engagement as social ethics, yet it does not discuss social ethics per se, as a discipline; we embark upon that now.

In recent years, medicine has begun to use the term *social ethics*, though in many cases it is gratuitous. For example, Miguel Escotet, in his article "Pandemics, Leadership and Social Ethics,"[3] writes:

> This Viewpoint [column] argues that the absence of worldwide social ethics is at the root of our present social, political, and economic crises. More to the point, the current COVID-19 pandemic is, in part, a consequence of insufficient scientific research, inappropriate education systems, and globally fragile health structures and human services.[4]

Escotet's article addresses "insufficient scientific research, inappropriate education systems, and globally fragile health structures and human services" but not social ethics. Other than its mention in the title and in this paragraph, the paper never again mentions or obliquely addresses social ethics. Escotet is by no means a singular example of employing the term *social ethics* nominally, then otherwise disappearing it.

Another issue is the use of the term *social ethics*, then embarking upon what is ostensibly a social-ethical analysis, without any explication of the foundations, nature, and scope of social ethics; that is, no guidance as to what the authors understand as *social ethics*. For example, Thomas Mappes, Jane Zembaty, and David

DeGrazia edited the anthology *Social Ethics: Morality and Social Policy*.[5] Known for their excellent anthology on biomedical ethics (which went to seven editions), *Social Ethics* is their last work. It includes chapters on abortion, euthanasia and physician-assisted suicide, the death penalty, sexual morality, same-sex marriage, pornography, hate speech, censorship drug control, addiction and medical use of cannabis, terrorism, human rights, torture, world hunger, poverty, economic justice, individual responsibility, animals, the environment, and global climate change; that is, a range of issues that are *au courant*, though not necessarily related. Each chapter presents articles with contrasting views, legal opinions, and a modest amount of discussion of policy, without hardcore analysis of social structures relative to the issues. Yet, the content of the book would indicate that, for them, *social ethics* consists of ethical reflection, combined with legal perspectives and opinion, in relation to clinical, social, and global issues. However, there are problems. The book does not contain a foundational discussion of the nature and scope of social ethics per se. Instead, it launches into chapters on specific issues. In addition there is no discussion of the reason specific issues were chosen. And, as well, a number of chapters are intimately related to the famous Hart–Devlin debate (for the moment we will defer that discussion), which the authors do not mention or address in the book. Indeed, Mill's work *On Liberty*[6] is discussed under the topic of pornography, rather than sexual morality where it figured prominently in the Hart–Devlin debate.

When we come to bioethical works per se, they are largely driven by concerns for what they term *social justice* or *rights*. In his article "The Social Ethics of Primary Care: The Relationship Between a Human Need and an Obligation of Society," [7] Edmund Pellegrino uses the term *social ethics* nominally, though he touches upon a social ethical issue. However, his is a rights-based argument rather than a social-structural critique or argument. He states:

> The need for primary care is a universal human need, that it imposes a claim on society and the professions, and that the claim is relative not absolute, but nonetheless a strong one in a democratic, affluent, technologically capable society like ours. This proposition will be developed in three steps: the first locates the moral center of primary care; the second defines in what sense it might be considered a right or obligation; and the third outlines the potential conflicts between such an obligation and others already binding on health professions and society.[8]

Pellegrino's concern is for *a relative right to primary care*, and for physicians' self-determination. He does acknowledge that physicians do owe a debt to society, that it is reasonable for people to expect society to provide primary care, that society owes a level of primary care to its people, and that there are other goods in addition to health that complicate the resolution of competing claims. The resolution of those competing claims "is seriously hampered by our collective inability as yet to define the acceptable conditions of social justice. Without such principles, it is not possible to choose rationally among competing claims."[9] He lays out the claims but, disappointingly, does not suggest means of resolution, or point to a direction society either might or should take; he leaves us with a philosophical cliff-hanger, theory without praxis.

Justice in Bioethics: (Social) Justice versus Social Ethics

Most of the bioethics literature that purports to address social ethics raises issues of *social justice*, customarily without addressing social ethics. For the most part, the majority of writers rely on the concept of justice, or more specifically the biomedical principle of justice as articulated in Tom Beauchamp and James Childress' landmark book *Principles of Biomedical Ethics*,[10] (now in its eighth edition). Beauchamp and Childress explicate the concept of justice specifically as *distributive justice*; that is the distribution of burdens and benefits in society, under conditions of scarcity (rationing).

In their first edition, Beauchamp and Childress acknowledge their focus on comparative distributive justice, defining it in terms of *desert,* rather than as *fairness*,[11] though doing so without discussion. *Justice as fairness* refers to the impartial and equitable treatment of individuals or groups, ensuring that they are treated justly and without prejudicial discrimination. John Rawls is the most famous of the exponents of justice as fairness.[12] What constitutes *fairness* and how it is to be achieved is the subject matter of competing theories of justice. *Desert*, in common language, means "what one deserves," but is more complex in its philosophical usage where there are *deservers* (generally, persons), *desert-bases* (grounds for desert), *desert* (the thing that the deserver deserves, such as reward, punishment, honor, recognition, censure, etc.). For example, the patient (person) needs (desert-base: need) nursing care (what the patient deserves); or the nurse-researcher (person) discovered X (desert-base: merit) and deserves to be nominated for Academy membership (the thing that the researcher deserves). Each of these features (deserver, desert, desert-base) receives considerable, granular discussion in the philosophical literature. Various desert-bases related to *justice* include need, merit, effort, social contribution, contribution to the marketplace (ability to pay), and equality. Beauchamp and Childress write that:

> One has acted justly towards a person when that person has been given what he is due or owed, and therefore has been given what he deserves or can legitimately claim.... What persons deserve or can legitimately claim is based on certain morally relevant properties which they possess, such as being productive or being in need. Similarly, it is wrong, as a matter of justice, to burden or to reward someone if the person does *not* possess the relevant property.... The more restricted expression "distributive justice" refers to the proper distribution of social benefits and burdens. Distributive justice applies only to distribution under conditions of scarcity, e.g., where there is competition for benefits.[13]

There are conditions that create competition where scarcity does not exist, such as maldistribution, that they do not address; and if distributive justice necessitates scarcity and competition, then it is ill-equipped to address structural issues of injustice where no scarcity or competition exists. Beauchamp and Childress further divide distributive justice into questions of macroallocation or microallocation. They discuss the *formal principle of justice* (historically attributed to Aristotle), that *equals shall be treated equally, and unequals unequally, in accord with their relevant differences*. The *material principles of justice* specify what constitutes a relevant difference, such as need, effort, societal contribution, merit, or that all are equal.[14] They rightly point out that the material principles represent various political systems. Because they chose *desert* rather than *fairness* (a choice that they acknowledge) they are left to justify the *material principles of justice*, not on the basis of rules generated by *justice* itself, but on the basis of the other principles they advocate, chiefly *autonomy* and its rule of *informed consent*. And yet, their other principles are self-reliant; that is, they rely upon an argument from within the specific principle itself for justification. In addition, they do not resolve the question of which material principle pertains to health-care access. From the material principles they move to *fair opportunity* without explaining its relationship to *desert*. They assert that fair opportunity (access) may not be denied on the basis of conditions for which persons are not themselves *responsible*, using the example of "mental retardation" (it's 1979) and access to special education. *Responsibility* presents a problem for distribution on the basis of *need*, as some *need* is, as they note, based on conditions beyond one's control (one's DNA), and some *need* is based on misadventure or stupidity, such as my cousin's broken arm from hang-gliding (yet he was not denied care). How then is *need* related to *fair opportunity*? Fair opportunity seems to precede need in their calculus. They follow with a brief discussion of John Rawls' *A Theory of Justice*[15] and conjecture that his theory might "provide a reason why some would argue that the principle of fair opportunity is in the end not a valid moral principle at all."[16] They proceed to a discussion of *macroallocation* and *microallocation* of benefits, and turn toward medical treatments. Macroallocation refers to "how much of society's resources should be exchanged for social goods including health-related expenditures."[17] They understand microallocation as "health professionals, hospitals, and other institutions determine which particular individuals shall obtain available resources."[18] They note that microallocation may be unjust at the point of *final selection* (choice of a specific patient) and that "it is easier to secure rules of initial inclusion and exclusion because they involve minimum standards, e.g., age and medical acceptability, and appear to be more objective and more easily applied than rules of final selection."[19] Indeed, final selection infrequently has rules and can easily become a form of illicit soft rationing by the practitioner. Rightly, justice should be applied at the macroallocation and meso-allocation levels, and the rules of mid-level i.e., *mesoallocation*, should govern final selection. Beauchamp and Childress extend their discussion of microallocation to the end of the chapter. By their eighth edition, the section on justice has doubled, and includes clearer sections including new (from the first edition) sections on traditional theories of justice (Utilitarian, Libertarian, Egalitarian, and Communitarian) and recent theories of justice (Capabilities theories and Well-being theories). Their critique of communitarianism is not unjust, but it does not do it justice.

In terms of the use of justice in bioethics, in her address upon stepping down from the presidency of the Hastings Center, Mildred Solomon writes:

> Justice has always been a prominent value in bioethics, but too often, we have relied on a very thin notion of justice, more focused on fair procedures in the allocation of scarce resources than on the structural inequalities that damage people's life options, health, and well-being.[20]... There are exciting movements in this direction across our field, with prominent bioethics scholars calling for attention to social justice and universities around the world focusing attention on population-level bioethics. Much has begun, but there is much more waiting to be done.[21]

Well, they should have read nursing ethics.

The purpose here is not an analysis or critique of Beauchamp and Childress' position on justice. To be fair, trying to stuff justice into 20 or even 45 pages is like trying to stuff a sleeping bag back into the pouch it came in—if it is done at all, it's a wrinkled mess. Rather, the purpose of this glimpse at Beauchamp and Childress is to make note of several things. First, what they offer on the principle of justice does not do justice to justice. Second, what they offer on the principle of justice is the entire meager substance of what most nurses know of justice when they attempt to extend it to practice. Justice, however, is *not* a bedside principle and should only ever be used at the macroallocation and mesoallocation levels. Third, their starting position is theoretical, top-down, non-contextual, and narrowly problem-focused on access to or cost of health care, rather than a critique of social structures (as Solomon notes, above). A top-down reasoning is a hallmark of a principalist approach. Fourth, while they align justice with health policy, focused on the allocation of (scarce) resources, they do not articulate a vision of *a good society* that justice or policy might aim toward or secure—as would the communitarians. Fifth, justice alone, or at least their vision of justice, is in itself inadequate to the task of social ethics and is incommensurate with the capacious vision of nursing ethics for a healthy society. And, finally, sixth, bioethics is increasingly misappropriating "social ethics" in ways that do not attach to the actual field of social ethics. This necessitates a consideration of social ethics, its origins, its ethos, its definition, and scope.

Social Ethics: What It Is

Bioethics has been inventing its own social ethics by drawing upon theories of justice, political theories, particularly contract theories, focusing on access to and cost of health care, with an eye to its application in health policy. There is little evidence in the American bioethics literature of a knowledge or awareness of the significant tradition of the social ethics movement, particularly as it coalesced in the late 1800s and early 1900s, or how it directly articulates with the origins of bioethics. However, European literature is more cognizant of the tradition and field of social ethics. Dutch philosopher in bioethics Martien Pijnenburg, in "Humane Healthcare as a Theme for Social Ethics," (2002) writes:

> *Social ethics...* is a reflection on the goodness and badness of social institutions created by men.... Social ethics includes reflection of collective values, prevailing views of men and society, social, cultural, historical roots and consequences for groups of citizens.... The social context is not, as is the case in individual ethics, taken for granted, but as an object of analysis and ethical judgement and to a certain, but for social ethics decisive extent, accessible for changes. Social ethics starts from the presumption that our social institutions and the way they are functioning are ultimately submitted to human responsibility. They are created and brought to existence by men to guarantee values and interactions that are considered as essential for the good life and the good society.[22]

In an earlier definition, Gibson Winter (1968) defines social ethics as

> issues of social order—the good, right, and ought in the organization of human communities and the shaping of social policies. Hence the subject matter of social ethics is moral rightness and goodness in the shaping of human society.... Ethical analysis takes place in order to approve and strengthen those institutions or aspects of a sector of the social system that sustain moral community, and in order to criticize, transform, or undermine those institutions or aspects of the social system that destroy such possibilities.[23]

Social ethics is about *social criticism and social change*. *Social criticism* is fundamentally ethical, though it draws upon the social sciences initially to substantiate, define, and parse the issues (as does Pragmatism). In contemporary times, it also draws upon critical theories not available in the early years of social ethics. *Social change* is often related to social policy but may also be wrought through activism and nongovernmental organizations, such as settlement houses, voluntary associations such as societies for the prevention of cruelty to children and animals, the Red Cross, and so on. In terms of health, social ethics is concerned with those factors that are essential to the health of society, that is, to a healthy society in which persons and the natural environment can flourish. Its starting point is not that of bioethics, when disease, illness, or trauma bring the person through the door of the medical system. Social ethics' starting point is substantially antecedent to the hospital bed. For example, bioethics begins at the emergency department door when an uninsured 13-year-old child of a destitute family is brought in for chemical burns incurred while working nights sanitizing meat-packing equipment and slaughterhouse floors.[24] Social ethics, however, would look at structural issues of poverty, child exploitation, the violation of child labor laws, *and* access to care for an exploited child. Social ethics is about the positive agenda of building a good society, as well as the negative agenda of identifying and changing the harmful aspects of society. As Pijnenburg's and Winter's definitions indicate, social ethics is about the critique of society, its values and social structures, including their historical roots, challenging what is not good, right, or fitting, targeting it for transformation, and reinforcing those social institutions and sectors of that society that sustain moral community. Social ethics is possessed of a reformist bias that is about substantially more than social justice alone; it is about a vision of and for good persons in a good society, human flourishing, welfare and well-being, dignity, respect, a welcoming community, equality, equity, safety, and more—and including social justice.

The Three Functions of Social Ethics

Social ethics has three essential moral functions: (a) reform within the group, (b) *epideictic* discourse, and (c) speaking the values of the group into society for its reform. The reformist bias of social ethics contends for change within a given community itself, in this case nursing, seeking to bring the reality into closer conformity to the ideal. The first function is to put our own house in order so that we may, without pretense or hypocrisy, communicate nursing values into society in ways that contribute to shaping social and health policy. The second function of social ethics, *epideictic discourse*, is a bridge function between the first and third functions.

Putting Our House in Order

Nursing ethics is a social ethics that is equipped to address social-structural injustices and issues. Even so, and despite its moral commitments, its execution has been unfaithful, and at certain points spectacularly so. It is not nursing's ethics, its values, ideals, and vision, that are so horribly defective or inadequate, but rather its implementation has been tragically flawed. Looking within requires that we engage in intentional self-examination to confront the blindness, injustices, and oppressions that exist within the profession, as well as nursing's complicity in perpetrating, perpetuating, or tolerating social injustices. Individuals have been excluded from nursing on the basis of race, ethnicity, religion, (dis)ability, gender, socio-economic status, and more. Progress or advancement within the profession has frequently been constrained for many. Additionally, some individuals are admitted to nursing educational programs who meet admission standards yet represent the antithesis of nursing values and ideals. Nursing has not consistently articulated a vision for a good society, or a healthy society, within the profession and within society. Nursing has failed at a number of junctures, and yet its ethics toolkit has what we need to do better and to do good.

Nursing's current reckoning with racism is one example of putting our house in order. The National Commission to Address Racism in Nursing was formed to lead the way.

> On January 25, 2021, leading nursing organizations launched the National Commission to Address Racism in Nursing (the Commission). The Commission examines the issue of racism within nursing nationwide focusing on the impact on nurses, patients, communities, and health care systems to motivate all nurses to confront individual and systemic racism.[25]

That work, now in progress, is multifaceted and will have multiple outcomes including policy statements. The ANA has recently adopted a statement on racial reckoning:

> On June 11, 2022, the ANA Membership Assembly, the governing and official voting body of ANA, took historic action to begin a journey of racial reckoning by unanimously voting 'yes' to adopt the ANA Racial Reckoning Statement. This statement is a meaningful first step for the association to acknowledge its own past actions that have negatively impacted nurses of color and perpetuated systemic racism.[26]

This is one example of the first function of social ethics. *Epideictic discourse* is the second function.

Epideictic Discourse

The language we write, speak, and hear, by which we lead others to act, is of a particular sort: it is referred to as *epideictic discourse. Epideictic* (meaning "to show") *discourse* refers to one of Aristotle's three species of rhetoric, and is a kind of public speech that "sets out to increase the intensity of adherence to certain values, which might not be contested when considered on their own but may nevertheless not prevail against other values that might come into conflict with them."[27] The function of epideictic discourse is to remind the hearers of their shared values and value structure in order to "increase the intensity of adherence to values held in common by the audience and the speaker... making use of dispositions already present in the audience in order to foster action upon those values."[28] Its intent is to evoke values, not emotion, in order to galvanize to action based on those values—rather than inciting to mob action, an important difference. Epideictic discourse reminds the group of its values and identity in its own communal life, within the society that it seeks to influence. It is *hortatory* (to exhort) and *paraenetic* (morally instructive) in nature and is a form of *moral suasion*. Examples of epideictic discourse in public address abound. See, for example, Jane Addams' "The Subjective Necessity for Social Settlements" (1892), Susan Anthony's "On Women's Right to

Vote" (1920), Eleanor Roosevelt's "The Struggle for Human Rights" (1948), Maya Angelou's "On the Pulse of Morning" (1993), or ANA's *A Suggested Code* of 1926 (remembering that it is now almost 100 years old):

> Heir throughout the ages of those who have nurtured the young, the weak and the sick, the mother, the kindly neighbor, the knight on the battlefield, the nun and the deaconess within or without enclosing walls—nursing emerges as a profession from its historic setting in an attempt to meet the present demands of society. The most precious possession of this profession is the ideal of service extending even to the sacrifice of life itself...[29]

Not to leave men out, consider Martin Luther King, Jr.'s "I Have a Dream" speech (1963), King George VI's "Radio Address" (1939), Winston Churchill's "We Shall Fight on the Beaches" (1940), or John F. Kennedy's "The Decision to Go the Moon" (1961).

Once one's own house is in order, and the inhabitants motivated to act, we move to the third function of social ethics: to represent the values and perspectives of the community to the larger society. This function still uses epideictic discourse, but this time upon society itself. It argues for change in society in accord with the moral values of the community at large and the nursing community. Social ethics is intrinsically political. It seeks to affect society, policy, and legislation to effect change in accord with, for us, nursing values.

To engage in social ethics is not without risk, as it challenges the status quo and thus poses a threat to those who benefit from and would preserve that status quo. Consider our nursing forebears who were jailed, beaten, tortured, and force-fed as they sought the enfranchisement of women. Consider Abraham Lincoln, Mohandas Gandhi, Jesus, Martin Luther King, Jr., Medgar Evers, Bantu Stephen Bico, Óscar Romero, Chico Mendes, Dian Fossey, Bérta Cáceres, Dom Phillips, and thousands of other activists for human rights, religious freedom, racial equality, the health of the natural environment, and other concerns, who have been murdered, assassinated, or executed. 'Tis a perilous thing to challenge the idols of privilege, power, prestige, position, and money, for they fight back, often without restraint or conscience.

The Coercive Force of Ethics: *Moral Suasion*

The law has teeth. It can fine, imprison, and even execute you. The coercive force of ethics is different: it relies on *moral suasion*, manifest in a range of degrees as peer pressure, perhaps ostracism, shunning, or exclusion, or, in some traditions, parents simply "guilt the kids" into obedience. Epideictic speech and *ars praedicandi* (the art of preaching, or moral and religious arguments) are not as persuasive in society as they once were. The coercive force of moral suasion was stronger in earlier times. For example, before the printing press was invented, when books were hand-copied, the scribes placed a curse or a blessing in the front of the book. These hand-copied books contained a blessing that the reader might profit, or a curse that a book thief, or someone who read the book with dirty hands, might perish. Blessings and curses were understood as *performative utterances*; that is, they accomplished what was spoken. Moral infractions or violations, simultaneously sins as well, were very high-risk behaviors. These scribal curses and blessings later became "book plates." This one, from the Monastery of San Pedro in Barcelona, Spain, is my favorite book curse:

> For him that stealth, or borroweth and returneth not, this book from its owner, let it change into a serpent in his hand and rend him. Let him be struck with palsy, and all his members blasted. Let him languish in pain crying aloud for mercy, and let there be no surcease to his agony till he sing in dissolution. Let bookworms gnaw his entrails in token of the Worm that dieth not [Satan] and when at last he doth go to his final punishment, let the flames of Hell consume him forever.[30]

When curses and blessings were believed to be performative utterances, and when moral infractions were dark sins, such a curse would likely dissuade those who were tempted to steal this book or read it with dirty hands. With this book curse, the fine for late return is entirely too steep—I would return it forthwith.

The village of Eyam, England, in the 1660s when the Great Plague raged through Europe, provides us with a more communal example of *moral suasion* (and another of my favorites). In September 1665, a tailor received a bolt of cloth infested with fleas carrying bubonic plague. When the pestilence remitted months later, 77 villagers were dead. In the late spring of the following year, the plague broke out again in the tiny village. The rich had already left, and now the commonfolk also decided to flee the village, even though they had nowhere to go. Their 28-year-old village rector (a Church of England clergyperson in charge of a parish), one William Mompesson, exhorted the villagers to quarantine themselves to protect the people of the surrounding county, Derbyshire, from the spread of the plague. He was persuasive. The villagers agreed to stay, knowing the heightened risk to themselves. The town was marked out by a circle of stones, painted white, in a half-mile radius, as a warning to keep away. Provisions and goods that the village needed were left just outside the perimeter of the stones. When the plague finally ended, 259 of 350 villagers had died. These villagers risked their own lives for the sake of others beyond their quarantine. This heroic act is celebrated each year in the English Midlands, in the same field in which young Rector Mompesson preached.

Moral suasion invokes a person's or community's moral nature or sense. The use of moral suasion is most effective with persons of good will, or your children. It is largely ineffective with persons bent toward criminality, severe self-interest, or untruth for it relies upon the person's acknowledgment of guilt or shame.

The Emergence of Social Ethics

There was considerable social ferment in the United States, Canada, and Great Britain as the nineteenth century became the twentieth century. In this period, there is a remarkable convergence of social forces as well as social issues. We have seen the cauldron of social issues that our respective countries faced. Maureen Flanagan writes:

> The impulse for reform emanated from a pervasive sense that the country's democratic promise was failing. Political corruption seemed endemic at all levels of government. An unregulated capitalist industrial economy exploited workers and threatened to create a serious class divide, especially as the legal system protected the rights of business over labor. Mass urbanization was shifting the country from a rural, agricultural society to an urban, industrial one characterized by poverty, disease, crime, and cultural clash. Rapid technological advancements... left many people feeling that they had little control over their lives. Movements for socialism, woman suffrage, and rights for African Americans, immigrants, and workers belied the rhetoric of the United States as a just and equal democratic society for all its members.[31]

Indeed, neither democracy, nor capitalism, nor the churches, were living up to their promise. Rural poverty, urban squalor—"Double, double toil and trouble; Fire burn and caldron bubble... Like a hell-broth boil and bubble." This was a new kind of hell-broth for immigrants, workers, racial and ethnic minorities, women, the poor, and all those at the bottom rungs of society for which they had no ladder.

Converging Movements

In this context we see (a) Progressivism and the rise of *voluntary associations*, some simply for affiliative purposes, but others for social activism targeting particular issues; (b) the development of philosophical Pragmatism and its social engagement; and (c) the rise of the social ethics movement. These are all intertwined—with nursing in the mix of it all—and this is the social ferment that births social ethics in nursing.

Progressivism and the Rise of Voluntary Associations (Associationalism)

Voluntary associations, especially those groups that affiliate for purposes of social reform, are important in American society in that they create political pressure for social and legislative change. For women—and nurses—voluntary associations were their only means of political action at their disposal, as they did not have a vote. The diplomat, political philosopher, scientist, and historian Alexis Charles Henri Clérel, Comte de Tocqueville, or Alexis de Tocqueville, visited the US in the

1830s. In *Democracy in America* (1833) he made a number of observations about the US and its formation of the political and civil voluntary associations essential to democracy (to prevent a "despotic influence of a majority"[32]). Of civil associations, he writes:

> Americans of all ages, all conditions, and all dispositions constantly form associations. They have not only commercial and manufacturing companies, in which all take part, but associations of a thousand other kinds—religious, moral, serious, futile, extensive or restricted, enormous or diminutive. The Americans make associations to give entertainments [fêtes], to found establishments for education, to build inns, to construct churches, to diffuse books, to send missionaries to the antipodes; and in this manner they found hospitals, prisons, schools. If it be proposed to advance some truth or to foster some feeling by the encouragement of a great example, they form a society [they associate]. Wherever at the head of some new undertaking, you see the government in France, or a man of rank in England; in the United States, you will be sure to find an association.[33]

Tocqueville's observation was that Americans distinctively took advantage of voluntary associations as a powerful and effective means of social action for a great variety of civic objectives, and as a form of self-governance through social corrective activism. Those civic objectives could, of course, have political consequences.[34] Voluntary associations were the means by which women and nurses wrought social change.

Women-Initiated Associations

Theda Skocpol, of the Civic Engagement Project of Harvard University, writes:

> Both class and gender transformations have affected U.S. associations. Most large voluntary federations from the 1800s through the 1960s were cross-class, single-gender affairs. Business and professional people joined together with white-collar folks and perhaps with more privileged farmers or craft or industrial workers. But it was predominately men or women, not both together, who formed most of these multi-purpose voluntary associations. For much of American history, segregated male and female roles provided broad, shared identities through which huge numbers of Americans could band together across regional and class lines.[35]

These gender-segregated associations, could also be, and not infrequently were, racially segregated.

*Activist Nurse Lillian Wald asks, "Have you ever seen a
starving child cry?"[36]*

Starving children don't cry,[37] something that nurses have painfully witnessed, and
by which they have been moved on behalf of children and poor families. Flanagan
discusses a number of the women-initiated, cross-class, voluntary associations that
represented women working on behalf of women, children, workers, and society,
somewhat in that order.

> Women organized in voluntary groups worked to identify and attack the prob-
> lems caused by mass urbanization. The General Federation of Women's Clubs
> (1890) coordinated women's activities throughout the country. Social justice
> Progressives lobbied municipal governments to enact new ordinances to ameli-
> orate existing urban conditions of poverty, disease, and inequality. Chicago
> women secured the nation's first juvenile court (1899). Los Angeles women
> helped inaugurate a public health nursing program and secure pure milk regu-
> lations for their city. Women also secured municipal public baths in Boston,
> Chicago, Philadelphia, and other cities. Organized women in Philadelphia and
> Dallas were largely responsible for their cities implementing new clean water
> systems. Women set up pure milk stations to prevent infant diarrhea and organ-
> ized infant welfare societies.[38]

In the Progressive mix, Florence Kelley, Louis Brandeis, and Josephine Goldmark argued for labor laws governing work conditions, minimum wages, and
work hours. Josephine Goldmark (1877–1950) was a labor activist who worked
against child labor, for an eight-hour work day, and for passage of the Keating–
Owen Act of 1916 and the Fair Labor Standards Act of 1937. From 1919 to
1923, funded by the Rockefeller Foundation, Goldmark researched US nursing
schools. Her research was published under the title *Nursing and Nursing Education in the United States* (1923). It examined nursing education, reorienting it
toward education and away from hospital service.[39] Goldmark lived, for many
years, at the *Henry Street Settlement*, which was originally founded as *Nurse's
Settlement*, by social progressive nurse-reformer Lillian Wald (1867–1940).[40,41]
It was associated with Jane Addams' Hull House Settlement in Chicago. There
was considerable interaction between and among settlements, all working toward social reform and assisting those in need. See, for example, Jane Addams'
book *Democracy and Social Ethics*.[42] Both Hull House and Henry Street Settlement were beehives of women social activist-reformers, intellectuals, and hu-
manitarians, including, nurses, social workers, artists, teachers and more—and
Lavinia Dock.

Women and nurses founded and ran an astonishing array of social reform associations, large and small, encompassing everything from worker rights to pure

milk, food, and water supplies. When the Sheppherd–Towner Maternity and Infant Welfare Bill was about to sunset and was up for re-authorization,

> The hostility of the male-dominated American Medical Association [AMA] and the Public Health Service to Sheppard–Towner and to its administration by the Children's Bureau, along with attacks against the social justice network of women's organizations as a communist conspiracy to undermine American society, doomed the legislation.[43]

This was not the first, nor the last, time that women and nurses would be on opposite sides of the medical establishment, the AMA, and be decried as communist. This is an example of an *ad hominem* logical fallacy, and scare tactic, to attempt to discredit an idea by attacking its author as communist. This same argument was used to oppose the creation of Medicare.

Much of the Progressive social reform of the period was driven by women, including nurses and social workers, through their voluntary associations and the organizations and agencies that they spawned. Some were racially segregated. Others, such as the Settlements, were not. Henry Street Settlement played a role in the formation of what would become the National Association for the Advancement of Colored People (NAACP).[44] Despite the extraordinary degree of women-led activism for reform, Flanigan notes:

> Much literature on the movements emphasizes male initiatives and fails to appreciate gender differences. The public forums movement promoted by men, such as Charles Sprague Smith and Frederic Howe, was a top-down effort in which prominent speakers addressed pressing issues of the day to teach the "rank and file" how to practice democracy. In Boston, Mary Parker Follett promoted participatory democracy through neighborhood centers organized and run by residents. Chicago women's organizations fostered neighborhood centers as spaces for residents to gather and discuss neighborhood needs.[45]

Her point is important for several reasons. First it shows what I term the "disappearing women phenomenon" where women's activity and accomplishments are "disappeared" from the historical record and credited to men. Second, it points to an observed gendered difference in approach—the men working top-down, giving directive lectures; and the women in the trenches with and alongside the persons they hoped to serve—seeing the starving child who cannot cry. Third, these Progressives have an emphasis on *democracy* that derives in part from the philosophy of Pragmatism of the period. And fourth, a collateral observation, that this same distinction between the "men's" top-down and the women's bottom-up "in the trenches" approach is, in part, a difference between bioethics and nursing ethics. Bioethics has largely developed from abstract, rationalist, European philosophical theories; nursing ethics derives from the tradition, narrative, and community of nursing, from its nursing practice and its lived, relational experience.

Though much less gender-specific, *associationalism* continues today, representing a full range of interest-focused groups. There are charitable, sporting, hobby, youth, political, honorific, and professional associations and many more, which includes the American Nurses Association, American Hospital Association, and the American Medical Association as voluntary associations. Some serve leisure and recreational purposes while others serve to address deeper structural issues of justice and fairness.[46]

While I initially called this a *convergence*, in reality it is messier than that. We have a hell-broth of social problems; an era of social reform called Progressivism; a rise of *associationalism* that generates voluntary associations that generate organizations and agencies; women's activism that involves women reformists, nurses, social workers, women attorneys, economists, and others acting with the skills of their respective fields or professions. Into this mix we will also find a dominant philosophy of Pragmatism, and the rise of the social ethics movement. We now turn to these remaining movements in succession.

Pragmatism: Philosophy in a Sweating World

Early modern nursing used the term *sweating* to describe the exploitation of nurses, their overwork, their hazardous and difficult work conditions, and low wages. Sweating, in relation to all workers, including child laborers, was a major issue of the Progressive era during which Pragmatism emerged. Pragmatism is a "Made in the USA" product, a philosophical movement of the later 1800s and 1900s. It dominated American philosophy until World War II, when (some have argued) an influx of refugee Continental philosophers brought analytic philosophy, causing Pragmatism to wane. However, Pragmatism has undergone a contemporary renewal, and is seen today especially in black, black feminist, black radical feminist, and feminist ethics reinterpretations.

Philosophy of Pragmatism

There have been a range of interpreters of Pragmatism, though the most prominent at the time of nursing's coalescence were Charles Sanders Pierce, and especially William James and John Dewey.[47,48] James, a philosopher, psychologist, historian, and physician, was a Harvard academic. John Dewey was a philosopher, academic reformer, psychologist, public intellectual, and professor at the University of Chicago. Both men influenced nursing and nursing ethics in terms of philosophical content, as well as in educational theory; that is, that nursing education should be informed and guided by a philosophy and theory, and not a haphazard, happenstantial agglutination of topics.

As a philosophy, Pragmatism emphasizes the practical consequences and usefulness of ideas; that is, that the value of an idea or belief lies in its practical consequences and how it helps us understand the world and act effectively within it. Pragmatism does not develop linearly, but rather develops through a series of arguments, developing several streams, including contemporary Neopragmatism.[49]

Pragmatists argued against philosophical rationalists' position that reason is the primary source of knowledge and that some truths can be known by reason alone, independent of sensory experience. Pragmatists argued that reason alone cannot provide a complete understanding of reality, and that practical consequences, history, context, culture, and lived experience are crucial for determining the truth or usefulness of ideas. The strengths of Pragmatism are that it emphasizes the interconnectedness of theory and practice, and rejects the separation of abstract ideas from their practical implications. It promotes a holistic understanding of knowledge and encourages active engagement with the world.[50] The weaknesses or critiques of Pragmatism are that it is subject to relativism and theoretical weaknesses, and that the emphasis on real-world consequences instrumentalizes ethics. In what Misak terms "the eclipse narrative," it has been asserted that Progressivism waned as analytic philosophy rose, though it began to make a comeback or renewal in the 1980s forward. Misak, a Canadian pragmatist philosopher, asserts:

> Wittgenstein's later philosophy... is also arguably a kind of pragmatism with its emphasis on the primacy of practice and meaning as use.... Pragmatist theses, arguments and concerns pervade the analytic philosophy that reigned in Oxford and Cambridge throughout the second half of the 20th century. Thus, the eclipse narrative fails not only as an account of the fortunes of pragmatism in the US, but also of the fortunes of pragmatism in England.... pragmatism was not marginalised or eclipsed in the post-Dewey period. Rather, pragmatism has been a constant and dominant force in professional philosophy in the US and elsewhere for nearly 100 years. As far as philosophical idioms go, pragmatism is among the most successful in the history of the discipline.[51]

In its early iterations, Pragmatism went hand-in-glove with Progressivism, and concern for the prevailing range of social harms and injustices, including the issue of women's suffrage. Bernstein writes:

> With Dewey... the social and political aspect came into the foreground.... democracy as a form of communal life in which "all share and all contribute" is central to [his] philosophic vision. While deeply skeptical of all "true believers" and never sympathetic with calls for "total revolution," Dewey [was] committed to a program of radical democratic social reform. The pragmatists were not apologists for the status quo. They were among the most relentless critics of American society for failing to realize its democratic promise.[52]

Modern nursing emerged within this ethos, one that informed and shaped early nursing, and within which nursing exercised its social ethics and practice. Pragmatism has continued to appeal to nursing for its engagement with real-world problems; its ability to engage with a complex, rapidly changing world; its emphasis on social contexts, power structures, and social inequalities; its compatibility with intersectional analyses; and that it bends toward activism. However, the ways in which Pragmatism continues to be furthered in nursing tend to focus on the theory—practice division, theoretical analyses, and concerns for research methodologies. There is little discussion in nursing of Pragmatism vis-à-vis ethics or social ethics despite its central role in early nursing ethics.[53,54,55,56,57,58,59,60]

Friends and Communities

Before moving to the first period of the social ethics movement, it is important to mention that while the Progressive Movement and Pragmatism were intertwined in terms of perspective, they—and nursing—were also linked by social connections, friendships, educational institutions, and personal experiences and commitments. John Dewey was on faculty at Teachers College (TC), Columbia University, which provided advanced education for graduate nurses who sought to be nursing educators. TC provided advanced education for Canadian as well as American nurses, thus helping to export Pragmatism to Canadian nursing. The settlement houses, Hull House and Henry Street Settlement, served as residential communities and places of congregation for nurses, social reformers, and social workers who were Progressivists and Pragmatists. Jane Addams, Lillian Wald, Julia Lathrop, Florence Kelley, Sophonisba Breckinridge, Ida Cannon, Mary Brewster, Anne Stevens, Francis Perkins, Margaret Sanger, Grace Abbott, Mary McDowell, and Isabel Robb were among the many leaders in nursing, social work, and social reform who were personally associated with one another. Lavinia Dock (known as a Progressivist, but not a Pragmatist) and Lillian Wald were part of the same circle of progressive reformers and social activists. They shared a passion for improving the lives of the poor, vulnerable, and marginalized populations, and worked together to advance their causes within the nursing profession and the broader social reform movement. Apart from the interconnectedness of these movements, what also stands out is the close communities of professional women who supported, challenged, sustained, and shared with one another.

The Rise of Social Ethics, in Three Periods

In addition to Progressivism and Pragmatism, the third major player in the milieu was a public expression of the developing academic field of *social ethics*, which is also tied to bioethics. Gary Dorrien's magisterial work *Social Ethics in the Making: Interpreting an American Tradition*[61] (which I commend) focuses on social ethics within the American setting, though social ethics also finds expression in the UK, Canada, Norway, Sweden, Germany, the Netherlands, Belgium, Austria, India, the Philippines, Brazil, Chile, South Africa, Nigeria, and other countries. In each of those countries, it was and remains theologically impelled. The *social ethics movement* had three periods, of which the *social gospel* (or *social gospel movement*) was the first, the *Christian realism period* was the second, and the third was that of *liberation theologies*.

The Social Gospel Period

The *social gospel* was a Protestant Christian theological teaching that formed the basis for a widely influential, international movement for social reform. Its academic arm was the discipline of *Christian social ethics*. Though it began as a Protestant Christian religious expression of Progressivism, it also included a Roman Catholic expression and grew to be reflected in Jewish and other traditions, collectively, as *religious social ethics*. Graduate degree programs (MA, PhD) in social ethics were (and remain) offered in university schools of religion, university schools of theology, and in religious seminaries.[62]

The social gospel movement arose in the late 1800s and early 1900s in the US, Canada, and the UK. As a movement, it was a response to the problems consequent to urbanization, industrialization, poverty, and the understanding that the Christian faith had a responsibility in the face of these problems, but had failed markedly in that responsibility. Its emphasis was on social action over dogma or doctrine; on reforming social structures that created social injustices, over evangelism and personal salvation; and on social activism over religious quietism and piety. It thus represented the more liberal wing of Christianity, and was (and remains) repudiated as "Godless Christianity" by the conservative side of the tradition.

Walter Rauschenbusch, along with Richard T. Ely, and Washington Gladden, were the social gospel's major proponents. Walter Rauschenbush was a seminary theologian, Baptist pastor, and, incidentally, grandfather of contemporary philosopher Richard Rorty, who served as pastor at a church in a New York slum known as "Hell's Kitchen." The neighborhood was home to Irish immigrants who were working-class poor, living under terrible conditions of poverty. Rauschenbusch was prompted to social activism by the social injustices he witnessed as he pastored the people, including the grinding poverty, squalor, and the funerals for children that he would conduct.[63] Rauschenbusch's most important works are *Christianity and the Social Crisis* (1907),[64] which influenced leaders in the movement, and *A Theology for the Social Gospel* (1917),[65] which rallied liberal Protestant churches to the movement. Rauschenbusch writes of six social sins:

> Religious bigotry, the combination of graft and political power, the corruption of justice, the mob spirit, militarism, and class contempt—every student of history will recognize that these sum up constitutional forces in the Kingdom of Evil.... They were not only the sins of Caiaphas, Pilate, or Judas, but the social sin of all mankind, to which all who ever lived have contributed, and under which all who ever lived have suffered.[66]

Rauschenbusch called for "the redemption of social life from the cramping influence of religious bigotry, from the repression of self-assertion in the relation of upper and lower classes, and from all forms of slavery in which human beings are treated as mere means to serve the ends of others."[67] He wrestles with the problem of evil, not as individual sin but as collective or sociopolitical evil. He writes that "if a group practises evil, it will excuse or idealize it, and resent any private judgment which condemns it. Evil then becomes part of the standards of morality sanctioned by the authority of society. This confuses the moral judgment of the individual."[68] He identified four evils, exercised by "super-personal entities" (society): militarism, individualism, [predatory] capitalism, and nationalism. The social goods that he juxtaposed against these evils were pacifism, solidarity, socialized democracy, and internationalism.[69]

Despite his concern for social reform, and his opposition to social structures that enslaved, we must not be blind to Rauschenbusch's more than problematic views on race, and US imperialism (Manifest Destiny). Miguel A. De La Torre[70] notes that while Rauschenbush worked against oppressive social structures and conditions, he also retained a paternalistic attitude toward persons of color and immigrants. He was also of a view that the US could lead to a better world order through the exercise of its power. De La Torre writes:

While Rauschenbusch saw himself living in a democracy, he failed to make the connection between what he was writing and the consequences of the emerging US Empire for the colonized... [he] believed that for the United States to be great it must enter the race of conquering foreign lands... the war Rauschenbusch supported signified the United States' entry into imperialism.[71]

Rauschenbusch, as with many historic figures, embodied both good and evil—as do nations—including this nation from which I write. The militarism that Rauschenbusch supported produced atrocities and massacres. While we grapple with the moral complexity of historic figures, we must also do so regarding the nations of our own birth or citizenship.

The social gospel movement and social ethics is also represented in the Roman Catholic tradition. In 1891, Pope Leo XIII published the encyclical *Rerum Novarum*.[72] The Catholic Church has a long tradition of social theology, but had not engaged with the consequences of the industrial revolution, the plight of workers, and predation by corporations. *Rerum Novarum* focuses on the economic context of that day in relation to

the vast expansion of industrial pursuits and the marvellous discoveries of science; in the changed relations between masters and workmen; in the enormous fortunes of some few individuals, and the utter poverty of the masses; the increased self-reliance and closer mutual combination of the working classes; as also, finally, in the prevailing moral degeneracy.[73]

The encyclical points to specific social ills perpetrated by unjust economic conditions allowed to flourish by the politics of the day. Pope Leo notes specifically that:

it has come to pass that working men have been surrendered, isolated and helpless, to the hardheartedness of employers and the greed of unchecked competition.

The mischief has been increased by rapacious usury, which, although more than once condemned by the Church, is nevertheless,... still practiced by covetous and grasping men. To this must be added that the hiring of labor and the conduct of trade are concentrated in the hands of comparatively few; so that a small number of very rich men have been able to lay upon the teeming masses of the laboring poor a yoke little better than that of slavery itself.[74]

Rerum Novarum shook up the Catholic world by directly taking on a potent political and economic issue. It explicitly supports the right of workers to form unions. It also takes a middle path by, also explicitly, rejecting both socialism and unconstrained capitalism. It affirms a right to private property, with a somewhat shaky justification in the law of nature. *Rerum Novarum* is the foundational text of modern *Catholic social teaching* (CST) and Catholic social ethics. It would subsequently be followed both by additional social encyclicals as well as a substantive and extensive body of CST.

There are many persons in the CST stream of the social gospel and social ethics, but John Ryan, priest and son of an Irish immigrant family, and the colorful Mary "Mother Jones" Harris stand out. Deeply influenced by *Rerum Novarum*, Ryan became the leading Catholic proponent and moral theologian for economic and social reform, and the leading Roman Catholic Progressive of the Progressive Era. With other Progressives (and nurses), he sought legislation that would regulate child labor, establish living wages, and regulate work conditions, provide national health insurance, regulate the free market, and more.[75] Mary G. Harris "Mother Jones" was born in Cork, Ireland. Her family immigrated to Canada then to the US during the Great Famine (1845–1852). Mary married but lost her husband and four children in a yellow fever epidemic. She moved to Chicago but lost her home and dressmaker shop in the Great Chicago Fire of 1871. She joined the Knights of Labor to help rebuild Chicago after the fire, and began organizing strikes and protests.[76] Her life was spent in organizing workers, in boycotts and strikes, in educating workers, in being arrested, tried, and jailed. She was accounted a gifted orator who used biblical allusions and stories to galvanize workers.[77] Mother Jones had concern for all workers, including child laborers, and young women workers, all of whom were subject to exploitation and hazardous work conditions. Mother Jones believed the government would always take the side of power, of the rich, and would punish and obstruct workers who sought to improve their wages, work conditions, and hours. It is worth noting that as one who believed women belonged in the home, Mother Jones ran afoul of suffragists.[78]

The Christian Realism Period

The social gospel movement had an idealistic edge, believing that society could be reformed toward justice. That vision proved to be naive and roseate—and quixotic. As an expectation of faith, activism could not be relinquished but it could be reformulated. Reinhold Niebuhr is the figure most identified with this shift, though Christian realism reaches back to Augustine of Hippo (354–430 CE). Christian realism is a political theology that arose following the unfathomable moral depravity of Hitler, Stalin, Mussolini, the Holocaust, concentration camps, stalags, and gulags. True to his theological roots Niebuhr believed that humankind is ever given "to tyranny and idolatry." Niebuhr pastored a church in Detroit during a period of race riots and labor disputes. Like Rauschenbusch and many others, he develops his theology within the fires of pastoral responsibility, in his case for a white working-class congregation. Christian realism seeks to address the complexities of human nature, humanity's potential for good as well as for tyranny and idolatry; the good or evil that can manifest in or be perpetuated by social and political systems; and the search for social justice in the world that a flawed collective humanity creates. Niebuhr understood that Christian ethical ideals and values would be in a fight cage with the moral vicissitudes of human systems, a match that would require balancing idealism with pragmatism. Evil would have to be confronted and even so may yet persist. He articulates his vision of Christian realism chiefly in two books, the first *Moral Man and Immoral Society: A Study in Ethics and Politics*.[79] This book's thesis it that persons are more likely to sin when a member of a group, than as an individual. The second book was *Christian Realism and Political Problems*.[80] While he recognizes the difficulties of achieving social justice in the face of intractable and perhaps immutable power, he nonetheless advocated tangling with social and political issues, undergirded by Christian social ethics, an understanding of human nature, a good dose of social science, and steadfast faithful commitment. This period is largely associated with one person, Reinhold Niebuhr. Subsequently, Presidents John Kennedy, Jimmy Carter, Barack Obama, Secretary of State Madeline Albright, and The Rev. Martin Luther King, Jr. all acknowledged Niebuhr's influence upon their own perspectives. Niebuhr was a white, middle-class, Christian theologian and pastor who lived, worked, and taught within the wider world, but had his being within the insularity of a white, middle-class life, pastoral, and academic world.

The social ethics movement was not limited to the US. Charles Kingsley, F.D. Maurice, Charles Gore, R.H. Tawney, and William Temple were key figures in the social ethics tradition in the UK. In the UK, the social gospel movement influenced the development of Christian socialism, the establishment of labor parties, and the pursuit of a wide range of social reforms.[81] It contributed to the expansion of social welfare programs and the promotion of economic justice in the UK and in other nations (e.g., Germany). The social gospel movement in Canada impacted social and political reforms, including the establishment of social welfare programs, labor rights, and universal health care. Tommy Douglas was one of its notable figures.[82,83,84]

The Niebuhrian period of social ethics is followed by a third, that of liberation theologies. Dorrien writes:

> For fifty years, social ethics remained a social gospel enterprise,… even in its
> minority streams that were not white, male, middle-class, or Protestant. In the

1930s the field pushed aside its optimistic, social gospel beginnings in favor of Reinhold Niebuhr's, sterner language of sin, power politics, transcendence, and realism, which held center stage for 30 years,... [until] the rise of liberation theology. All three of these movements held high, a vision of social transformation... Niebuhrians judged that the social gospel sold out the struggle for social justice, because it was too middle-class and idealistic to be a serious force in power politics. Liberationists judged that Christian realism sold out the struggle for social justice because it was too middle-class, idealistic, white, male dominated, nationalistic, and socially privileged. But liberation theology was too marginal, and radical in US American society, to make much of an impact upon it; meanwhile, social ethics produced offshoots with small followings in every direction today.[85]

The third period of social ethics, that of liberation theologies, seeks to overcome the lacunae of Niebuhrian realism and its embeddedness in American dominant culture. The liberation theologies, for there are many, bring non-white, non-male, non-Western voices into the mix. By doing so, they have a greater power to expose and address social oppressions that afflict racial, minority, and impoverished communities.

Liberation Theology

Leaders in the social gospel and Niebuhrian periods of social ethics had access to the works of Marx, Weber, Durkheim, the founders of sociology; and members of the Frankfurt School, and others who critiqued society and social structures, though doing so within their own European and American cultures. Critical theories as we have them in our toolkits today, had not yet arisen. Post-colonial, intersectional, feminist, critical race, queer theories, and liberation theologies would come to the fore and would critique the failings of earlier social ethics and articulate a potent corrective to the preceding eras of the social ethics movement. They would become a means of addressing the structural oppressions that exist today.

Liberation theology, with roots in Catholic social teaching, emerged primarily within the Latin American Roman Catholic Church in the 1960s and 1970s. Catholic theologians and educators Gustavo Gutiérrez (Peru),[86] Leonardo Boff (Brazil),[87,88] Paulo Freire (Brazil),[89] Juan Luis Segundo (Uruguay),[90] and Jon Sobrino and Ignacio Ellacuria (El Salvador) have been influential in the movement, with Gustavo Gutiérrez considered the founder. Liberation theology was also taken up in Protestant circles, by Rubem Alves (Brazil, Presbyterian) and José Míguez Bonino (Argentina, Methodist).

Liberation theology seeks to address social, political, and economic oppression, from a theological perspective, particularly in the context of poverty and marginalization. Liberation theologians emphasize the biblical teachings on justice, liberation, and solidarity with the poor and oppressed which, in the Latin American context, gave rise to the principle of "a preferential option for the poor." The term can be traced to the 1968 Latin American bishops' conference held in Medellín, Colombia. The conference focused on social issues of poverty and injustice and advocated for a preferential option for the poor as a response to oppression. This moral notion was further developed and expanded upon in the subsequent papal encyclicals *Populorum Progressio*[91] (1967), by Pope Paul VI, and *Sollicitudo Rei Socialis*[92] (1987), written by Pope John Paul II on the 20th anniversary of *Populorum Progressio*. John Paul II writes on the moral "duty of solidarity" with the poor:

> the originality of the Encyclical [*Populorum Progressio*] consists not so much in the affirmation, historical in character, of the universality of the social question, but rather in the moral evaluation of this reality. Therefore, political leaders, and citizens of rich countries considered as individuals, especially if they are Christians, have the moral obligation, according to the degree of each one's responsibility, to take into consideration, in personal decisions and decisions of government, this relationship of universality, this interdependence which exists between their conduct and the poverty and underdevelopment of so many millions of people. Pope Paul's Encyclical translates more succinctly the moral obligation as the "duty of solidarity;" and this affirmation, even though many situations have changed in the world, has the same force and validity today as when it was written.[93]

These encyclicals, as with the wider social ethics literature generally, call for specific actions to prevent, correct, and ameliorate the social evils and injustices that they address within the context of CST. Latin American liberation theology that extends CST is not the only liberation theology: it has correlates in other nations such as Minjung theology in Korea, founded by theologian Ahn Byung-Mu,[94] and Dalit liberation theology in India associated with theologian/pastors Arvind P. Nirmal, M.E. Prabhakar, and Vedanayagam Devasahayam. Minjung and Dalit liberation theologies are among a group of Christian postcolonial theologies. Latin American theology has tended to be the best known, but there are black, feminist, womanist, Mujerista, Native American, ecojustice, and other liberation theologies as well. These liberation theologies arise within the lifeworld and lived experience of their community and undertake to address ethical concerns that affect that community.

The term *liberation theology* was independently coined by both Gustavo Gutiérrez and James Cone (1938–2018) in 1968. Liberation theology has five attributes:

> Liberation theologies employ action-reflection (praxis-oriented) methodologies in response to particular forms of oppression, normally consisting of five elements: 1) identification with particular forms of oppression and suffering, 2) prophetic critique of that condition, 3) social analysis of the causes of oppression and suffering, 4) biblical and theological engagement to address that suffering and overcome that oppression, and 5) advocacy of structural change

toward a greater approximation of justice. Liberation theologies engage in intentional reflection upon particular experiences in which these five elements interact dynamically according to the forms of suffering and oppression specific to particular populations, historical experiences, and contexts.[95]

Nursing is, at present (and much overdue), examining its history of racism and the structures of the profession that disadvantage persons of color. This makes the work of James Cone, Cornel West, and Miguel A. De La Torre particularly relevant to both nursing as a profession and to nursing ethics. Cone, a theologian, published *Black Theology and Black Power*,[96] *A Black Theology of Liberation*,[97] *God of the Oppressed*,[98] *The Cross and the Lynching Tree*,[99] and a number of other works. His books lay out the distinctiveness of the black experience, black theology, the struggle for civil rights, and a wrenching indictment of the white church for its willing participation in racist structures or its failure to speak out and take action against racism. Cone dug deeply into the black Christian community experience, writing: "I was on a mission to transform self-loathing Negro Christians into black-loving revolutionary disciples of the Black Christ."[100] Booker T. Washington, W.E.B. DuBois, Reverdy Ransom, Ida B. Wells-Barnett, Martin Luther King, Jr., and James Cone were of the successive line and lineage of the black social gospel–social ethics stream, concerned for its application to structures of racism as experienced by black Americans.[101] Cone influenced Bantu Stephen Biko, Desmond Tutu, Alan Boesak, Cornel West, a number of womanist theologians, and others.

Cornel West continues the social gospel–social ethics tradition today, with a reformulation of American Pragmatism. While his most influential works have been *Race Matters*[102] (1993) and *Democracy Matters*[103] (2005), for our purposes it is his book *The American Evasion of Philosophy: A Genealogy of Pragmatism* (1989) that is of particular import for nursing ethics. In this book he addresses the American resistance to analytic philosophy, in favor of Pragmatism. He acknowledges the contributions that Pragmatism has made to American thought, but also understands its limitations. What West offers is a vision of Pragmatism, influential at the start of modern nursing, and Progressivism that weds philosophic discourse to cultural criticism and cultural change through political engagement, that (breathe here) brings the social gospel, the black social gospel, black liberation theology, and religious social ethics together to bear upon the seemingly intractable American problem of racism.

A number of black theologians have described racism as a form of self-worship, and self-deification, that distorts and scars the soul of the racist person while harming the othered persons. That is, racism harms both the oppressor and the oppressed. Martin Luther King, Jr., James Baldwin, Malcolm X, and Frantz Fanon all draw this connecting line. For those within the Christian tradition, and many religious traditions, there can be no greater incrimination than to understand that one's racism is the sin of idolatry. This is the power of religious discourse within any religious tradition—the power to convict and to command *metanoia*, a turning around, a turning away from, one's idolatries.

Contemporary social ethicist, Miguel A. De La Torre, extends the social ethics tradition with access to critical theories. He writes:

The underlying problem with Eurocentric ethics is that moral reasoning is done from the realm of abstraction. Ethics is less concerned with "what you do" than "how you think."... Why must people of color in general, Latina/os specifically, follow Euroamerican ethical analytical paradigms, when engaging in moral reasoning?... [he] analyzes twentieth-century Eurocentric ethics to expose its indistinguishability from middle-class respectability and conformity, as well as its complicity with empire, and thus its inherent tendency to oppose marginalized communities.... Almost all the best-known ethicists of the twentieth century were white males. Specifically, they were white males embedded within a social location that informed, shaped, influenced, and constructed their worldview. Regardless of how progressive we wish to consider these ethicists, they remain a product of the empire to which they belong, reflecting the racism and ethnic discrimination of their time that continues to make empire possible. True, they may have challenged the empire, critiqued the empire, and even called for profound reform, but in final analysis, they contributed to the undergirding racial and ethnic assumptions that provided justification for the empire because they failed to recognize their complicity with the overarching power structures that make empire possible. They call for justice without challenging the dominant culture's retention of its power and privilege. The end result is a "kinder, gentler" form of oppression.[104]

He does not entirely overturn what has gone before, but instead redeems what can be redeemed, and brings forward new ways of seeing, thinking, and acting. Not unlike nursing ethics, his claim is:

Liberative ethics argues that theological and theoretical reflections are derived from praxis, turning on its head the Eurocentric deductive, ethical paradigm, which begins with theory as "truth," and then moves to praxis as the implementation of that truth. As liberative ethicists point out, the truth, believed by the dominant culture, is a construct, reflecting the bias and prejudices of that culture, which, consciously or unconsciously, developed ethical paradigms that are complicit with empire and fall short of calling for radical changes in how wealth, power, and privilege are disbursed.[105]

In place of the Eurocentric deductive ethical paradigm, De La Torre calls for "an ethics of civil initiative," distinguishing it from civil disobedience. In reconstructing ethics, he calls for an ethics *en lo cotidiano*, an ethics *de nepantla*, an ethics *para la lucha*, an ethics *en conjunto*, an ethics *de acompañamiento*—concepts that are some decades old that De La Torre calls on *la comunidad* to expand and develop into new ethical paradigms "based on a radical activism focused on the liberation of Hispanics from the prevailing dominant social structures."[106]

Nursing has a strong ethical tradition, based in praxis, and yet today it lives in the gated community of a white, Eurocentric, largely male, rationalist bioethics that does not hear the voices of those at the margins—or perhaps even nursing. If nursing were to return to its own ethics, to hear the voices outside the gates, it would avail itself of untold resources that would help nursing bring to realization the values and vision that it holds for a good society, a healthy society. But we need to be willing to hear what is challenging, disturbing, and perhaps even indicting.

De La Torre offers nursing a methodology that is unexpectedly compatible with nursing ethics. His intent is to formulate an ethics that encompasses the Latina/o lifeworld as it is experienced by the community, including its experiences of structural oppressions and marginalization. To bring this to life, he calls for ethics *en lo cotidiano* (in the everyday) that is "unapologetically anchored in the autobiographical stories and testimonies of the disenfranchised,"[107] an ethics of daily relationships and social relations.[108] He notes that ethics uses fictional case studies to teach a principle and its nuances; the "case studies are created not as a guide for participating in community-changing praxis, but to test ethical concepts and analytically push the limits of moral reasoning."[109] His notion of *nepantla* is one of an ethics "with a preferential option for those living on the hyphen in Hispanic-American," of the poor, "the culturally oppressed and socially dispossessed," as persons between marginality and acceptance, regarded as neither truly Latino nor as truly American.[110] In his development of an ethics *para la lucha* (for the struggle) he takes a cue from Ada María Isasi-Diaz who writes of Latinas:

> An anthropology developed out of the lived-experience of Latinas centers on a subject who struggles to survive and who understands herself as one who struggles.... Of course the centrality of struggle as a constitutive element of the everyday lives of Latinas, of Latinas' self-construction, can be understood and grasped only against a background of oppression due to specific historical injustices that are the cause of great suffering. But in listening carefully to grassroots Latinas, one find that what locates in life is not suffering but *la lucha* to survive. To consider suffering as what locates us would mean that we understand ourselves not as moral subjects but as one acted upon by the oppressors.[111]

The concept of an ethics *en conjunto* "means 'in conjunction with,' or 'conjoined in,' implying not only the coming together but also the integration and intimacy involved in such a sharing," as a deep collaboration.[112] An ethics *de acompañamiento* "is a praxis of being present alongside disenfranchised latina/o *communidades en lo cotidiano* and *en la lucha.*" These are ethical concepts that together create a beginning social ethics drawn from within *la commmunidad,* the Latina/o community, to address issues of oppression and marginalization. These concepts, he notes, are not static, but evolve over time and context as the life of the community changes.

De La Torre's reconceptualization of social ethics for his Latina/o community is a voice that nursing needs to hear as it addresses racism within nursing across decades and into the future. His methodology has something profound to teach nursing ethics about uncovering and addressing particular oppressions. It also has a wisdom for nursing to consider for itself. For example, there is much written about moral distress in nursing, but in Ada María Isasi-Diaz's construct above, "To consider suffering [moral distress] as what locates us would mean that we understand ourselves not as moral subjects but as one acted upon by the oppressors." Nursing does not, of course, experience the pervasive and brutal oppressions bound to race, poverty, or minority status in this country, and has in fact historically participated in those oppressions. But nursing can in humility learn, and needs to learn, and to act by hearing the voices of those who are oppressed, marginalized, neglected, or forgotten.

Hearing Voices

Despite the contributions of theologians to the genesis of bioethics as a field, bioethics has largely secularized in a way that also engages in prejudice against religion—even while roundly condemning most other forms of prejudice. A fundamental principle of liberation theology is to cause the unheard to be heard, to give voice to those who have been marginalized structurally. As nursing explores its own history of racism, it has not yet drawn upon indigenous ethics, black social ethics, womanist ethics, black theology, feminist theology, or black liberation theology, all of which provide trenchant religiously suffused analyses of racism and ethnicism in American culture, and propose avenues for effecting change.[113,114] Nursing needs to hear, attend to, and welcome these religious voices. So too, bioethics.

Social Ethics across Religious Traditions

The concept of *religion,* as it is understood in the contemporary Western context, does not directly translate to all cultures or to some non-dominant cultures within Western societies. In religious studies, the notion of religion-as-a-Western-construct is largely understood as a reflection of the rise of modernity and the Enlightenment in the West that led to the secularization of public life and the differentiation between religious and secular domains. This secular framework influenced the perception of religion as a personal or private matter, distinct from political and social life and, at least overtly, separable. However, many non-Western cultures have their own ancient and suffusive belief systems, often predating the Western concept of religion. These non-Western systems encompass various if not all aspects of life, including daily life, health, spirituality, morality, marriage and family, community, society, law, governance, that is, the whole of life, and are not separable from the general culture and its way of being.[115,116,117,118] For example, "In the Tongva language [California Native American language], no word exists for nature, because we are not separate from it."[119] In other languages, no word exists for religion, or charity, because its speakers are not separate from it. This is important for our purposes in that access to ethics in some traditions comes only through the larger and prior category of their theology.

Every major religious tradition has a religious social ethics, many of which were active in American society at the time of the social gospel movement forward, and many of which had an activist as well as an academic arm. The Jewish tradition has a long history of social ethics, enacted through individual congregations as well as through organizations. Lillian Wald, a Jewish nurse-social activist, is a good exemplar of her tradition. Wald founded the Henry Street Settlement, and her work in public health, among the post, in establishing visiting nursing, in women's suffrage, and more, is representative of Jewish (and nursing) social ethics. There is also a journal of *Socially-Engaged Buddhism*, though of more recent vintage, and there are social teachings in Islam. This is to say that most major religions have social teachings, with a view of the good society and the responsibilities of individual adherents to work toward the common good and a good society.

Jewish ethics and bioethics has a rich social-ethical tradition of Jewish ethics and bioethics. I would refer the reader to David Novak's *Jewish Social Ethics*, and his *The Jewish Social Contract: An Essay in Political Theology*; also, Belkin's *The Obligation of the Jew to Social Justice*, as well as Elliot Dorff's books on bioethics. Islam offers books on social ethics as well such as Sachedina's *Islam and the Challenge of Human Rights*, Rizvi's *Social Ethics in Islam*, Al-Atram's *Ethical Foundations of Social Justice* and Al-Jayyousi's *Islamic Perspectives on Sustainable Development: Justice and Responsibility*. The Buddhist tradition offers us Sulak Sivaraksa's *The Socially Engaged Buddhist*, Damien Keown's *Buddhist Bioethics*, and Kotler's *Engaged Buddhist Reader*. There are a number of books in the Native American tradition, including superlative books on environmental ethics. See Nerburn's *The Wisdom of the Native Americans,* Nelson's *Original Instructions: Indigenous Teachings for a Sustainable Future*, and Oliver and Heldke's *Living Justice: Indigenous Reflections on Philosophy, Cosmology, and Ethics*. I also suggest *Indigenous Bioethics: Decolonizing Bioethical Theory and Practice* edited by Link and Taylor. I strongly urge a familiarity with other cultural and religious approaches to bioethics. The reader is also referred to the series on *Health and Medicine* in a number of religious traditions, published by Crossroad, with some reprinted by Wipf and Stock in Eugene, Oregon. The series covers 22 religious traditions, including Judaism, Islam, Catholic, Orthodox, Methodist, Buddhist, Christian Science, Lutheran, Evangelical, Reformed, and more.

While social ethics has been tied historically to religious traditions, its concerns, methods, values, ideals, and aims, much like yoga, it can be embraced without aligning with the religious grounding that generated it. In addition, social ethicists who come from specific traditions work together, across religious traditions, and collaboratively with those who do not align with any religious or spiritual tradition.

The Invisible Influence of Social Ethics in Nursing

Contemporary nursing literature has not attended to the social ethical elements that were formative in shaping nursing, its ethics, and its social ethics. The effects of the social ethics movement are far-reaching but under-researched. For example, Lilliam Wald (1867–1940) founded Henry Street Settlement (1893 to present). Annie Warburton Goodrich (1899–1954) taught at Teachers College, Columbia University and was director of the Henry Street Settlement Visiting Nurses Association, eventually to become the first dean of Yale University School of Nursing (1923). As noted in Chapter 2, Annie Goodrich's book *The Social and Ethical Significance of Nursing: A Series of Addresses* drew concepts from the social ethics tradition, and quotes from Dewey's *Reconstruction in Philosophy*,[120] *Experience and Nature*,[121] *The Quest for Certainty*,[122] and his articles in *The New Republic*, "American Education and Culture,"[123] and "Individuality, Equality, and Superiority."[124] She also quotes his definition of *art* (without a citation).[125] Virginia Henderson (1897–1996) received her BS and MA from Teachers College, Columbia University and began her public health nursing career at Henry Street Settlement (1921), and later became a Visiting Nurse in Washington, DC. After teaching at Teachers College, in 1953 she moved to Yale University School of Nursing where I had the good fortune of being in personal conversations with her on topics in religion and theology, social ethics, and ethics in nursing in the later years of her career at Yale. She was, at that time, working with faculty of Yale Divinity School. Though she wrote mostly on the individual nurse, Henderson was infected by social ethics influences from her student years. In a personal reflection, given as a speech, she writes:

> In those days not even lip-service was given "patient centered care," "family health service," "comprehensive care," or "rehabilitation." But there was, for me, an influence in those early student days that negated the mechanistic approach [taught by physicians]. Annie W. Goodrich... whenever she visited our unit, she lifted our sights above techniques and routines. With her broad experience in hospitals, in public health agencies, and educational institutions, she saw nursing as a "world-wide social activity," a creative and constructive force in society. Having a powerful intellect and boundless compassion for humanity, she never failed to infect us with "the ethical significance of nursing,"[126]

Henderson, influenced by Progressivism, Pragmatism, and the social ethics movement as well as her Henry Street, visiting nursing experience—and Annie Goodrich—was an advocate of publicly financed, universally accessible health services.[127] There is an under-researched lineage of the social ethics movement that persists in nursing to this day. These influences are present but not explored and are unacknowledged in nursing generally and in bioethics as well.

Social Ethics Links to Nursing Ethics and Bioethics

We have reached back to the era of Pragmatism, Progressivism, the social gospel, religious social ethics, Catholic social teachings, and liberation theologies because they intermingle with early nursing, have continuing influence (however subliminal or covert), and have direct descendants of these movements involved in the founding of bioethics and its subsequent development.

Several bioethicists, some deceased but many still active, have been influenced by these movements. Specific influences may vary, but here are a few ethicists or bioethicists (and a few of their works) who have drawn inspiration from these movements:

- Lisa Sowle Cahill: *Bioethics and the Common Good* (2005); *Genetics, Theology, Ethics: An Interdisciplinary Conversation* (2005); *Theological Bioethics: Participation, Justice, and Change* (2005); *Sex, Gender, and Christian Ethics* (1996).
- Daniel Callahan: *Setting Limits: Medical Goals in an Aging Society* (1987); *False Hopes: Why America's Quest for Perfect Health Is a Recipe for Failure* (1998); *Abortion: Law, Choice and Morality* (1972); *Enhancing Human Traits: Ethical and Social Implications* (1998); *The Roots of Ethics: Science, Religion, and Values* (1981); *What Price Better Health?* (2006); *Hazards of the Research Imperative* (2003); *Roots of Bioethics: Health, Progress, Technology, Death* (2012).
- H. Tristram Engelhardt, Jr.: *Bioethics and Secular Humanism: The Search for a Common Morality* (1973); *The Foundations of Christian Bioethics* (2000); *Global Bioethics: The Collapse of Consensus* (2006); *After God: Morality & Bioethics in a Secular Age* (2017); *The Foundations of Bioethics* (1996).
- James Gustafson: *Ethics in Human Reproduction* (1983); *Ethics from a Theocentric Perspective* (1981); *Casuistry and Modern Ethics: A Poetics of Practical Reasoning* (2003).
- Stanley Hauerwas: *A Community of Character: Toward a Constructive Christian Social Ethic* (1981); *Vision and Virtue: Essays in Christian Ethical Reflection* (1974); *Responsibility for Devalued Persons: Ethical Interactions Between Society, Family, and the Retarded* (1982); *Suffering Presence: Theological Reflections on Medicine, the Mentally Handicapped, and the Church* (1986); *Abortion Theologically Understood* (1991); *God, Medicine, and Suffering* (1994); *Living Gently in a Violent World: The Prophetic Witness of Weakness* (with Jean Vanier) (2008).
- Albert Jonsen: *The Abuse of Casuistry: A History of Moral Reasoning* (1988); *Clinical Ethics: A Practical Approach to Ethical Decisions in Clinical Medicine* (1982); *Bioethics: Beyond the Headlines* (2005).
- Richard McCormick: *How Brave a New World: Dilemmas in Bioethics* (1980); *Doing Evil to Achieve Good: Moral Choice in Conflict Situations* (1978); *Health and Medicine in the Catholic Tradition: Tradition in Transition* (1984); *Ambiguity in Moral Choice* (1977).
- Ruth Macklin: *Mortal Choices: Bioethics in Today's World, (1987)*; *Mortal Choices: Ethical Dilemmas in Modern Medicine* (1988); *Against Relativism: Cultural Diversity and the Search for Ethical Universals in Medicine* (1999); *Double Standards in Medical Research in Developing Countries* (2004); *Ethics in Global Health: Research, Policy, and Practice* (2012).

- Paul Ramsey: *The Patient as Person: Explorations in Medical Ethics* (1970); *The Ethics of Fetal Research* (1975); *Ethics at the Edges of Life* (1980).
- Rosemary Radford Ruether: *Gaia and God: An Ecofeminist Theology of Earth Healing* (1994); *Women Healing Earth: Third World Women on Ecology, Feminism, and Religion* (1996); *Integrating Ecofeminism Globalization and World Religions* (2005); *Sexism and God-Talk: Toward a Feminist Theology* (1983); *Christianity and Ecology* (2000).
- Allen Verhey: *Theological Voices in Medical Ethics* (1993); *From Christ to the World* (1994); *On Moral Medicine* (1987); *The Christian Art of Dying* (2011).

The social gospel movement is a lived social ethics movement that produced a body of social ethics literature, such as *Rerum Novarum*, is linked to early nursing social ethics, and has foundational ties to bioethics. A number of nursing leaders, including in bioethics, have come from the social ethics tradition (myself included), or have been influenced by it, though I must leave it to them to be self-disclosing.

There is, however, another piece to fit in that relates to social and health policy. Social ethics is ultimately political, for social criticism challenges the status quo and social change presses for changes in social structures. The Hart–Devlin debate was one of great significance and attention in the discipline of ethics, but is not discussed in the field of bioethics. In terms of social policy considerations, and nursing participation in policy formation, the Hart–Devlin debate must be given attention.

The Hart–Devlin Debate and the Legislation of Morality

There is an important context to the H.L.A. Hart–Lord Patrick Devlin debate of the 1950s and 1960s. It is a jurisprudential debate between legal philosophers over the legislation of morality. The debate focused on whether the law should enforce particular moral norms, and to what extent the law should intervene in or criminalize the private affairs of individuals. The debate revolved around the UK Wolfenden Report, more formally titled *The Report of the Departmental Committee on Homosexual Offences and Prostitution*.[128,129] The report was published in the United Kingdom on 4 September 1957, after a number of well-known men, including Alan Turing, Oscar Wilde, Lord Montagu of Beaulieu, Anthony Grey, Michael Pitt-Rivers, John Gielgud, and Peter Wildeblood were convicted of homosexual offences. The *Guardian* published an excellent retrospective (2007) on the context and the Report.[130] At issue was the decriminalization of "homosexual acts" and prostitution (though prostitution did not receive the same degree of attention). Allegations of homosexuality itself (as opposed to "homosexual acts") could and did result in prosecution. Journalist Geraldine Bedell, in 2007, writes:

> Smiling in the park could lead to arrest... being in the wrong address book could cost you a prison sentence... hundreds of thousands of men feared being picked

up by zealous police... often for doing nothing more than looking a bit gay... arrests often seemed to have an arbitrary, random quality... there would be intermittent trawls through address books of suspected homosexuals, with the result that up to 20 men... accused of being a "homosexual ring," even though many of them might never have met.... In the mid-1950s, there was an atmosphere of a witch-hunt.... In 1989, during the Conservative campaign for family values, more than 2,000 men were prosecuted for gross indecency, as many as during the 1950s and nearly three times the numbers in the mid-Sixties.[131]

The Wolfenden Report advocated the decriminalization of sexual activity conducted in private between men. Lesbians were not included in the legislation bearing upon homosexuality.[132] The report saw the role of criminal law as *not* extending to intervention "in the private lives of citizens, or to seek to enforce any particular pattern of behaviour, further than is necessary to carry out the purposes we have outlined."[133] Those purposes were "to preserve public order and decency, to protect the citizen from what is offensive or injurious, and to provide sufficient safeguards against exploitation and corruption of others."[134] Patrick, Baron Devlin, strenuously disagreed. As Peter Cane notes:

> Although Devlin did not express it as straightforwardly as he might have, his basic point was that the criminal law is not (just) for the protection of individuals but also for the protection of society—"the institutions and the community of ideas, political and moral, without which people cannot live together." For that reason, he argued, the sphere of the criminal law should not, as a matter of principle, be limited to regulating conduct that has direct adverse effects on identifiable individuals.[135]

Herbert Hart responded in rebuttal, drawing upon John Stuart Mill's *principle of harm* which you will know from his work *On Liberty.* Mill's oft-quoted principle is that "The only purpose for which power can rightfully be exercised over any member of a civilized community against his will is to prevent harm to others."[136] Mill's principle of harm, or more specifically interference with another's autonomy if it would be exercised to harm another, received considerable attention from Beauchamp and Childress' first edition (1979) of *Principles of Biomedical Ethics*,[137] but disappears by the eighth edition (2019).[138] Yet, the notion of interference in personal autonomy, and Mill's principle of harm remain important to any discussion of legislation, particularly legislation that would criminalize private behavior. That is, it has become increasingly important in the US in terms of proposed laws that would criminalize reproductive decisions, same-sex marriage, gender transitioning, and more, not simply for the persons making these decisions, but for those who assist in any way, whether as a health professional or a bus driver. Hart's argument held sway. Twenty years after H.L.A Hart's *Law, Liberty and Morality* (1955)[139] and Lord Devlin's *The Enforcement of Morals* (1959),[140] Joel Feinberg published a four-volume work on the topic, *The Moral Limits of the Criminal Law* (1984).[141] This is an intricate controversy that is not directly relevant to day-to-day nursing, but is of surpassing importance to those in nursing who devote their professional energies to ethics, policy, and legislative issues—and to nurses who vote. In the current US context, both civil legislation and criminal law have come into issues of reproductive rights, gay marriage, transpersons' participation in sports and use of public restrooms, and more. Here, issues are both private (e.g., use of birth control—and legal notions of a right to privacy), and public (e.g., transwomen's participation in women's sports). Thus, the issues have become even more tangled in recent decades. The Hart–Devlin debate remains as relevant today as it was in the 1950s and 1960s, and deserves greater nursing attention, particularly as it has had unequal application in issues related to global health. It is time now, however, to stop pulling items out of the closet and to close the door for another day.

Conclusion

Bioethics and its nursing representative know naught of the social ethics movement or the social gospel, and yet descendants of social ethics, in black, white, Latina/o, indigenous, Asian, religious, and secular communities, have ties to the birth of bioethics itself. The histories of bioethics have failed to draw from the distinctive American context of these traditions. Given that social ethics' lineage traces to religion, and that bioethics became secularized (if not inhospitable to religion), it is understandable that bioethics does not embrace social ethics, relying instead on a thin notion of justice, and without a larger notion of a good society toward which to aim. In effect, bioethics has become a moated castle. Religious, liberationist, and social ethicists' voices moved or were moved out of the bioethics community, and with intersectional and postcolonial theories, and minority ethics voices, stand at the portcullis; they have not been re-admitted, to the detriment of bioethics and the people it is intended to serve.

Nursing's origins have imbued it with a different way of being in the world. Nursing lived its practice in the trenches, with and among the people it served. Tenement buildings, settlements, factories, schools, flophouses, rural communities on horseback, nursing went everywhere where nursing was needed. It saw the world as it was and had a robust vision for health and human flourishing, human dignity, and nursing as caring.

An archaic use of the word *conversation* refers to one's way of being in the world. Both senses of conversation, as a way of being, and as an exchange of ideas and communication, need to be brought to bear upon the problems that ethics grapples with today. The world of nursing care has a large repertoire of wisdom to bring to bear, if it would but do so, in addressing today's intractable social problems. Lillian Wald, Lavinia Dock, Mary Burr, Isabel Robb, Cornell West, Martin Luther King, Jr., James Cone, Oren Lyons, Jack D. Forbes, Søren Kierkegaard, Gustavo Gutiérrez, Philip Deloria, K. Tsianina Lomawaima, Aristotle,

Alasdair MacIntyre, Charles Taylor, Paul Ramsey, Pope Leo XIII, Elizabeth Anscombe, Iris Murdoch, Mary Midgley, Philippa Foot, Miguel De La Torre, Kari Martinsen, and a host of others are available to join nursing's conversation. Nursing must seek out the full community of voices, including those forgotten, those unheard, those shunned, those silenced, those marginalized, and those who speak in a whisper or not at all. Nursing ethics needs the full, inclusive, community of discourse in conversation.

Unlike bioethics, social ethics, of itself and in nursing, has always had a vision of the good society, of human flourishing, of social justice, of dignity, respect, and the common good. And, as importantly, it has been rooted in nursing experience, nursing relationships, in the realities of nursing practice. Any attempt to reform society from the top-down, based on non-contextual, rationalist abstract principles will only perpetuate its distance from the lives lived by the people. Any attempt to reform society without a vision of the good society is doomed as directionless. The world needs nursing's vision; this is no time for nursing timidity or reticence. To return to the intrepid Lavinia Dock, she writes:

> This [ANA nursing] society, as one body, would often be astonished at the actual extent and weight of its influence if its whole latent and at present unsuspected power were actually to be systematically exerted in an intelligent and energetic manner.[142]

It is time for this latent power to be asserted. It is time for nursing ethics, the native flower of nursing soil, to reclaim and renew its heritage and vision, and for its voice to ring aloud in the corridors of hospitals, in the halls of legislatures, and in the streets of society. We are nursing: it is time to roar!

Notes

1 American Nurses Association, *Code of Ethics for Nurses with Interpretive Statements* (Silver Spring, MD: American Nurses Association, 2001).
2 American Nurses Association, *Code of Ethics for Nurses with Interpretive Statements* (Silver Spring, MD: American Nurses Association, 2015).
3 Miguel A. Escotet, "Pandemics, Leadership and Social Ethics," *Prospect* 49, (2020): 73–76. DOI: 10.1007/s11125-020-09472-3
4 Ibid., 73.
5 Thomas Mappes, Jane Zembaty, and David DeGrazia (eds.), *Social Ethics: Morality and Social Policy*, 8th ed. (New York: McGraw-Hill, 2012).
6 John Stuart Mill, *On Liberty* (London; Longmans, Green, Reader and Dyer, 1859).
7 Edmund Pellegrino, "The Social Ethics of Primary Care: The Relationship between a Human Need and an Obligation of Society," *The Mount Sinai Journal of Medicine* 45, no. 5 (Sept.–Oct. 1978): 593–601.
8 Ibid., 593.
9 Ibid., 5.
10 Tom Beauchamp and James Childress, *Principles of Biomedical Ethics* (Oxford: Oxford University Press, 1979).
11 Ibid., 169.

12 John Rawls, *Justice as Fairness* (Cambridge, MA Belknap/Harvard University Press, 1971).
13 Beauchamp and Childress, *Principles*, 169.
14 Ibid., 179.
15 John Rawls, *A Theory of Justice* (Cambridge, MA: Harvard University Press, 1971).
16 Beauchamp and Childress, *Principles*, 187.
17 Ibid., 188.
18 Ibid., 189.
19 Ibid., 193.
20 Mildred Z. Solomon, "Recalibrating Bioethics for the Reality of Interdependence: The Challenge of Collective-Impact Problems," *Hastings Center Report* 53, no. 3 (2023): 3–5, 4. DOI: 10.1002/hast.1483
21 Ibid., 6.
22 Martien Pijnenburg, "Humane Healthcare as a Theme for Social Ethics," *Medicine, Health Care and Philosophy* 5 (2002): 245–252.
23 Gibson Winter, *Social Ethics: Issues in Ethics and Society* (New York: Harper & Row Publishers, 1968), 6.
24 US Department of Labor, "More than 100 Children Illegally Employed in Hazardous Jobs, Federal Investigation Finds; Food Sanitation Contractor Pays $1.5m in Penalties" (2022). https://www.dol.gov/newsroom/releases/whd/whd20230217-1
25 National Commission to Address Racism in Nursing. https://www.nursingworld.org/practice-policy/workforce/racism-in-nursing/national-commission-to-address-racism-in-nursing/
26 American Nurses Association. *Our Racial Reckoning Statement.* https://www.nursingworld.org/practice-policy/workforce/racism-in-nursing/RacialReckoningStatement/
27 Chaïm Perelman and Lucie Olbrechts-Tyteca, *The New Rhetoric: A Treatise on Argumentation*, trans. John Wilkinson and Purcell Weaver (Notre Dame, IN: University of Notre Dame Press, 1969), 51.
28 Ibid., 51.
29 ANA, "A Suggested Code," *American Journal of Nursing* 26, no. 9 (1926): 600–601, 599.
30 Marc Drogin, *Anathema! Medieval Scribes and the History of Book Curses* (Totowa, NJ: Allanheld, Osmun, & Co., 1983), 88.
31 Maureen Flanagan, "Progressives and Progressivism in an Era of Reform," *American History* (published online, Aug. 5, 2016). DOI: 10.1093/acrefore/9780199329175.013.84
32 Alexis de Tocqueville. *Democracy in America*, Vol. II, trans. Henry Reeve (New York: D. Appleton & Co., 1899), 591.
33 Ibid., 593–594.
34 Jason Kaufman, "Three Views of Associationalism in 19th-Century America: An Empirical Examination," *American Journal of Sociology* 104, no. 5 (1999): 1296–1345. DOI: 10.1086/210176.
35 Theda Skocpol, "Building Community Top-down or Bottom-up? America's Voluntary Groups Thrive in a National Network," *Brookings*, September 1, 1997. https://www.brookings.edu/articles/building-community-top-down-or-bottom-up-americas-voluntary-groups-thrive-in-a-national-network/
36 Jacob Krain, "Lillian Wald, American Jewish Success," *The Jewish Magazine.* http://www.jewishmag.com/51mag/wald/lillianwald.htm
37 Nicholas Kristof, "Starving Children Don't Cry," *The New York Times*, Opinion Section (Jan. 2, 2021). https://www.nytimes.com/2021/01/02/opinion/sunday/2020-worst-year-famine.html
38 Flanagan, "Progressives and Progressivism." DOI: 10.1093/acrefore/9780199329175.013.84
39 Josephine Clara Goldmark, *Nursing and Nursing Education in the United States* (New York: Macmillan, 1923).

40 Kathryn Kish Sklar (March 1, 2009), "Josephine Clara Goldmark." Jewish Women: A Comprehensive Historical Encyclopedia. Jewish Women's Archive. Retrieved October 23, 2014. https://jwa.org/encyclopedia/article/goldmark-josephine-clara

41 Hillary Howard, "The Mystery of this Dusty Book, Signed by Amelia Earhart and Eleanor Roosevelt," *The New York Times*, Aug. 23, 2019. https://www.nytimes.com/2019/08/23/nyregion/henry-street-settlement-lillian-wald.html

42 Jane Addams, *Democracy and Social Ethics* (New York: Macmillan, 1902).

43 Maureen A. Flanagan, "Progressives and Progressivism in an Era of Reform," *American History* (Aug. 2016). DOI: 10.1093/acrefore/9780199329175.013.84

44 Library of Congress, "NAACP: A Century in the Fight for Freedom." https://www.loc.gov/exhibits/naacp/founding-and-early-years.html

45 Maureen A. Flanagan, *America Reformed: Progressives and Progressivisms, 1890s–1920s* (New York: Oxford University Press, 2007), 10.

46 Cruz, Estefanía. "Asociación de Jóvenes Inmigrantes y el futuro del liderazgo latino en Estados Unidos: capital social y compromiso político de los *dreamers,*" *NorteAmérica*, 11, no. 2 (July–Dec. 2016), 165–191.

47 Douglas McDermid, *The Varieties of Pragmatism: Truth, Realism, and Knowledge from James to Rorty* (London: Continuum, 2006).

48 H.S. Thayer, *Meaning and Action: A Critical History of Pragmatism*, 2nd ed. (Indianapolis, IN: Hackett, 1981).

49 Israel Scheffler, *Four Pragmatists: A Critical Introduction to Peirce, James, Mead, and Dewey* (London: Routledge & Kegan Paul, 1986).

50 Cornel West, *The American Evasion of Philosophy: A Genealogy of Pragmatism* (Madison, WI: University of Wisconsin Press, 1989).

51 Cheryl Misak and Robert B. Talisse, "Pragmatism Endures," *Aeon* (Nov. 18, 2019). https://aeon.co/essays/pragmatism-is-one-of-the-most-successful-idioms-in-philosophy

52 Richard Bernstein, "The Resurgence of Pragmatism," *Social Research* 59, no. 4 (Winter 1992): 813–840.

53 Gweneth Hartrick Doane and Colleen Varcoe, "Toward Compassionate Action: Pragmatism and the Inseparability of Theory/Practice," *Advances in Nursing Science* 28, no. 1 (Jan. 2005): 81–90.

54 Christine Hallett, "Pragmatism and Project 2000: the Relevance of Dewey's Theory of Experimentalism to Nursing Education," *Journal of Advanced Nursing* 26, no. 6 (Dec. 1997): 1229–1234. DOI: 10.1046/j.1365–2648.1997.00423.x

55 Sara Dolan, Lorelli Nowell, and Graham McCaffery "Pragmatism as a Philosophical Foundation to Integrate Education, Practice, Research and Policy across the Nursing Profession," *Journal of Advanced Nursing* 78, no. 10 (Oct. 2022): e118–e129. DOI: 10.1111/jan.15373

56 Deborah S. Thoun, Megan Kirk, Esther Sangster-Gormley, and James O. Young. "Philosophical Theories of Truth and Nursing: Exploring the Tensions," *Nursing Science Quarterly* 32, no. 1 (2018), 43–48.

57 Lorelli Nowell, "Pragmatism and Integrated Knowledge Translation: Exploring the Compatibilities and Tensions," *Nursing Open* 2, no. 3 (Nov. 2015): 141–148. doi.org/10.1002/nop2.30

58 Naoya Mayumi and Katsumasa Ota, "Implications of Philosophical Pragmatism for Nursing: Comparison of Different Pragmatists," *Nursing Philosophy* 24, no. 1 (Jan. 2023): 1–10.

59 Eun-Ok Im, "Properties of Situation-Specific Theories and Neo-pragmatism," *Advances in Nursing Science* 44, no. 4 (Oct.–Dec. 2021): e114–e126.

60 Peter Allmark and Katarzyna Machaczek, "Realism and Pragmatism in a Mixed Methods Study," *Journal of Advanced Nursing* 74, no. 6 (June 2018), 1301–1309.

61 Gary Dorrien, *Social Ethics in the Making: Interpreting an American Tradition* (Chichester, UK: John Wiley & Sons Publishing/Blackwell Publishing Ltd, 2011).

62 Schools of religion focus on the academic study of religions and may or may not be aligned with a particular religious tradition. Schools of theology generally teach from within a particular religious tradition. Seminaries prepare both clergy and theologians from within a particular religious tradition.

63 Dorrien, *Social Ethics*, 15.

64 Walter Rauschenbusch, *Christianity and the Social Crisis* (New York: Macmillan & Co., 1907).

65 Walter Rauschenbusch, *A Theology for the Social Gospel* (New York: Abingdon Press, 1917).

66 Ibid., 249–250.

67 Ibid., 142.

68 Ibid., 119.

69 Ibid.

70 Take note of the middle initial "A" in his name, as Miguel de la Torre (no "A"; 1786–1843) was a Spanish Governor of Puerto Rico and served in the Spanish–American War. De La Torre's book is an excellent example of identity-rooted social ethics, and to be commended.

71 Miguel A. De La Torre, *Latina/o Social Ethics: Moving Beyond Eurocentric Moral Thinking*, (Waco, TX: Baylor University, 2010), 9–10.

72 Pope Leo XIII, Encyclical: *Rerum Novarum* (May 15, 1891). https://www.vatican.va/content/leo-xiii/en/encyclicals/documents/hf_l-xiii_enc_15051891_rerum-novarum.html

73 Ibid.

74 Ibid.

75 John A. Ryan, *A Living Wage: Its Ethical and Economic Aspects* (New York: Macmillan Co. 1906). https://archive.org/details/livingwageitseth00ryan).

76 AFL-CIO, "Mother Jones," https://aflcio.org/about/history/labor-history-people/mother-jones

77 Elliott Gorn, *Mother Jones: The Most Dangerous Woman in America* (New York: Hill & Wang, 2001).

78 Gail Collins, "America's Women," The Illinois Labor History Society (2003): 287–289. www.kentlaw.edu/ilhs/majones.htm; photo from George Meany Memorial Archives.

79 Reinhold Niebuhr, *Moral Man and Immoral Society: A Study in Ethics and Politics* (New York: Charles Scribner's Sons, 1932).

80 Reinhold Niebuhr, *Christian Realism and Political Problems* (New York: Charles Scribner's Sons, 1953).

81 M. Loveland, *British Christian Socialists and the Gospel of Socialism, 1848–1905* (Leiden: Brill, 2000).

82 Rick Helmes-Hayes, "The Perfect Sociology, Perfectly Applied: Sociology and the Social Gospel in Canada's English-Language Universities, 1900–1930," 44th Sorokin Lecture. Saskatoon: University of Saskatchewan (Feb. 7, 2013). https://artsandscience.usask.ca/sociology/documents/44th%20Annual%20Sorokin%20Lecture.pdf

83 N. Gartrell, *The Social Gospel and Labour in Canada: The United Church of Canada and the Ontario Labour Movement, 1900–50* (Toronto: University of Toronto Press, 2009).

84 Andrew Ives, "Christians on the Left: The Importance of the Social Gospel in the Canadian Social Democratic Tradition," *Revu Lisa* IX, no. 1 (2011): 188–204. https://journals.openedition.org/lisa/4169

85 Dorrien, *Social Ethics*, 674.

86 Gustavo Gutiérrez, *A Theology of Liberation: History, Politics, and Salvation*, rev. ed. (Maryknoll, NY: Orbis Books, 1988).

87 Leonardo Boff, *Ecclesiogenesis: The Base Communities Reinvent the Church* (Maryknoll, NY: Orbis Books, 1986).

88 Leonardo Boff, *Church: Charism and Power – Liberation Theology and the Institutional Church* (New York: Crossroad, 1986).

89 Paulo Freire, *Pedagogy of the Oppressed*, trans. Myra Bergman Ramos (New York: Herder & Herder, 1970).

90 Juan Luis Segundo, *The Liberation of Theology* (Maryknoll, NY: Orbis Books, 1976).

91 Pope Paul VI, *Populorum Progressio* (Mar. 26, 1967). https://www.vatican.va/content/paul-vi/en/encyclicals/documents/hf_p-vi_enc_26031967_populorum.html

92 Pope John Paul II, *Sollicitudo Rei Socialis* (Dec. 30, 1987). https://www.vatican.va/content/john-paul-ii/en/encyclicals/documents/hf_jp-ii_enc_30121987_sollicitudo-rei-socialis.html

93 Ibid.

94 Ahn Byung-Mu, Yung Suk Kim, and Jin-Ho Kim (eds.), *Reading Minjung Theology in the Twenty-First Century: Selected Writings by Ahn Byung-Mu and Modern Critical Responses* (Eugene, OR: Wipf and Stock Publishers, 2013).

95 Craig L. Nessan, "Liberation Theologies in America," *Oxford Research Encyclopedia of Religion* (Oxford: Oxford University Press Academic, 2017). doi.org/10.1093/acrefore/9780199340378.013.493

96 James Cone, *Black Theology and Black Power* (Maryknoll, NY: Orbis Books, 1969).

97 James Cone, *A Black Theology of Liberation* (Maryknoll, NY: Orbis Books, 1970).

98 James Cone, *God of the Oppressed* (Maryknoll, NY: Orbis Books, 1975).

99 James Cone, *The Cross and the Lynching Tree* (Maryknoll, NY: Orbis Books, 2011).

100 James Cone, *Said I Wasn't Gonna Tell Nobody: The Making of a Black Theologian* (Maryknoll, NY: Orbis Books, 2018), 94.

101 Gary Dorrien, "Recovering the Black Social Gospel" (Harvard Divinity Bulletin, Summer/Autumn 2015). https://bulletin.hds.harvard.edu/recovering-the-black-social-gospel/

102 Cornel West, *Race Matters* (Boston: Beacon Press, 1993).

103 Cornel West, *Democracy Matters: Winning the Fight against Imperialism* (London: Penguin Publishing Group, 2005).

104 Miguel A. De La Torre, *Latina/o Social Ethics: Moving Beyond Eurocentric Moral Thinking*, (Waco, TX: Baylor University Press, 2010), 4–5.

105 Ibid., 118–119.

106 Ibid., 88.

107 Ibid., 71.

108 María Pilar Aquino, *Our Cry for Life: Feminist Theology from Latin America* (Maryknoll, NY: Orbis, 1993).

109 De La Torre, *Latina/o Social Ethics*, 70.

110 Ibid., 72.

111 Ada Maria Isasi-Diaz, *En La Lucha, In the Struggle: A Hispanic Women's Liberation Theology*, Minneapolis: Fortress Press, (1993): 168 as cited in De La Torre, *Latina/o Social Ethics*, 74.

112 De La Torre, *Latina/o Social Ethics*, 76.

113 Cornel West, *The American Evasion of Philosophy: A Genealogy of Pragmatism* (Madison, WI: University of Wisconsin Press, 1989).

114 Dorrien, "Recovering the Black Social Gospel."

115 Talal Asad, *Genealogies of Religion: Discipline and Reasons of Power in Christianity and Islam.* (Baltimore, MD: Johns Hopkins University Press, 1993)

116 Richard King, *Orientalism and Religion: Post-Colonial Theory, India, and "The Mystic East"* (London: Routledge, 1999).

117 Tomoko Masuzawa, *The Invention of World Religions: Or, How European Universalism Was Preserved in the Language of Pluralism* (Chicago: University of Chicago Press, 2005).

118 Wifred Smith, *The Meaning and End of Religion* (Minneapolis, MN: Fortress Press, 1991).

119 Craig Torres, *Tending Nature: Indigenous Land Stewardship* (PBS Television Series, 2021). https://www.pbs.org/video/indigenous-land-stewardship-ap7s1s/

120 John Dewey, *Reconstruction in Philosophy* (New York: Henry Holt and Company, 1920).

121 John Dewey, *Experience and Nature* (London: Allen & Unwin, 1929).

122 John Dewey, *The Quest for Certainty* (London: G. Allen and Unwin, 1929).

123 John Dewey, "American Education and Culture," *The New Republic* (July 1, 1916).

124 John Dewey, "Individuality, Equality, and Superiority," *The New Republic* (Dec. 13, 1922).

125 Goodrich, *Social*, 294. Quote from John Dewey, "Significance of the School of Education," *Elementary School Teacher*, 4 (1904): 441–453.

126 Virginia Avenal Henderson, *The Nature of Nursing: Reflections after 25 Years* (New York: National League for Nursing, 1991).

127 Virginia Henderson, *The Nature of Nursing: Reflections after 25 Years*, 32–33.

128 UK Parliament. *The Report of the Departmental Committee on Homosexual Offences and Prostitution* (London: Parliament, 1957). https://www.parliament.uk/about/living-heritage/transformingsociety/private-lives/relationships/overview/sexuality20thcentury/

129 Human Rights Watch, "This Alien Legacy: The Origins of 'Sodomy' Laws in British Colonialism" (December 17, 2008). https://www.hrw.org/report/2008/12/17/alien-legacy/origins-sodomy-laws-british-colonialism

130 Geraldine Bedell, "Coming Out of the Dark Ages," *Guardian* (June 24, 2007). https://www.theguardian.com/society/2007/jun/24/communities.gayrights. See also: Adam Mars-Jones, "The Wildeblood Scandal: The Trial that Rocked 1950s Britain – and Changed Gay Rights," *Guardian* (July 14, 2017). https://www.theguardian.com/books/2017/jul/14/against-the-law-the-wildeblood-scandal-the-case-that-rocked-1950s-britain-and-changed-gay-rights

131 Bedell, "Coming Out of the Dark Ages."

132 Rebecca Morgan, *The Lesbian Paradox: Homophobia, Empire, and the Law in 1950s Britain* (June 11, 2020). https://rebeccajanemorgan.medium.com/the-lesbian-paradox-homophobia-empire-and-the-law-in-1950s-britain-4ea1b7732b0d

133 Report of the Committee on Homosexual Offences and Prostitution, Cmd 247, 1957 (UK), Paragraph 13.

134 Ibid.

135 P. Cane, "Taking Law Seriously: Starting Points of the Hart/Devlin Debate," *Journal of Ethics* 10 (2006): 21–51, 22. DOI: 10.1007/s10892-005-4590-x

136 J.S. Mill, *On Liberty*, ed. G. Himmelfarb (Harmondsworth: Penguin Books, 1974), 68.

137 Beauchamp and Childress, *Principles of Biomedical Ethics*, 56–64.

138 Ibid.

139 Herbert L.A. Hart, *Law, Liberty and Morality* (Stanford, CA: Stanford University Press, 1955).

140 Patrick Devlin, *The Enforcement of Morals* (Oxford: Oxford University Press, 1959)

141 Joel Feinberg, *The Moral Limits of the Criminal Law: Harm to Others*, 4 vols., New York: Oxford University Press, 2010.

142 Lavinia Dock, "The Duty of This Society in Public Work," *American Journal of Nursing* 4 no. 2 (Nov. 1903): 99–101.

11

VOICES AND VIGNETTES

This book is a career-culminating work that necessarily comes at the end of my career, where the evolution of my thoughts can be seen, and at a time when I can now be embarrassed by what I wrote in my salad days, or perhaps last year. I had the great and wondrous opportunity to work with those nurses (and theologians, philosophers, physicians, and attorneys) who were early into bioethics and its application to nursing and health policy. On the other hand, at the end of my career, I have also lost a number of those cherished colleagues, to eremitic retirement, frailty, death, or cognitive decline. I give particular mention to several of my ethics friends in Canada as well as Latin and South America who are missing from this chapter. In a sense, I waited too long, but could have done none other. All of the persons represented here have made distinctive contributions in different domains of nursing ethics and have thoughtful personal stories to tell. I had originally intended to intersperse these personal vignettes throughout the book, but came to the conclusion that they should be gathered into one chapter, even if a long chapter.

This chapter is a celebratory party of guests—the voices of 11 of my ethics friends and colleagues across the years. These are personal, not academic, reflections as the authors share the stories of their careers and passions for nursing and ethics as they entered the field of bioethics in the late 1960s and onward. These voices do represent some global spread, but not to the degree that I would have wished given the passage now of some 50 years. Most of these persons are at or beyond retirement age, so are able to look back across their lives and across the field of bioethics as it emerged. So as not to be directive, and to allow a maximum of freedom, the request to these persons was deliberately vague and open-ended. There is no attempt to homogenize their contributions, but rather to leave their voices as they are. To quote my rabbi friend, "May they be for you a blessing."

DOI: 10.4324/9781003262107-12

Anne Davis: Remembering My Post-Doctoral Kennedy Fellowship in Medical Ethics, at Harvard University, Cambridge, MA, 1976–1977

Getting There

While waiting for the elevator at the University of California at San Francisco School of Nursing, where I was a faculty member teaching Psych-Mental Health Nursing, a colleague noticed a flyer about the Kennedy Fellowship in Medical Ethics and brought it to me, saying, "This might interest you." I applied immediately after talking with the dean and the department chair. Over 200 people had applied that year; 12 were flown to Washington, DC for an interview, and they (The Joseph P. Kennedy, Jr. Foundation) awarded four fellowships. I was one of the recipients. The minute I heard that I had a fellowship, I organized my housing and got a season ticket to the Boston Symphony Orchestra. My Fellowship was to Harvard University, Cambridge, Massachusetts.

The summer preceding the fellowship, I had met Mila Aroskar at the Kennedy summer intensive session on bioethics at Georgetown University in Washington, DC. She, too, was going to Harvard on a Kennedy Fellowship. The foundation awarded four fellowships a year, two to nurses, and two to physicians. The fellowship could be taken at either Harvard University or at Georgetown University where the fellows would engage in studies, their own research in bioethics, and more. We talked with a physician who previously had been at Harvard as a Kennedy fellow. This conversation helped us organize our course of study.

Being There

Mila and I met with William Curran, an attorney on the faculty of the School of Public Health, who ran the Kennedy Fellowship Program with Drs. Stanley Reiser and Arthur Dyck. All of Harvard was open to us. We took courses in the Medical School, Law School, Philosophy department, School of Public Health, and the Divinity School. We were also on the Ethics Committee at Children's Hospital. It was a new and emerging field and this was medical ethics in action (later to become biomedical ethics, then bioethics, but not just yet).

It was all wonderful, but something was missing in terms of nursing. Over lunch, I said to Mila, "We need something to pull all this knowledge together. We need structure. Let's write a book." Mila's response was, "Anne! We don't know enough to write a book." A long discussion ensued and we did write a book. As I said then, we are not writing the great American novel, but a basic textbook for nurses.

One Problem

A problem arose one day and William Curran asked me to come to his office. Mrs. Eunice Kennedy Shriver, head of the Kennedy Foundation, had called and wanted the fellows to focus their studies on mental retardation or what is now called developmental disability. I was upset by the idea of dropping everything so that the funding would continue and I made this very clear. Another faculty member in the program said to me, "Anne, think of the nurses in the future who want to study in this program." I shot back, "I am." Mila and I were the first nurse educators to be Kennedy fellows as it had only been open to medical doctors. As I left Bill Curran's office, he asked what I planned to do. I said I would let him know after I thought about it.

The next day I wrote a Progress Report with three sections: (a) statement of my intent and the goals in my application for the fellowship, (b) my work accomplished to date according to those goals, and (c) my work to accomplish by end of fellowship according to those goals. I gave my Progress Report to Bill Curran's secretary, saying, "No word is to be changed before he mails it to Mrs. Shriver." Bill Curran asked Mila to write a Progress Report, then he sent them both off and that was the end of that.

Some Final Words

The Kennedy Foundation had a huge impact on the development of bioethics as a field of study and a clinical reality. I am grateful that I was awarded a Kennedy Post Doc Fellowship. That experience, and the career it led to, enriched my life and provided me with a way to help students and practicing clinical nurses to cope with bioethical issues they confront. I am now going on 93 years old, and I wonder daily what the future bioethical issues will be. I suspect I cannot even imagine!

Christine Grady: Consensus with Compassion and Caring in Trying Contexts

I was the second child in a large, Irish Catholic, lower-middle-class, suburban family, which emphasized attention to the less well-off and contributions to society. Growing up in the 1960s, I was aware that opportunities for women were limited. Always a science nerd and interested in helping others, I chose to study nursing in college, despite some pushback from certain family members.

Nursing was a perfect choice for me—interesting and challenging both intellectually and emotionally. Being a nurse allowed me to seize opportunities and learn and grow. Yet, my nursing education and initiation began in the 1970s—tumultuous times characterized by questioning established rules and institutions. Hence, I constantly questioned and pushed the envelope in terms of what nurses were able and allowed to do. I was always advocating for change—from refusing to wear my white cap at nursing school graduation, to challenging physicians when I felt they didn't really "see" the patient or I was uncomfortable with their medical decisions, to spearheading curricular innovations at schools of nursing, pushing for different policies or norms at the hospital unit or institutional level to support patients, and seeking a voice at larger health-care tables.

My first nursing position out of college was on a fast-paced neurology/neuro-surgery unit at the Massachusetts General Hospital. We cared for patients ranging in age from 16 to well over 60 with acute onset multiple sclerosis, glioblastomas and other brain tumors, para or quadriplegia from accidents, and other devastating conditions. I observed courage, defeat, and defiance in the face of overwhelming prognoses. I wondered how much the will to fight mattered in terms of patient outcomes and wondered how to help people die well. Subsequently, I worked as a nurse in community hospitals where my responsibilities ranged from caring for people with acute and chronic illnesses and injuries, to delivering babies, staffing the ambulance, and being "in charge" of the entire hospital. I wondered about how institutional decisions were made and priorities set, how resources should be distributed, and what should count as expertise. Later, I worked on an NIH-funded Clinical Studies Unit caring for adults and children undergoing experimental bone marrow transplantation—all were very ill, their care and course were extremely complicated, and almost everyone died. I wondered about the value and limits of research, why we spent so much on trying to save people instead of on keeping people healthy, and again how we ought to help people and make decisions at the end of life. Still later, I volunteered for one of the first home hospice programs in the US and questioned how we support patients and their families during and after terminal illnesses. I decided to study public health and enrolled in a master's program in community health nursing.

My practicum was in a daycare facility for patients with chronic mental illnesses, some of whom had been released into the community after spending decades in state institutions. I wondered about the responsibilities of society to care for vulnerable people and the (often unanticipated but sometimes negative) consequences of policy decisions seemingly made in good faith. I taught public health nursing in California and wondered and worried about the limits of our health-care system, especially in reaching youth and people in remote locations. Working in Brazil with Project Hope intensified my interest in many questions about allocation of resources and health-care systems, as I witnessed poor children not receiving desperately needed care, health-care professionals sometimes shirking their moral obligations to patients, the consequences of haphazard allocation decisions, and the challenges of providing nursing care sometimes without water, or electricity, medications, or needed supplies. I came to the National Institutes of Health around the same time as HIV/AIDS (although it wasn't yet called that). In those early years, I cared for so many young, previously vibrant men in the prime of their lives who were suffering from a new, very scary, seriously debilitating, usually fatal, and frequently ostracizing illness that we were trying desperately to learn about. I wished that we knew better how to protect people, to treat them, and to help them at the end of their lives. I worried about tensions between individual interests and the public health, about stigmatization and sometimes violence, about family conflict and the contours of family. I wondered about the limits of health-care providers' obligations when faced with substantial but uncertain risk, about when, if ever, it was okay for health-care providers to refuse to care for certain patients, about the crucial importance of research and the ethical landmines that it sometimes posed, about the need for honest communication about the unknowns and the value of sharing information.

These experiences I had providing nursing care and teaching nursing were extremely rewarding. I did not appreciate that many questions which troubled me or things I wondered about were questions of ethics. Although nurses and physicians and other health-care professions have had a long-standing professional ethics, "bioethics" and its language and methods really only emerged in the late 1960s and 1970s in the US. In the various places I worked during those years, I was not aware of ethics committees or any persons devoted to ethical issues. I was well aware of efforts to promote women's rights, civil rights, gay rights, and question things. But it was only later that I learned that the Hastings Center and the Kennedy Institute of Ethics were formed around this time, and that the Karen Ann Quinlan case and the Tuskegee syphilis study were in the news. I gradually realized that I would benefit greatly by learning more about bioethics to help me think about and address many of the issues that I cared about. While still working as a clinical nurse specialist primarily focusing on HIV/AIDs, I went back to school for a PhD in Philosophy. Although it was not all smooth sailing, and I had moments of almost existential crisis, the philosophy PhD put me in a good position to seek bioethics opportunities.

In the late 1990s, the NIH Clinical Center formed a new Department of Bioethics. I was one of the first to apply to work there. The NIH Bioethics Department provided opportunities for me to grow in many ways. I had support to do my own bioethics research. I served as an attending on the Bioethics Consultation service. I mentored bioethics fellows from a wide range of disciplinary backgrounds. I appreciated being involved in providing ethics education and consultation to nurses as well as to patients, clinicians, researchers, and others. My nursing background and skills served me well as a bioethics consultant and researcher, in ways distinct from some of my bioethics colleagues. I felt that I had an advantage when talking and listening to patients, families, and caregivers not only because I had a sort of insider understanding of what they were experiencing, but also because I had some practice fostering these kinds of relationships. At the same time, being a nurse sometimes presented obstacles. On more than one occasion, I was asked about my credentials by a skeptical consult requestor. For one of my early research publications, I was advised to remove RN from my title (I didn't). When I applied to be the Head of the Department, the search committee struggled with whether or not a nurse could or should run the department instead of a physician (I got the job). During many years in the department, I have had the opportunity to collaborate and learn from others who are smart and engaged but have different disciplinary backgrounds. Over time, I also seized opportunities to engage in cutting-edge topic areas and to represent bioethics as a nurse-bioethicist on committees and working groups of various kinds. In 2022, I was still head of the Department of Bioethics and have had many opportunities to participate in activities of national importance.

Starting in 2010, I had the privilege and honor of serving as a Commissioner on the US Presidential Commission for the Study of Bioethical Issues (PCSBI). As I see it, inviting me to be a commissioner checked several boxes—a bioethicist, a nurse, a woman, and a federal government employee. Of the six US National Bioethics Commissions appointed since 1974 by either the concurrent US President or the US Congress, this was the first bioethics commission to allow inclusion of federal government employees, and only the second bioethics commission that had a nurse as a commissioner (Dr. Retaugh Dumas served on the National Bioethics Advisory Commission, 1996–2001). For six years, as a Commissioner, I worked alongside my fellow commissioners and a talented staff to tackle timely and complex issues as requested by the US President and the US Secretary of Health and Human Services, as well as issues that were at the top of people's minds at the time.[1] My perspectives (and possible biases) that evolved from my work as a nurse and a bioethicist were brought to bear in several ways. One example was the report we did on the sexually transmitted disease (STD) studies conducted in Guatemala in the late 1940s, an egregious example of research deemed "ethically impossible." As Commissioners, we agreed to proceed cautiously in judging people and studies by standards and norms that were not all in place at the time. My familiarity with research ethics and the principles for what makes research ethical were valuable to our evaluation of these studies. My familiarity with the many regulations, guidelines, and literature that have emerged since that time was also helpful in assessing the strengths of oversight and safeguards operating today that greatly reduce the possibility of such unethical research happening again. The Commission's report about Ebola raised some issues reminiscent of my experiences caring for patients with HIV. When we considered testimony from nurses and doctors working in West Africa with Ebola patients, I was proud to be a nurse and humbled by their courage and moral compass. My patient care and research experiences also were useful when the Commission considered the issue of capacity to consent as part of our report on Neuroethics and the BRAIN initiative. When the Commission undertook a project on incidental findings, my experiences with how patients receive and understand information were useful to our deliberations. My experiences with patients and teaching nursing students helped me to contribute to one of the important roles of a commission like PCSBI, to be responsive to the public and to strive to inform and reassure them about timely and challenging ethical issues.

In mid-2022, the world is in its third year of a devastating global pandemic from COVID-19. Nurses have been an essential backbone of the pandemic response, caring for so many sick and dying patients, vaccinating millions, and educating the public, among other things. Nurses, and other health-care professionals, have been doing all this under conditions of uncertainty, fear, scarcity, evolving information, and rampant divisiveness. They are frustrated, tired, and distressed. Yet, they keep showing up, providing quality care under challenging circumstances, and saving lives. The ethical challenges inherent in nursing care during a pandemic are many, some familiar and some novel. Nurse-ethicists have an important role in supporting ethical decision-making and resources for practicing nurses and nurses in training, and all of us have to work together to apply lessons learned to improve and assure ethical workplaces, support nurses and the health-care workforce, and prepare for future pandemics. We have certainly learned that the exigencies of a pandemic with a novel, highly transmissible, and pathogenic virus put considerable strain on the systems in place to provide needed patient care. We have learned that health-care providers need support, more than we usually provide, but as importantly we need to bolster the systems in which health care is delivered. We have learned how valuable bioethics can be to making decisions that consider both data and values for individual patients, families, and clinicians, as well as for organizations and society. Bioethics can valuably help in anticipating and in dealing with the consequences of decisions made and omitted, help us learn to disagree but still come to a workable consensus, and remind us how important it is to show compassion and caring for each other.

Emiko Konishi: Doing Nursing Ethics in Japan

I am enjoying my time and space in an apartment for retirees. My story begins with a short conversation with a nursing student, Maki, who works part-time on weekends at our dining room.

Maki, a Nursing Student

One Saturday morning when we sat down for breakfast, Maki came to serve. I said, "Hi, Maki, I didn't see you for a while, how are you?" She replied with no smile, "Clinical, one more week." I had known from her that she was a second grader at a three-year vocational nursing school run by a city medical association. "But," she continued, "assignments are overwhelming, our scary teacher checks my performance all the time, and worse is, during the clinical weeks, we must live in the hospital dorm because of the Corona virus. No food is provided, so we eat only cup Ramen we buy from the vending machine, and we are not allowed to go home for a rest." Her clinical experience appeared to be far from enjoyable. Maki said further, "I may not be able to continue school." Hearing this, the word "sustainability" came to my mind—sustainability in nursing will possibly be at risk. In Japan, while BSN programs are steadily increasing in number, more than half the licensed fresh graduates are from diploma schools. What could I do for her?

Bioethics Conference

On that day, I attended an online conference of the Japan bioethics association. It included three symposia on ethics consultation and clinical ethics committee (CEC). The speaker groups, bioethicists, and nursing scholars together, had started to provide community outreach consultation for home-care nurses and care-workers. This is a remarkable change. When several Japanese hospitals began to have CECs in the early 1980s, the typical focus was on big "difficult cases" such as brain death and removing life support from coma patients.[2]

In its 30-year history, something has been overlooked by this bioethics association—something very important to nursing, such as Maki's experience. There had been no focus on the voices of nurses or nursing students, or on the dailyness or trivialness of life. Issues surrounding health workers' work environment or students' learning environment have rarely been on the agenda. Environment is where virtuous nurses and other professionals are produced and nurtured.

Japan Nursing Ethics Association

In 2008, a small group of nurse educators and practitioners established the Japan Nursing Ethics Association (JNEA). From San Francisco, Dr. Anne Davis sent us a message, "Start small and grow." Now, JNEA has grown to have 850 members, of whom half are practicing nurses and several are bioethicists, and has continued to hold annual conferences and publish its journal every year.

Among JNEA's past discussions that ranged from clinical to social issues, taken up here is an article in our ethics journal.[3] The authors, all clinical teachers, presented stories about their students who were practicing in hospital wards. One of the stories is quoted here:

> It was the first clinical practice for Yumi, a first-year nursing student. Mrs. C was Yumi's patient with aphasia. Yumi did not impose herself, but shared time with Mrs. C, looking out the window and sometimes folding origami. From other people's perspective, Yumi was doing nothing. However, when Mrs. C was with Yumi, her face was peaceful and lively. Nurses in the ward were saying, "To see them sitting side by side makes us feel peaceful, too." For patients with aphasia, nurses usually rely on tools such as character boards or simple sign language to gain quick and efficient communication. Whereas Yumi just relied on time, so slowly, thus establishing communication and a warm relationship with the patient. At the end-of-the-week meeting, a nurse said, "Yumi, we know you were devoting time for the patient in order to understand what the patient wanted to say. We do not have that time, and so we are using this lack of time as an excuse. You have made us realize that we have forgotten the importance of an effort— effort that you were making in order to know the patient."

In the article, the authors say that teachers and nurses have much to learn from what students see, feel, and think.

Teaching and Learning Nursing Ethics in Japan

From 1995, Anne taught nursing ethics for six years at my former school Nagano College of Nursing[4] and then she came to Japan several times to give lectures in many places until 2015. During this time, a network of "Anne sensei's children" was gradually formed and its size is still growing.

In her lectures, Anne often suggested to us, "Japanese nursing must decide its own ethics content and methods of teaching nursing ethics. You have a unique culture." Perhaps I could say that Anne's suggestion has partly been responded to by the following: 1) establishing JNEA in 2008, and 2) publishing a nursing ethics textbook. The first edition of this book[5] was the earliest nursing ethics textbook in Japan in that all the authors were Japanese nursing professionals, most of whom being "Anne's grown-up children." It is wonderful that several other nursing ethics textbooks have been published recently by bioethicists and nursing scholars. However, unlike those other textbooks where principle-based ethics is the core, our textbook has independent chapters from the beginning on (a) the Japanese value of harmony (Wa); (b) East Asian values of politeness (Rei), family (Ie), filial piety (Oya koukou), and face (Mentsu); and (c) virtue ethics in the East and the West. Also included are many case studies and stories from nurses' practice fields. In the more recent editions,[6] the content has been widened to include an independent chapter on ethics of care; more social issues such as domestic violence, poverty and prisoners; and more international issues including assisting nursing in developing countries and care for international patients.

To teach nursing ethics in class, paying special attention to Japanese culture and values, is most challenging. From our perspective, the "West" is more logical and expressive, so it is relatively easier for Japanese teachers to give Western knowledge to students. Indeed, bioethics principles such as autonomy, do good, and do no harm appear in the national nurse-licensing exam every year. Whereas, the "Japan" style is more tacit, and there is a meaning in what is left unsaid.

For my seminars with master students and practice nurses, I find the following phrase by Jonhstone[7] to be most helpful. "Unlike other approaches to ethics, nursing ethics recognizes the 'distinctive voices' that are nurses, and emphasizes the importance of collecting and recording nursing narratives and stories from the field."

I encourage students to write narratives. Their examples are problems arising from nurses' "thin understanding" of bioethics principles, the autonomy principle in particular; nurses' actions or no actions due to unconscious influence of Japanese values on nurses, such as politeness, modesty, and tacit understanding of other people's feelings; nurses' uncertain feelings about what to do; and sometimes nurses' joys. Sharing the stories in class, students are often in tears and my class becomes a kind of moral space. Then we get back to related chapters of our ethics textbook.

From my teaching and learning experiences in class, I think the following two things are important: (a) Students need to know Western bioethics principles because these are common language in the Japanese health care, related laws and guidelines. But teachers must be careful so that students do not understand these principles superficially, the autonomy principle tends to have such pitfalls. Narratives, stories, and case studies are helpful tools against this problem. (b) Moral distress is important but risky to teach at the beginning. Once students learn this term, they are tempted to explain problems as moral distress and go no further. But I know Japanese nurses, who do not know this concept, are making efforts to find a way out of the action barriers. Such nurses are resilient and polite in order to protect patients. Japanese traditional values illuminate their behaviors.

Back to Maki

That Saturday, I gave Maki a copy of the clinical teachers' article mentioned above and another student's narrative:

> On my 4th day of practice, my patient Mr. A suddenly became unconscious and was connected to a respirator. At Mr. A's bedside, I could do nothing but gaze at the patient and rub his cold arms and legs all that day. I was doing the same thing until the evening of the next day. Feeling depressed and miserable that I was doing nothing for the past two whole days, I came back to the nurse station. But my teacher, showing me the printout of Mr. A's ECG monitor, said, "Hiro, see this, during the time you were in Mr. A's room, his irregular and weak pulses improved. You have done the core of nursing, even experienced nurses cannot do such a great thing, you are fantastic!" My teacher made me aware of my worth, which I did not notice. He taught me that I did good for the patient. I was really saved.

Final Words

Two weeks later, Maki came back to the dining room. She reported to me, "I read it all! I learned that there are so many good teachers and nurses. Sure, I will become a nurse."

Perhaps those stories had touched her heart, although she may not be mature enough to see that ethics was residing in those stories. But I look forward to seeing her practicing as a nurse in the near future. Then, she will surely think about nursing ethics and say that "I am glad I am a nurse."

In an editorial of our ethics journal, Miki Ono, one of Anne's children, writes, "Nursing ethics is home for nurses to come back to, confirm who they are, and go back to work."[8]

Pamela Grace: Stumbling onto Nursing Ethics: A Road Less Traveled

A nurse and midwife in England, my mother loved her job but came by it the hard way. Her protective working-class parents thought that a nurse's work was too arduous and steered her toward secretarial work in a mill in Manchester. She hated it and, after a few years, rebelled and signed up for nurse training at Hope Hospital in Salford, before telling them what she had done. It was the beginning of World War II. The hours were long as she told it: 72 hours per week with a half day off, lectures after night shift, and many seriously wounded among the patients to care for. As luck would have it, she ended up on a ward that cared for prisoners of war and had many a tale to tell of good and bad behavior. An SS officer who bullied his subordinates, and a kind young Italian soldier who, unasked, helped the other patients and cried at night for his family. Her hospital was bombed during the Blitz of Manchester in 1941; the nurses' home suffered a direct hit, and 14 nurses were killed. According to family lore, some vulnerable patients were evacuated to Wales, and she was sent with them, so missed the hospital bombing. But in an era before easy access to phones, her family did not know this and thought her among the dead until she returned three days later.

I enjoyed the tales she told, and as teenagers my sisters and I were co-opted to help at various events on the geriatric floor where she was the senior sister (nurse manager). We got to see discipline, kindness, and compassion in action. However, I was not sure I wanted to be a nurse. For a brief period, I thought I would be a medical doctor, but a profound lack of studiousness, a distaste for the classroom, and a disinclination to do homework led to the headmistress of my academic high school 'suggesting' my parents remove me from school. This was not uncommon in the UK at that time. Only the most studious finished the last two years and went on to university; the remainder were steered towards practical occupations.

This was the beginning of my stumble into opportunities that directed my career. Luckily, I could sign up for pre-nursing work as a cadet nurse. Which meant I worked two to three days per week in my local hospital and attended classes in the technical college the other days. I loved it! I had hated my very academic and rather dryly taught classes in high school and being confined to a classroom all day long.

Cadet nurses in the UK during that era rotated through all of the hospital departments to see how they worked. We assisted physical therapists, X-ray technicians, autoclaved instruments for theater, made up the unguents in pharmacy, and so on. On the wards we fed patients, helped them walk, changed flower water, and buttered bread for afternoon tea. All things that might seem mundane, but offered opportunities for countless interactions with patients, and a sense that one was needed. After two years, I was accepted into a nurses' training school in a large hospital in Liverpool, and the real work began. This education, which resembled that of the US diploma schools, was in many ways a trial by fire. We staffed the wards and were often expected to know what we had not yet been exposed to, a problem that puzzled me. Also, there was an accepted bullying of younger students by older students, staff nurses, and sisters. Not everyone engaged in this behavior and there were wonderful role models. But it did not make sense to me, and I could see how such attitudes interfered with good patient care. I vowed that as I moved up the hierarchy, I would not be one of those who bullied. It just did not make sense to me to expect people to know something that they had not been exposed to. For example, in the first few months, I was sent to get a sphygmomanometer and I had no idea what that was but was afraid to ask. Luckily, my second place to look was the general supply closet where the shelves were labeled.

All of this is to say that the environments in which nurses worked could be troubling, and avenues to express concerns did not exist. Not all of the wards were difficult places to work, however. I was also privileged to work in some areas where there was a sense of camaraderie that put patients at ease (wards in the UK at that time were the long open Nightingale type)—thus I knew things could be different.

A few years post-registration, I applied for an assignment in the US, not meaning to stay, yet here I am. The US has been good to me in terms of educational opportunities that I might not have been afforded in the UK, given my earlier rather sketchy educational history. However, I continue to have concerns about the US health-care (non-)system, in which my students now work. It leaves a lot to be desired in terms of justice, access, and equity.

Florida was the site of my first nursing position in the US. I found the work environment radically different from what I had experienced in the UK. For example, there was a lot more documentation as well as more restrictions on what nurses could do independently. I came to understand this was in part a response to legal pressures and worries about lawsuits that were rising during this time, but also had to do with the way health care is financed in the US. Nevertheless, the cumbersome paperwork and need to get "orders" for even the most mundane things such as evaluating when a post-op patient could be safely allowed out of bed, or when stitches could be removed, I felt hampered care. Also, I still encountered difficult situations where I saw that patients were not receiving the care they needed or had delayed care so long that they were in dire straits. Additionally, support for nurses was, for the most part, lacking. To be fair, I was recruited in an era of a severe nursing shortage and often found myself responsible for more patients than I could possibly handle well. There seemed to be an acceptance of this as status quo. But it was exhausting, frustrating, and I often felt inadequate to the task. Surely, if this was expected, it must be possible. Thus, there was something wrong with me. I should be able to work faster and more efficiently. But how does one keep track of 50 patients with only two licensed practical nurses and two aides for assistance? Granted, in the 1970s, there was not so much technology as currently. However, patients were still very sick and deserving of attention. Logically, prevention of potential crises is almost always better than trying to manage them at their peak.

I decided a change to working in an intensive care environment was in order. These specialty areas were becoming more prevalent and seemed better staffed. Also, I wanted to improve my skills and be able to better handle emergencies. As I moved around the US, taking different assignments in critical care environments, I thought that my discomfort with complex, sometimes conflictual patient care problems would lessen. Instead, I found so many more problems where my voice on behalf of a patient was not heard or patients and their families would be pressed to agree to interventions that it seemed to me were not in their interests. However, in the 1970s and 1980s, ethics resources were scarce; there was a general sense that patients should go along with recommendations, and nurses should know their place in the hierarchy and accede (this was not true of all the settings in which I worked). This was medical paternalism in action, although not exactly the legal concept of *parens patriae*, from which contemporary ethical ideas of paternalism are derived. *Parens patriae* is the doctrine that holds there is a responsibility of governments to protect the most vulnerable in society. The medical paternalism that I encountered was the predominant idea that a treating physician knows better than the patient what clinical interventions and/or courses of treatment are appropriate for that patient and pertained even when the patient obviously had decision-making capacity as we define it now. Medical paternalism tends not to take into account the patient's context, desires, and preferences. At the risk of over-generalizing, medical paternalism as practiced in earlier decades focused more on the possibility of physical cure, or improvements in vital signs rather than patient wishes and preferences. I saw a few nurses who would speak up to articulate patient wishes and these were my role models. Many, although by no means all, of these nurses had furthered their education. They had baccalaureate or master's degrees and were confident about the boundaries of their knowledge.

Thus, I determined to pursue a Baccalaureate of Science in Nursing (BSN). Unfortunately, I was not initially accorded any course credit towards a BSN, so I limped along a bit at a time. I took content challenge exams, studied to exempt myself from some liberal arts courses via the College Level Exam Program (CLEP), and so on until I eventually graduated. These studies broadened my understanding of the world, enhanced my critical thinking abilities and my appreciation that the characteristics of individuals are significantly influenced by their background, and subsequent experiences. Their stories matter for the courses of action (or inaction) they take. Nurses can often provide a map, resources, and aids in their quest for better health or relief from suffering, but we have to know something about their goals or life trajectory. Navigating the increasing complexity and tangles of contemporary health-care environments can be difficult even for experts. We also have to tap into the resources of others. To effectively do this, we have to know how to cogently articulate the problem in order to propose solutions that will be heeded by the medical team, or at least tried.

In many ways, then, my baccalaureate studies introduced me to sociopolitical complexity. I determined that a graduate degree in nursing would provide further sophisticated thinking skills and it did. I became an Adult Nurse Practitioner (APN) in primary care. However, I discovered more problems in these settings, especially in rural West Virginia and Tennessee where I practiced. The lack of good primary care often led to more severe disease and impairment than needed to have occurred.

One elective course taken during my master's degree program provided an "aha!" moment. This was a bioethics course. I have described the profound effect the class had on me elsewhere and attributed the insights gained to philosopher Dr. Mark Wicclair, professor for this course. The beginning analytic and philosophical tools I gained led to me pursuing a PhD in philosophy with a concentration in medical ethics at the University of Tennessee, Knoxville. At the time (early 1990s), this program was remarkable for having both a full philosophy curriculum and a health-care ethics practica. A significant proportion of graduates of this program went on to have careers as ethics educators and clinical ethicists under the guidance of Dr. Glenn Graber, director of the applied ethics portion of the curriculum. Two of my philosophy student peers (most of whom were half my age) remarkably became nurses after completing a PhD in philosophy—the value of practical experiences was not lost upon them.

So this rather extensive background provides context for my interest in viewing nursing ethics as its own entity. I thought I would find the answers to my questions about how to address the issues most often faced by nurses during my PhD studies. However, what I found was that the focus in the ethics part of the course work was on difficult bioethical-type conflicts, the sort that require a team approach to resolve. The questions I raised did not seem to be considered as important; as one faculty told me, "Those issues are just not as juicy." Yet from my perspective, many of the issues that rose to the level of bioethical crises could have been avoided with better and earlier communication and the input of nurses, patients, and families. When I brought these insights to the fore, I was told to remove my nurse's hat and put on a philosopher's hat. Of course, I could not do that for the obvious reason that it was my nursing experiences that led me to study the role of philosophy in addressing nursing practice problems.

Further, and during this time, I was fortunate to teach in the College of Nursing (CON) at the University of Tennessee, Knoxville (UTK) and continued to work part time both as a nurse practitioner in UTK-CON's Veterinary Occupational Health Service and as a staff nurse in the coronary care unit (CCU) of a local hospital. This combination strengthened my emerging belief that nurses are not always well served by the bioethics community. This is because the problems we face are only rarely dilemmatic or complexly conflictual in nature. Problems in nursing contexts are, for the most part, encountered on a more frequent basis and include such things as being unable to access resources needed for optimal patient care, encountering family members who pressure the patient to choose certain interventions they do not want, or inadequate staffing that has put us in crisis mode. By crisis mode, I mean we do not have time to provide for patient comfort needs but must focus on handling the most critical or life-threatening events. Additionally, we were confronted with the fact that the life stories of many patients revealed a prior lack of access to care or to needed assistance and inadequate home support.

All of these circumstances contributed to my realizing that nurses have professional responsibilities to provide the care that the profession ostensibly exists to provide, and that we need to view our responsibilities as not just concerned with immediate patient care, but also how patients got to this stage of their ill health. In my case, this presented as caring for patients with cardiovascular problems, some leading to amputation, and learning how many had not had good primary care management or preventive care because of lack of access. This struck me as a grave injustice. It led me to explore the idea that professional advocacy cannot just be about speaking up in the moment but must also be concerned with root causes of poor health. As Fowler argues, this has historically been one of nursing's concerns and we need to keep this as a focus for the discipline. Otherwise, we are neither serving individuals nor society well.

I had been interested for some time in the issue of advocacy and how nurses were urged to be advocates for their patients. Yet it was not clear what this meant or how far nurses should risk themselves to "advocate" for those in their care. The importance of exploring this concept, how it had come to be adopted as a nursing tenet—as amorphous as the term is—eventually led to my dissertation, which constituted a philosophical analysis of advocacy and its meaning for health-care practice generally and nursing practice specifically. To be clear, this was not a concept analysis in the nursing sense. At the time, I was not even aware of concept analyses as used in nursing. It was an in-depth look at the legal, popular, and health-care literature to parse elements of the idea of advocacy. It resulted in an understanding of the risks to nurses and patients of relying solely on one of the various existing definitions as found in the literature.

Ultimately, what resulted was a caution about using the term advocacy to exhort nurses to act when the definitions, scope, and limits were not clearly articulated and risks to the nurse accounted for. Advocacy, from this exhaustive review, is best understood as professional responsibilities to act to provide the human "good" promised by a given health-care profession, via their disciplinary understandings and implicit or explicit codes of ethics. When we can act to get an individual what they need in the moment but intractable barriers exist, then we have to work with others to overcome them, and this may require addressing problematic policies and even negative sociopolitical circumstances. Thus, advocacy viewed as professional responsibilities to meet nursing goals is a broader concept than is often understood and is derived from the field of inquiry that is nursing ethics. Protecting, promoting, and restoring health and relieving suffering are the historically derived goals of nursing internationally. When there are obstacles to our work, then we have concomitant responsibilities to individuals and society to strive to overcome these. Nurses and the profession more generally exist to meet an unmet social need. If we can no longer do this, then we have obligations to be transparent about what is and what is not possible and why. A tenet of moral philosophy is that we cannot hold someone ethically accountable if they have no action choices—it is a logical impossibility. The ethical objectives of nursing practice are essentially professional advocacy. It is acting to overcome barriers to the provision of the good promised at the individual, unit, policy, or societal level depending on the root cause or causes of the barrier.

I recognize controversy remains about what constitutes a profession and why the idea of profession is important. However, I have argued elsewhere that, for lack of a better term, identifying a group of persons who provide a critical human service, have specialized education, skills, and some level of autonomy over practice as a profession permits society to hold them accountable for delivering their services.

In turn, this leads to consolidation of the idea that nursing ethics is its own field of inquiry about the who, what, and why of nursing. In concert with prior scholars, we can understand nursing ethics as being "inquiry into the boundaries of practice, the appropriate knowledge base for that practice and apt characteristics of members."[9,10,11,12] As noted elsewhere and articulated slightly differently, nursing ethics is "the study of what constitutes good nursing practice, what obstacles to good nursing practice exist, and what the responsibilities of nurses are related to their professional conduct."[13] Nursing ethics necessarily intersects with the ethics of other health-care professions which, similarly, is the field of inquiry about the roles and responsibilities of that group, their clinicians as well as the education necessary to develop ethical practitioners who can fulfill the goals of the profession. I do not see bioethics as a professional ethics per se, although health-care professionals necessarily have an interest in bioethical problems and their resolution. Bioethics is the field of inquiry about the impact of bioethical technologies on human beings.

In conclusion, I feel fortunate that my life meanderings led to gaining the tools to explore the origins and locus of problems that I and other nurses face in practice. The tools of philosophy have helped me be clearer about what nursing ethics is and how to continue to develop nurses who can practice ethically in spite of obstacles, understand when remedies are beyond their singular abilities to address, and know how to access resources and/or collaborate with others as these are needed.

Miriam Hirschfield: Human Rights and Nursing at WHO

Ethics and human rights—my personal beliefs and commitment have their very early roots in my mother's anguish over the death of her first child, a three-year-old, a week after Hitler marched into Vienna. Who cared for a hospitalized Jewish child then? In March 1938, fascism and racism destroyed her world, threatening not only the livelihood, but life itself of her family and community. Her personal anguish of loss fused with realizing the frailty of a democracy and the failings of human decency. She had not understood it was coming: "We did not care for politics, so politics cared for us." My father was incarcerated for being a Jew, but they were lucky, unlike millions of others. They managed to leave and become refugees.

An early lesson and an early demand: remaining silent in the face of injustice is evil. Social inequality and racism are evil—at age 80 today, my mother is still present as a daily yardstick. My parents returned to Vienna after World War II. Anti-Semitism and racism and the memory of the Holocaust were all present, while my brother and I were privileged children—loved by "well-to-do" parents, who had been able to build a new livelihood in New Zealand.

A left wing-Zionist youth movement added the "ideological layer" to the emotional; learning through simulated trials on ethical dilemmas related to opposing the Apartheid regime or the use of the atom bomb—discussions of adolescents developing a "Weltanschauung."

I chose nursing school, not out of a calling, but the understanding that it did not demand the discipline of university study, which I lacked at the time. And it promised a profession after only three years, enabling me to leave Vienna and emigrate to Israel. In June 1967, I lived the Israeli victory of the Six-Day War in the ICU of a large public hospital—18- and 19-year-old soldiers, dying or crippled for life, brought by helicopters from the Golan Heights. No joy over Jerusalem reunited could blind me to the insanity of war.

Realizing how little I knew, I took advantage of an opportunity that arose to study oncology nursing at New York University (NYU) and Memorial Sloan Kettering (formerly James Ewing Hospital) in New York. It was the first time I understood that nursing was a serious intellectual and emotional challenge. Dr. Norma Owens, the inspiring black nurse who headed the program, Inga Thornblad, a wonderful clinician and teacher, and Hiroko Minami, a student colleague, became my mentors—yes, I had been lucky to blindly choose our profession. It would enable me lifelong learning, helping me to find meaning and "my way."

Tel-Aviv University had opened a post-basic nursing program, and I was accepted. An early assignment was a paper on "What do I believe?" related to nursing, an assignment to clarify basic values—equity, respect for person, and discussing dilemmas. I was working as a staff nurse, then a clinical instructor, so real-life examples were plentiful. Reva Rubin and Jeanne Quint-Benoliel, visiting professors, opened special windows.

In 1972, Professor Anne Davis came to Israel to present in an international conference; we met. I had been accepted to the University of California, San Francisco (UCSF) for a master's program. Anne subsequently became my lifelong mentor and later friend.

I returned to Israel to fulfill my teaching obligation, then returned to UCSF to study toward a Doctor of Nursing Science (today a PhD) degree. Professors Anne Davis and Pat Underwood (nursing), Anselm Strauss (sociology), Margaret Clark (medical anthropology), and Maida Turner (aging and human development), as well as American and international student colleagues, were deeply influential to me.

Returning to Israel, my work life was divided between teaching at Tel-Aviv University and later creating a nursing baccalaureate program by uniting six diploma schools (a human relations challenge!) and working with the Kupat Holim Clalit Health Fund, at the time the major health-care provider in the country, to develop long-term care services for the whole country. Dr. Lea Zwanger—a nurse who had fought in the Palmach (the underground movement to gain Israel's independence), politically committed, opinionated, demanding, and with humor—was a different role model and boss.

We planned educational and research projects with the primary health-care nurses in Kupat Holim's clinics. They "suddenly" became aware of demented older persons living in their catchment areas and that families were caring for them. It had not been on their radar. My dissertation had been on family caregiving of demented elderly persons. Together with Baruch Ovadia, responsible for social work in Kupat Holim, we held courses for the "long-term care teams," which had been created after the 1973 Yom Kippur War. Thousands of dependent patients were then "referred to the community" to free hospital beds for wounded soldiers. The teams' role was advice and guidance of the primary care teams throughout the country.

We taught and practiced teamwork, case management, and counseling and also needed medical involvement. So, Dr. Hava Sroka, a neurologist, joined us. She mentored students while they worked with her to support the family caregivers of her patients.

We knew that our fund was essentially a medical insurance scheme. We believed that our aging members deserved our care, even for long-term problems not legally covered under medical insurance, and were ready to bend rules of eligibility. When a national committee to prepare a new law on "long-term care" was set up, I represented nursing in the university and the sick fund on the committee. Questions of "What does justice require?" as the rights of patients, caregivers, and intergenerational families' responsibility, versus population solidarity, occupied our discussions.

At one of the international nursing conferences, I heard Professor Astrid Norberg on feeding of demented patients. At the evening reception, I explained to Astrid that Swedish solutions would be unacceptable in Israel. "Why not? We should explore!" she responded, which was the beginning of an international seven-country research project on (force) feeding end-stage dementia and terminally ill cancer patients. Astrid is the lead nurse researcher in the field; Anne Davis led the American group.

Meanwhile, I became a consultant to a World Health Organization (WHO) group in Manila on "Health care of the elderly," learning from the experienced Dutch consultant Dr. Zonnenfeld. A consultancy on the "Assessment and planning of health care services for the elderly" in Fiji followed in 1983. My longtime friend Dr. Tamar Berman, a sociologist, advised me: "You ask everyone, individuals and then in groups. You always return to them to share your findings and ask them if they agreed, ask them what you have not understood, or what you have misunderstood; over and over again." My final report to the Fiji minister of health recommended: "Establish a long-term care fund, based in law, while your demographics still make it economically feasible." A New Zealand economist Denis Rose helped me determine a way of easily financing such a proposal. The minister decided, "Alas, it is not a priority." Fiji, as with so many developed countries (mine included), decided to wait for such legislation until it was much too late for many persons, patients, and family members alike, who would have needed the support.

Another WHO consultancy ended in bitter disappointment. For more than three years, I worked with Austrian nurses in Graz, Styria, on a demonstration research project on how to care for patients in the community, old persons who had been in long-term care facilities for years and even decades. All was ready for implementation when we received notification to stop the project; the hospital lobby feared losing large insurance funds.

In 1989, the Israeli Ministry of Foreign Affairs submitted my CV as a candidate for the WHO Chief Scientist Nursing position. I did not consider it a realistic possibility. Years before, Hiroko Minami (now a highly regarded nursing professor in Japan) and I had approached WHO in Geneva, to inquire about job offerings in the nursing division. We were dismissed out of hand.

I was selected for the post, but I had finally settled in Tel-Aviv and felt at home. I loved my work and thought it was important. Should I again uproot? The offer was hard to reject. I accepted and a steep, lonely learning curve began. While being aware of bureaucratic requirements and the challenge of interdisciplinary and international work, nothing had prepared me for WHO. In the first month, in a large meeting, I was told that I was remiss in not mentioning "primary health care and health for all"; when asked to give a keynote on the health of children, I told my boss that I was not knowledgeable on children's health. His response: "In this job you are expected to know it all." Well, I learnt, not all, but how to get around knowing less. Asha Singh Williams, an Indian colleague and friend, took me under her wing with Swiss nursing colleagues giving support—Dr. Rosette Poletti and Dr. Annemarie Kesselring, who took me for hikes on weekends.

The nursing position in WHO is a difficult one. You have only a secretary and in order to make a difference you must work through all the other divisions, mainly physicians, who do not consider nursing important. The International Council of Nurses (ICN) was an important partner. I found it crucial to build links with the regions. The regional nurse advisors became a wonderful team: Dr. Sandra Land and Maricel Manfredi in the PAHO/AMRO office in Washington, Jane Salvage in the EURO office in Copenhagen, Dr. Enaam Abu Youssef in the EMRO office in Alexandria (not thrilled to work with an Israeli, but wonderful once I was in post), Dr. Sally Bisch and then Dr. Duangvadee Sungkhobol in the SEARO office in New Delhi, and, not least, Kathy Fritsch in the WPRO office in Manila.

Among many projects of my eight years in the nursing position was a letter to the world chief nurses to do all in their power to stop female genital mutilation (FGM) and forbid nurses and midwives from participating. A bureaucratic feat was creating a two-person committee (myself and my assistant director general) where all the new WHO job vacancy notices would come to me. I could then discuss it with the respective division director, asking to change the requirement from "medical doctor" (a major barrier for nurses in applying to posts) to "technical officer," thus opening positions for nurses. I worked 12-hour days and worried about what I was accomplishing. I remembered the words of my Israeli colleague: "If you would come to work on my ward, I would know within a week if you are any good; if you would come to work in my hospital, it would take me a year; in that position—who can ever tell?"

In January 1998, Director General Dr. Hiroshi Nakajima appointed me Director, Division of Human Resources Development/Capacity Building. Dean Margretta

Styles had declared at the ICN Quadrennial Conference in Los Angeles that, "Once a nurse will fill that WHO position, nursing will have made it." Well, it had not made the difference for nursing. On a personal level it did make a difference, as my opinions suddenly carried weight—the same opinions, but now expressed by "the director" and not by "the nurse."

In early 1999, the new Director General, Dr. Brundtland, asked all of WHO HQ directors to resign from their positions and tell her what they wanted to work on. I chose "home-based and long-term care."

Thus, my most productive three years at WHO began. With the help of experts from around the world, we managed to publish more than ten reports/books, from case studies in poor countries on caregiving to HIV/AIDS patients, to textbooks on long-term care (LTC) in industrialized and developing countries. Betty Havens from Canada and the Jerusalem Brookdale Institute were my prime LTC expert advisors.

The two publications closest to my heart were global forecasts of need for LTC in all 192 member states. The "dependency needs" statistics were based on the Global Burden of Disease data, which included LTC needs throughout the life cycle. The information on the WHO website gave countries that might have the political will for action the needed information, with the trends reliable, if not the actual data. One of my greatest disappointments and sadnesses was that the information was deleted from the WHO website after I retired from WHO.

The other publication, still available on the WHO website, is "Ethical choices in long-term care: what does justice require?" Working with philosopher Daniel Wikler on "ethics" in WHO and a group of nurses, physicians, philosophers, anthropologists, and sociologists from around the globe, we made an effort to answer questions of how to re-think and address the challenge of future long-term care; what is (a) fair to the persons requiring care? (b) fair to the family caregivers? (3) fair to the care workers? and (d) fair to "care-work" exporting and "care-work" importing countries?

Over these years, I had the privilege of choosing and working with colleagues and teams from around the world, who knew far more on each and every specific topic, than I did. Collaboration pays off.

With my 60th birthday in December of 2002, I had to retire. Dr. Ruth Levin, a longtime friend, convinced me to join her on faculty at Yezreel Valley College in Israel's periphery. My task would be to establish a new baccalaureate nursing program.

We soon realized that our main challenge was to ensure "cultural safety" (a concept developed by Maori nurses, taking power differences in cultural relationships into account) for our students and faculty. About half our students were Palestinian (Arab) Israelis, with the other half a mix of different Jewish Israeli identities (kibbutz members, immigrants from the former Soviet Union, etc.). Classes and seminars in ethics and communication courses, jointly led by nurse clinicians and psychologists, became the backbone of the program. The ongoing qualitative evaluation, led by Dr. Daniella Arieli, an anthropologist, showed us that we faced a serious challenge with relationships between Jews and Arabs, within the larger reality of ongoing violent conflict and war. Working on these issues became our major focus, led by Professor Victor Friedman, an organizational psychologist.

In hospitals, I saw Ethiopian Jewish immigrant women solely in roles of cleaning (my mother's job in England and New Zealand as a refugee) and as nurse aides. I realized that their educational background had not prepared them for a university/college entrance exam. So, we started a preparatory program, got full scholarships, and planned extensive academic and social support. Within years, we had a large group of Ethiopian Jewish immigrant students with their own leadership group, who passed the national licensure exam. This "Opportunity for Success" program has by now more than 60 graduate nurses. It is an initiative I am proud of.

All through the last 45 years, my brother, Dr. Yair Hirschfeld, a historian, worked in backbench diplomacy, seeking a just solution with our Palestinian neighbors. The Oslo Accords was a personal accomplishment. His work has informed me over the years on the broader political issues related to our conflict.

WHO had asked me to edit a special issue of the Israeli–Palestinian journal *Bridges* on nursing. This began a more than 20-year collaboration and friendship with Dr. Amal Abu Awad, at the time a young Palestinian nurse educator. We began mutual exchange visits of groups of nurses. Upon their request, I found volunteer nurses from a Scottish WHO Nursing Collaborating Center to teach a large group of Palestinian nurses, hoping to enter PhD studies, statistics, and research methodology.

At ICN's 25th Quadrennial Congress in Melbourne, I was able to represent the Israeli Nurses Association and welcome, in our name, the Palestinian Nurses Association to ICN. It remains the only international organization that Palestinians could join without a struggle.

Dr. Nurith Wagner, a longtime friend and our leading Israeli nurse ethics expert, convinced me to join Nurses of the Middle East (NME). Following meetings and yearly conferences, enabling mainly Palestinian and Israeli nurses to meet, Dr. Dominique Egger, a former WHO Swiss colleague and partner, facilitated a series of workshops where together Palestinian and Israeli nurses identified common problems, seeking ways to address them. Two of the major issues identified were nurse referrals (some 40,000 Palestinian patients were hospitalized yearly in Israel) and infection control. Nurith and I remain active with "Physicians for Human Rights, Israel," their ethics committee, their fights for social justice, and access to health care for Palestinians, asylum seekers and migrants, and for human rights and quality health care for prisoners.

Most recently, the NGO Rozana together with the NME received a large USAID grant to work with nurses from six Palestinian and six Israeli hospitals to advance quality of care. In October 2022, Nurith Wagner and I, as a team, received a wonderful gift, the Thai Nursing Royal Srinagarindra Award; we received it for our career-long work in ethics and human rights. Alas, with the recent political developments of populism, growing fascism and racism, continued work on human rights for all is a growing challenge facing nursing—and facing all of us.

Peggy L. Chinn: A Personal History of Racism

Like so many other nurses, I grew up in a white Christian family with a strong emphasis on the evils of all things labeled as a "sin." Of course, the notion of "sin" is not unique to those who are born and raised "white," nor is it limited to those who are raised "Christian." But the conception of what is labeled as a "sin," or even what is learned from birth as the difference between "right" and "wrong," does have wide variations from family to family, from culture to culture, and even from nation to nation. In my upbringing, it was a sin, among many other things, to dance or to play cards—restrictions that puzzled me from an early period of my life and, of course, I learned to see in a different light as I became an adult!

My parents chose to become Baptist missionaries when I was in the second grade, and so our family traveled to Hilo, Hawaii, with the express purpose of bringing salvation to the "heathen." My parents hailed from Georgia and Tennessee, and never hesitated to convey in words and in actions their sense of superiority and "goodness" as the white missionaries, compared to the people of the town. There were no Hilo residents of African heritage in this predominantly Asian and mixed-race residents' town, many of whom immigrated to support the growth of the sugar cane fields that surrounded the town. However, during our trips to visit relatives in the mainland every three years, my sister and I learned the horrendously evil ways of the segregated Jim Crow South. From my parents' point of view, there was nothing odd, much less evil, about the way things were. When I questioned my parents as to why there were separate churches for black and white people, my mother's answer was "because they [implicitly referring to black people] like it that way."[14] Even to my 11-year-old mind, this seemed like a woefully inadequate response, but I did not know how to take the matter further.

It was in this complex exposure to what we might now call "diversity" that my sister and I were immersed in learning about the world of "us" and "them." Embedded in this was the notion of "good" and "evil." We were the people of God, the good people. On the mainland, we were the white people who lived on one side of the town where things were organized in neat rows of well-to-do bungalows. In Hawaii, we were the *haole* (white) family who preached the gospel of Christianity to save the world; we were the good *haole* family, living in a Hilo neighborhood dominated by Japanese, Chinese, Filipino, Hawaiian, and mixed-race families— people who needed to be "saved." We grew up as residents of a magical tropical island nation. But we knew nothing of the invasion of the Islands by white missionaries who brought salvation and stole the land, the economy, and dismantled the proud Hawaiian constitutional government. We knew of the influence of the white whalers who brought the carnal pleasures of sin to the Islands, but only as a matter of passing amusement.[15]

Every three years, we had the experience of visiting relatives in the southeast area of the US mainland, who lived in all-white neighborhoods with black families just blocks away in starkly contrasting communities of poverty, or very close to it. We learned, in the words and actions of our elders, that "those people" were not only "different" and "other"—they were viewed as lacking the character required to be in better situations; they were sinners—some of them worthy of being saved, but many simply not worthy of even that degree of concern.

As a child, I noticed the hypocrisies of pious white people who on Sunday claimed to love their neighbors, but who by Wednesday were embroiled in frightening domestic wars that left bruises and scars on the bodies of wives and little children. I noticed and wondered about the fact that all of the *haole* children, and the children of Chinese physicians and Japanese dentists, who even in the "melting pot" of Hawaii, were segregated in classrooms with fewer children, better books to read, and the ample supplies of art material that were lacking for children whose parents were laborers, store clerks, custodians—some Japanese but mostly Filipino, Portuguese, Hawaiian, and other Pacific Islanders.

What I did not notice until much later in adulthood was the fact that our grade-school curriculum only taught the history of Hawaii and the United States from the perspective of the white colonizers; we had no lessons about the Japanese and Chinese people who, in fact, were the majority of the population in our little town of Hilo. We learned to sing the beautiful Hawaiian songs composed by Queen Liliuokalani[16] phonetically—we could sing and recite the Hawaiian words but were never taught the language.[17] We did not know the meaning of the words we sang. We learned next to nothing about the Queen's remarkable life, her worldwide influence, her amazing majesty.[18] We learned very little about the original inhabitants of the Islands other than the "reports" of the white missionaries and the explorer Captain James Cook[19] who "discovered" the Islands in 1778. We learned nothing of the stories of the European whalers who, about 40 years after Cook's first visit, began to have a significant influence as biological fathers of many and, for some, fathers who integrated as members of Hawaiian families.[20]

Consider the fact that my family arrived in the Islands in 1949—just 52 short years after Liliuokalani's government was overthrown, and the US government seized control of the Islands. I, along with three other *haole* kids with US mainland roots and over 30 Asian kids with Japanese, Chinese, Filipino, and Hawaiian roots, learned nothing of this history. We learned to feel pride in reciting the pledge of allegiance to the US flag every morning at the start of the school day. There was barely any mention in all of grade-school as to how we came to be reciting that particular pledge, much less the erasure of the family and cultural histories that unfolded during those 52 years that formed who we were as 1st, 2nd, 3rd, 4th, 5th, and 6th graders, typically between the ages of 5 and 11.

Top all of this off with one other fact: none of our teachers in those grades were from the US mainland, nor were they *haole*. Yet the curriculum they taught was exactly what most mainland elementary schools were teaching. They were "local" women, mostly of Chinese, Japanese or mixed-race heritage. One or two teachers in the school had *haole* names due to marriage to a mainland *haole* man. I presume now that most of them had earned their teaching credentials from the University of Hawaii in Honolulu—the only location at the time that offered education degrees. A few might have attended mainland (mostly California) colleges because of spouses who enrolled in professional degree programs not available in the Islands at the time (medicine, dentistry, law). What they learned in becoming teachers also, in all likelihood, had no content related to their own histories or the histories of their people.

Recalling now the impressions I formed growing up, I am appalled and deeply offended. It has taken a lifetime for me to tap into the evil that is racism. In my childhood experience, there were no discussions of racism, even though the civil rights movement was beginning to stir on the mainland—a fact we never even learned about. In the Islands, we often spoke of the "melting pot" of Hawaii, where presumably there was no discrimination—despite the very visible and obvious fact that people of Hawaiian heritage were isolated in relatively rural, poverty-ridden towns where there were essentially no employment opportunities and the regional high schools were out of reach for many of the teens in the area. Most of the professional people in the larger towns and the city of Honolulu were predominantly Chinese, along with the minority well-to-do *haoles*; the grocery and retail industry was dominated by Japanese people. School segregation was institutionalized in the heritage of two prominent private schools in Honolulu. In 1842, the missionaries established Punahou School for their children[21]—a school that still allowed only a 10 percent "quota" of non-*haole* children when my son's father was admitted to kindergarten a century later in 1942.[22] In 1882, a comparable private school—Kamehameha School—was established for boys of Hawaiian heritage, with girls admitted seven years later.[23] When I entered the public Riverside School in Hilo, I went to the "English Standard School" for children who could speak "proper" English, located across the street from the "other" school for children who did not speak much English, or who spoke "pidgin" English (regardless of their actual academic ability).

It was not until I was in my 30s, living in Buffalo, New York, that I began to consider the very real dynamics of discrimination and disadvantage based on the social construction we know as "race." My personal history growing up in Hawaii and marrying into a Chinese/Hawaiian family was a unique background, but it did not give me any special insights related to racism, and in fact instead ingrained in me the assumption that a person's skin color (or race) does not matter. And it did not prepare me for life in a large northeast working-class city segregated into residential and social black/white neighborhoods. I became a member of a collective of progressive white women who were connected to the Women's Studies program at SUNY-Buffalo and who established and ran Emma: Buffalo women's bookstore. We talked about race and racism, and we held community programs featuring women of color who authored foundational feminist literature on racism, history, and experience of people of color. Yet our collective remained all white, a fact that we failed to confront throughout the ten-year life of the collective.

This fundamental, visible, and glaringly obvious fact of unquestioned and unexamined segregated whiteness is not unusual. It is, in fact, the profile of nursing as a profession. I, along with all of my white colleagues over my long career, have simply taken this fact for granted. Yes, we engage in bemoaning the lack of diversity in nursing, but without motivation to seriously question why this is the case. We have failed to face this fact as the ethical/moral issue that it is. Our failure contributes to and perpetrates the unjust inequities that render disadvantage for many, including a significant number of people of color, and secures advantage for the relatively few—mostly those who are white.

The pillars that support this injustice include: 1) individual racist attitudes and actions, 2) institutional policies that normalize continued discriminatory practices, and 3) persistence of social/political norms that sustain white privilege. It is time for white nurses to recognize that it is a fundamental responsibility of white people to resist and dismantle each of these pillars. Lectures, training seminars, and book clubs are the dominant "go-to" approaches to do so, but these efforts have very limited potential. It is time to leave the passive spaces of listening to admonitions about racism, and become active participants as anti-racist citizens. There are doable actions that I believe white nurses must engage in if we seek justice and intend to resist and dismantle the status quo; here is a basic overview of what is possible.

Make a personal, conscious decision to become anti-racist, and become well-informed with both depth and breadth of understanding. It all starts with your own decision and commitment. Educate yourself by reading and discussing the abundant ideas that are now on the web and in books and journal articles. Write your own "accountability statement" to clarify and codify your commitment. Find an "affinity group" to build support for one another's commitment to become anti-racist. You can refer to the "Overdue Reckoning on Racism in Nursing"[24] project in forming your own course of action.[25] In particular, our "Principles of Reckoning" provide a roadmap for what we believe to be meaningful action. We also provide a rich list of resources[26]—books, articles, webinars, and other resources that you can tap into.

Form partnerships between white nurses and nurses of color actively engaged in challenging racist policies and practices, with meaningful personal and interpersonal relationships between people of color and white people. Read and cite nursing literature by nurses of color, and connect with the authors to learn more about their work. Form actions together with nurses of color around health-care concerns that you share in common. Go to places and spaces where nurses and other people of color are engaged, and learn to take their lead as you become part of a community. Robin DiAngelo provides a brilliant explanation of what this means in her "Accountability Statement":

> Building relationships across race will require most white people to get out of their comfort zones and put themselves in new and unfamiliar environments. This is different from our usual approach in which we invite Black, Indigenous

and Peoples of Color into committees, boards, and places of worship—groups white people already control. We often do this when we have done no work to expand our own consciousness and developed no skill or strategy in navigating race. In effect we are inviting Black, Indigenous, and Peoples of Color into hostile water, then we are dismayed and confused when they choose to leave.[27]

Build platforms that center voices of nurses of color, with visible evidence that these voices are being recognized and followed. Understand that white privilege typically is seriously misused. Indeed, white privilege exists and cannot be denied, but it can be used to end racism. Rather than decry or, worse yet, deny the privilege of being white, white people can make conscious choices to use privilege in ways that begin processes of change. One approach is to restructure and remake spaces and places where change is possible—where white voices have typically dominated and prevailed. Examine each of the spaces in which you live and work, and start making change in even the smallest of ways, with the intent to build inclusive policies and practices. Follow through in ways that are not simply inclusive in the sense of being present, but inclusive of active leadership and participation. When you are planning a program, or an event, or even a single class lecture or learning activity, seek the leadership of people of color. Together, build in the visibility of nurses of color and assure that their voices are heard. Learn about barriers that in the past have excluded nurses of color, and join with nurses of color to seek to dismantle those barriers. Retain a strong dose of humility in doing this work; when you falter, acknowledge what happens and get to work to change what happens in the future.

There is no universal "how to" in overcoming racism. But this is not simply an academic project. Becoming anti-racist requires action. It is possible, indeed it is imperative, to forge our own paths in the direction of ending racism. The actions you take, and how you take action, must be your own creation. If we all do whatever we can do to resist and dismantle racism, I believe we will make significant change!

Verena Tschudin: On Founding the Journal *Nursing Ethics,* and the Human Rights and Nursing Awards

One day in 1992 or 1993, the day before going on holiday, I was bringing a manuscript to the Royal College of Nursing in London and by chance met there the editor of several of my books. The building was full of people attending a conference and there was nowhere to sit. My friend and I knelt down against a wall and then she asked me if I would be willing to edit a journal on ethics in nursing that her publisher would like to start. I provisionally agreed, saying that the holiday would present a good time to think about it.

My first action was then to contact my friend Professor Geoffrey Hunt to ask his opinion. He was very hesitant, trying hard to persuade me that this would not be a success. Suddenly, he changed his mind and suggested that I go ahead and he would be my assistant editor. The deal was done, and some 30 years later *Nursing Ethics* still has the same bright yellow cover and seems to be much read and needed. The editor is now Ann Gallagher, Professor and Head of Department of Health Sciences, Brunel University, London.

While working together, Geoff came up with the idea of establishing an awards system for nurses who do outstanding human rights work as part of their work, without any acknowledgment. Thus, the Human Rights and Nursing Awards were conceived and started as a novel event during the yearly conferences we also started, then at the University of Surrey.

The Human Rights and Nursing Awards were first given in 2001 to three people. Subsequently, they were given in 2003 and 2005, but only to two people each time. In 2005, a group of anonymous donors guaranteed a yearly sum for the Awards, thus making it possible to give the Awards every year; therefore, the next Awards were given in 2006 and yearly since then. In 2014, an anonymous donor set up an investment for the Awards so that a yearly sum (approx. £20,000) from interest can be used for the Awards.

The Human Rights and Nursing Awards are now presented to any nurse in recognition of an outstanding commitment to human rights and exemplifying the essence of nursing's philosophy of humanity to further their work.

The criteria for the Awards are that "The contributions and accomplishments of the nominee must be of international significance to human rights and that the contributions of the nominee have influenced health care and/or nursing practice." A short overview of some of the awardees follows, although each one of them deserves more attention. Their citations are on the website. I feel hugely privileged to have the chance to know so many outstanding nurses and people over time, while getting them through the selection and to the place where the Awards were given. Every nurse has the possibility to join their ranks.

2001

Karla Schefter, Germany/Afghanistan: She established and still runs (after 35 years in 2022) the best and entirely free-to-users hospital in Afghanistan. This continues with the new Taliban regime since August 2021.

Glenda Wildschut, South Africa: Her special interests were violence, trauma, and torture rehabilitation. She helped to develop a reparation policy for genocide survivors in Rwanda, a reconciliation process in Guinea Bissau, and a church response to the proposed truth commission in Sierra Leone.

Christine Schmitz, Germany/Médecins sans Frontières (MSF): Her focus was mainly in acute crisis areas. Her most striking experience has been the mission in the Bosnian enclave of Srebrenica. Together with an Australian doctor, she witnessed the enclave's brutal taking by the Bosnian-Serbian army in July 1995. The deportation of women and children and the killing of 8,000 men remain in her memory. Her testimony at the Court of Human Rights in (approx. 2015) was crucial.

2003

Cathy Crowe, Canada: She called for homelessness to be declared a national disaster on the same scale as floods and earthquakes.

Mpho Sebanyoni-Motihasedi, South Africa: She established a hub of care and counselling, skills development, training for caregivers in 80 villages, support groups for grannies, volunteers in the district, and 15 satellites in rural communities at a time when the word "AIDS" was totally taboo in South Africa.

2005

Fidelis Mudimu, Zimbabwe: At the time, the government regularly raided houses, beat up people at night, and destroyed houses and livelihoods. It was dangerous to visit the victims, as he could easily be killed, too. He ran an organization of nurses to "rescue" the victims from their houses and get medical care for them.

2006

Nurses at the St John's Eye Clinic, Gaza: Hanan Zaálan, Fouad Najjar, Ghazi El Baba, Mohamet Barakat, Abdallah El Baba: This group of nurses at the only eye clinic in Gaza worked (then) in situations of heavy bombing, raids, and lack of communication and any equipment. They were not given visas to collect the Award; the matron of the main hospital in Jerusalem collected the award on their behalf.

2008

Emmie Chanika, Malawi: She served as an officer in the Malawi Red Cross; on a commission to investigate the deaths of four politicians; initiated and founded the Prison Reform Committee; set up a blood donor scheme; served on the Malawi Housing Corporation; is a paralegal officer; and has been the Executive Director of the Civil Liberties Committee (CILIC) for many years. She said that all this was only possible because she is a nurse.

Sister Teresita Hinnegan, USA: At the age of 80, and after retiring from a long academic career at the University of Pennsylvania School of Nursing, she established safe houses for women who experienced violence and abuse, believing that the structures that condone any violence against women have to be challenged at all levels.

2009

Kathy Mellor, UK: She is a neonatal nurse practitioner, working in countries where health care is severely compromised by lack of education and limited resources: Nagorno-Karabakh, Armenia, Mongolia, Russia, and Nigeria. She created the well-known early discharge program for preterm babies and established "Kangaroo care," now used worldwide.

Branka Rimac, Croatia: During the civil war in 1995, she cared for wounded people in no-man's land, crossing borders at will. She has since become a leading nurse throughout Europe, establishing links and associations between countries and regions.

2010

Robert Simons, Netherlands: He was Chairperson of the International Federation of Health and Human Rights Organizations (IFHHRO), developing its remit and including human rights and advocacy training for health professionals throughout the world, with regional partners in Uganda, India, and Peru.

2011

Ana Luisa Aranha, Brazil: She created and ran a series of restaurants in hospitals and government establishments for nursing, medical, and other staff to work interchangeably together with mentally ill people to enable them to gain employability.

Thabsile Dlamini and Masitsela Mhlanga, Swaziland: This was then the country with the highest HIV/AIDS occurrence, and nurses died from the disease or left the country. These two nurses established special clinics for nurses with HIV. The pair came briefly to the attention of the international nursing press in 2000. Nurses in rural health facilities were being attacked by robbers looking for money. Some members of parliament suggested that nurses should carry arms to work for protection, but they refused, stating that arms would deter the public from seeking health care, and demanded that the government provide protection.

2012

Barbara Parfitt, UK and Bangladesh: She worked in a dozen countries to promote empowerment for women, women's rights, and the health-care rights of people who are sick, poor, or dying.

Soodabeh Joolaee, Iran: She had single-handedly established ethics teaching in Iran among nurses and doctors, and became the country-wide reference person on any ethical issues.

2014

Rula al-Saffar, Bahrain: She started and ran a campaign to free all medics and prisoners of conscience. In 2012 and 2013, she was nominated as one of the most influential Arab personalities.

Sister Jyoti Rosamma, India: She was then working among the poorest people in North India, helping them to set up their own businesses and using herbal remedies for their communities.

2015

Eileen Greene, Canada: She started and supported HIV care at Katutura Hospital, Namibia, by creating schooling and soup kitchen opportunities for the impoverished community living around the hospital.

Will Pooley, UK: He was nursing in Sierra Leone through the Ebola outbreak in 2014. He caught the disease, but returned to Sierra Leone to continue working when he was well again.

2017

Martha Turner, USA: She has done exemplary ethics work in the US Armed Forces and still works in many countries, especially Vietnam. She is the co-writer of the ANA's new *Code of Ethics*.

Bernadette Glisse, Belgium: She worked in Cambodia, first among refugees from the war in Vietnam, and was later asked to introduce human rights practices for prisoners throughout the country.

2018

Alice Leahy, Ireland: She is a nurse and former Chairperson of the Sentence Review Group and a former Irish Human Rights Commissioner. She founded the Alice Leahy Trust, providing health and related services to people who are homeless and vulnerable. It was said of her that if a homeless person died, they were at least known to God and Alice.

Miriam Kasztura, Switzerland: She worked around the world with Médecins Sans Frontières, and is on their board of directors. She is also heavily involved with the enforcement of human rights in underserved populations in Switzerland whose health-care needs are not met. She is pioneering nurse-led primary care consultation services for assessments, and health-promotion interventions for university students and employees.

2019

Yusrita Zolkefli, Brunei: She was nominated for her outstanding initiatives, both in education and practice, which inspired nurses to embrace ethics and law as part of their daily working life. Nurses learn how to know their beliefs and convictions and those of people with whom they disagree. This is vital for the work of advocacy for nurses. Her work has ensured that all nurses throughout Brunei have the opportunity for ethics education, understand the language of ethics, and use it.

Dorcas Gwata, Zimbabwe and UK: She migrated to the UK from Zimbabwe in 1991, first working as a cleaner, then as a care assistant. She is now a visiting Global Mental Health Lecturer at the London School of Health and Tropical Medicine and King's College. Dorcas works as a volunteer with AFRUCA (Africans United Against Child Abuse) and is a strong advocate on safeguarding issues for African children across communities affected by female genital mutilation, human trafficking, modern slavery, and witchcraft branding.

2020

Lisa Brown Gibson, Canada: She has been instrumental in the advancement of the rights of people with mental illnesses and addiction. She founded the Workman Theatre Project in 1987, now the oldest and largest multidisciplinary arts and mental health company in Canada, supporting artists professionally to achieve their highest potential.

Elisabeth Nishimwe Samvura, Democratic Republic of Congo (DRC): She is head nurse of the neonatology department at Heal Africa Hospital, Goma. The area has suffered nearly continuous conflict since 2003 and from ongoing Ebola. She focuses on family-centered care, encouraging bonding within the families, reducing the anxiety and post-traumatic stress often experienced by parents in neonatal units. She is recognized as a foremost expert in the delivery of neonatal care in conflict situations.

2021

Kerri Nuku, New Zealand: She is of Tainui descent and is driven by a concern for prevailing ethnic inequalities. She is particularly noted for her partnership working with and seeking to improve the health status of all people in New Zealand through inclusive participation in health and social policy development, and is a collaborator in the United Nations Universal Periodic Review and the World Health Organization (WHO) Human Resources for Health Project.

Suman Shrestha, Nepal: He moved to the UK in the 1990s to complete his professional and postgraduate nursing studies. In 1994, Suman opened the first center in Nepal caring for children and adults with intellectual and physical needs, and he remains a key supporter on regular visits. Suman has also been instrumental in the development of critical care both in the UK and in Nepal, and has led on UK national initiatives concerning the management of sepsis and established the strategic redeployment of nurses into critical care working during the COVID pandemic. Suman's achievements in Nepal are all the more remarkable as they are completed on a voluntary basis and dependent on his own fundraising.

2022 [Author's Addendum]

Deanna Mezen, UK: As nurse at one of the largest male prisons in Europe (Featherstone near Wolverhampton), she was the lead for palliative care where she developed the practice standard Dying Well in Custody that provided for a humane, dignified death with adequate and timely medication, psychosocial support, open cell door, and the presence of family and friends. She transformed the care culture within the prison for those at the end of life, making compassion and excellence of care a normative expectation. She has been an advocate for the men whom society has imprisoned, for veterans in custody suffering PTSD, and is the lead in a Healthcare in the Transgender support group.

Ricardo Ayala, Belgium/Chile: A civil and human rights activist and professor of ethics, he has worked for civil rights for those without voice in Chile: for indigenous women, for homeless persons, and for sexual minorities. He has worked for police reform, and against gender-based violence particularly in relation to workplace violence against trans nurses. His current endeavors include seeking to expand health coverage for marginalized communities in Ecuador and Belgium. Ricardo is committed to the role of the nurse in relation to human rights and politically informed nursing practice constructed within a socio-cultural and socio-historical background.

2023

Ruggero Rizzini, Italy: A nurse from Pavia in northern Italy, he received the award in recognition of the exceptional contributions that he has made to the development of health and social care in Pavia, Italy and in Guatemala, Central America. He has worked in Italy and Guatemala to raise awareness of the needs of society's most vulnerable persons. He has worked in St. Gertrudis slum in Guatemala with an emphasis on nursing and health care by opening facilities that promote well-being.

Ukraine mental health nurses: Thirty-two nurses from the community mental health teams in Ukraine received the award in recognition of their work in developing mental health services in the country. They were commended for resilience, courage, and resourcefulness for developing new ways of practicing under wartime conditions.

The variety of work done by the nurses who received the Human Rights and Nursing Awards is as remarkable as the people themselves. The money that goes with the Awards is to be used to further the work done by the recipients, but is given as a personal gift, in conjunction with the journal *Nursing Ethics*, and the recipients are invited to travel to the venue where the yearly ethics conference organized by Brunel University, London takes place to receive the Awards. The coordinator of the Human Rights and Nursing Awards and the members of the editorial board of *Nursing Ethics* constitute the selection committee.

Elizabeth Peter: Drawn to Feminist Ethics and Its Promise

While hard for me to believe, 35 years have passed since my commitment to nursing ethics began. In 1987, I was studying philosophy at York University while working part-time as a nurse at what was then a provincial psychiatric hospital, the Queen Street Mental Health Centre. (This hospital is now part of the Centre for Addiction and Mental Health.) While riding the railway to York one morning, I began to read *In a Different Voice* by Carol Gilligan,[28] which described "women's" moral orientation. I was immediately struck by how Gilligan's work resonated with nursing, with its emphasis on care, relationality, and particularly. She contrasted the ethic of care with the ethic of justice, characterizing the latter as being focused on impartiality, duties, and principles in a context of relationships of non-interference. I felt an excitement that there was a perspective that could better inform and articulate nursing ethics than deontology or utilitarianism could. I was now on a mission.

During my graduate studies, I continued to explore care ethics but increasingly encountered scholarship that critiqued these perspectives. While care ethics emphasizes the moral imperative of reducing human suffering and maintaining relationships, caring relationships have the potential to be exploitative or unfairly partial. Feminist ethicists at that time, such as Claudia Card and Rosemarie Tong, argued that the ethic of care may grow out of and perpetuate "women's" unrecognized and often exploited caregiving, leading to further powerlessness. In addition, the growing body of empirical research exploring Gilligan's claims indicated that most people use both care and justice considerations in their moral reasoning.

As a consequence of these critiques, I found myself becoming more drawn to feminist ethics as an approach for nursing ethics. In fact, to this day, I cannot really separate my commitment to feminist ethics from nursing ethics more generally. I initially was drawn to Annette Baier's work on trust. Her approach combines both love and obligation, which are similar to the ethics of care and justice. From Baier's perspective, in relationships of love, we trust others not to harm us, and in relationships of obligation, we trust others to recognize and fulfill obligations. Baier's work was attractive because it is relationship-focused, with the notion of trust implying interdependence.

As a feminist ethicist, I believed Baier's approach could also help draw awareness of the devaluation and invisibility of nursing, which is partially the result of the practices of nurses being associated with so-called "women's work." My recognition of the lack of esteem given to nurses by the public and health-care professionals, including nurses themselves, and the recognition of the responsibility nurses carry, often without a comparable degree of decision-making power, only further reinforced my commitment to nursing ethics using a feminist lens. Simultaneously, I also came to understand the potential power of nurses in part by reading the work of Sandra Lee Bartky about a feminist consciousness that encompasses a consciousness of both weakness and strength. Feminist ethics as a way of doing ethics helps us question the status quo, making it possible to work toward a better world for all. It is in this potential for change that my commitment to nursing ethics and feminist ethics continues even to this day.

My reflections on ethics and nursing have intensified over the last four years as a result of my responsibilities as the primary caregiver of my sister and parents, all of whom have had serious health problems. I have spent countless hours in hospitals and have done my best to navigate community services, all the while reflecting on love, inevitable losses, aging, the importance of human caregiving, and the potential of nursing ethics. The professional in me has also observed both the strengths and serious shortcomings of the Canadian health-care system. Most important, however, what used to be more of an intellectual appreciation of the importance of nursing has become a deep emotional appreciation of the significance of nurses' work and the values that inform it. I have been very lucky until now to have had only a very passing need for nurses, but now I rely on them constantly because of my family's dependence on them.

It's absolutely clear to me that nurses have the potential to have an incredible impact on the overall well-being of the lives of people, not only because of their knowledge and skills, but also the values that they enact. The excellent care I have witnessed has often included a deep attentiveness and respect. Yet, upon occasion, I have come across nurses and other health-care professionals who have treated my family members as merely bodies in a bed. It concerns me that only about half of the nurses I have encountered introduce themselves, making it difficult to know who is responsible for care and making nursing less visible than physicians and rehabilitation therapists. This lack of introduction is troubling because of what it signifies. It may mean that nurses consider themselves so insignificant and inter-changeable that they do not think it important to introduce themselves. It may also reflect that the importance of the nurse–patient relationship, often viewed as the foundation of nursing ethics, is only important in theory.

While nurses may go to work believing they are insignificant, they are not. Those nurses who have the capacity to not only be clinically competent but to engage with people with at least some genuine and personalized care are essential. The smallest gesture can be deeply memorable and can help reduce the sense of helplessness in a system that can be depersonalizing for patients, families, and nurses. These encounters make me wonder what accounts for the range of behav-iors and approaches. No doubt factors such as excessive workloads and exhaustion could play a role when practice is less than ideal, but there could be more. What role does, or did, ethics as an academic field have on their work? It's possible that when nursing ethics is taught, we have not adequately described ways in which values can be enacted. The practical application in the everyday likely needs more articulation so that abstract concepts can inspire realistic actions in the context of nurses' difficult working conditions.

It may also be that some nurses have not developed a robust moral identity as a nurse. Attention to moral identity formation is receiving increased attention in moral philosophy and moral psychology, with moral identity being viewed as the bridge between knowing the right thing to do and acting. I would argue that moral identity also has the potential to give us a sense of power and connection as a group of care providers who have played an important role in hospitals and the community for decades. Nursing ethics can be a part of that moral identity formation, especially if those who teach it and write in the area pay attention to not only the contributions of bioethics, but also those of nursing. We need to recognize that bioethics as a discipline has its roots in philosophy, medicine, and law, but that nursing ethics predates this and can offer ways of understanding that can be important to how we view ourselves.

While the historical importance of care and nurse–patient relationships is broadly recognized, Marsha Fowler's work has also brought to light the lengthy history that nurses have had working toward social reforms to address unjust social structures that lead to health disparities. Nursing ethicists recognize that it is important to embrace a social ethics. Feminist ethics is one approach that can help us be critical of the societies and health-care systems in which we live and work by creating a lens through which we can examine and address the social forces that create disparities and diminish the importance of care. Some of these forces also prevent nurses from delivering care according to their ideals and can lead to excessive moral distress.

For example, in Canada there is an extreme shortage of long-term care (LTC) beds not only because there is a lack of physical structures, but also because there is a lack of staff. As a result, hospitalized people who need LTC but cannot access it are what used to be called "bed blockers" because there is nowhere for them to go. While today in Canada the terminology has been sanitized, with these patients now being called "alternative level of care" (ALC) patients, the stigma has not gone away. My mother is such a patient. I have been reminded on several occasions that she is occupying an acute care bed and that I should take her home even though she has had two recent strokes and requires total nursing care. In a strange twist of fate, our family is now living out an extraordinarily distressing set of circumstances that I have written and spoken about many times. Like other family caregivers, if we were to take her home, I would need to leave my paid employment, we would need to renovate a part of our home, hire additional help for the round-the-clock care she requires, and find a way for her to be periodically transported out of the house to see a physician, if we would be lucky enough to find someone who would take her as a patient. No doubt, shifting care to families, especially women, saves the system money, but it is very costly financially and socially for families. With great ambivalence, I am now on the record as "refusing" with everything that implies.

Our situation, in which we are certainly not alone, reflects multiple societal factors that have led to the lack of attention to the LTC and home-care sectors, including the deep-rooted devaluation of care work, sexism, ageism, and neoliberalism. Because of the disproportionate number of deaths in LTC during the pandemic, the conditions for those receiving care and working in these settings have become increasingly visible and hopefully, the impetus for change. Nurses need to be cognizant of not only the ethical issues that exist at the bedside, but also those of the broader systems in which they work to be a part of that change. I believe nursing ethics can play a part by providing a lens for the analysis and articulation of the ethical problems that exist not only in LTC, but also in many areas of our health-care systems.

I try to remain hopeful, but critically hopeful, that nursing ethics will maintain a presence in all areas of activity that comprise what we call nursing. Its lengthy history can be the inspiration for the development of the moral identities of nurses. There is realistic hope for the future of nursing ethics because there is an increasingly large cadre of nurses globally with an excellent education in nursing ethics. I look forward to their contributions and how they will leave their marks on the history of nursing ethics.

Patricia Benner: Practice as a Way of Knowing, in Its Own Right, Rather than a Mere Image of Theoretical Thinking

In 1981, I was working with Professor Richard Lazarus at University of Berkeley, studying stress and coping in aging in the community, which was new to Professor Lazarus, whose research was primarily experimental laboratory work. We were studying mind–body relationships related to stress appraisals and coping. I suggested that I enroll in some mind–body philosophy classes to clarify our language and understandings, and this was life-changing for me as an experienced nurse, having worked in ICUs, emergency departments, and home health-care nursing for 18 years. I went to the UC Berkeley Philosophy Department and spent the next seven years there! Equally important is that all my doctoral students took philosophy courses from Professor Bert Dreyfus at UC Berkeley, and we would have a seminar to discuss the philosophy class in relation to nursing practices. The teaching assistants frequently commented that the most interesting research and philosophical questions came from the graduate nursing students. Bert Dreyfus waived all philosophical class prerequisites for nursing graduate students, stating, "For reasons I don't understand, the nursing students end up with the best understanding of Heidegger." Students often talked about needing this new philosophical language to describe their practice of nursing.

In the Philosophy Department, I began by studying Kierkegaard, with Hubert L. Dreyfus and his brilliant TA, now Dr. Jane Rubin, friend and colleague and author of the definitive dissertation on Kierkegaard. From Kierkegaard, I now had a language and an understanding of "lifeworld" and the role of indirect discourse (first-person-experience narratives). Kierkegaard used letters between people living in different lifeworlds (organized by concerns, practices, habits, meanings and social relationships, and more) to convey their ways of being in the world; first-person accounts of the narrators' experiences in their lifeworld, their self-defining commitments, meanings, and how they managed the stress and anxieties and everyday coping and comportment, complete with insights, blind spots, meanings, and more. This kind of understanding from inside a person's lifeworld, is the coin of the realm for understanding and explaining meanings, practices, habits, skills, and relations within persons' lives. For example, in Kierkegaard's writings, the Aesthete correspondent (aesthetic sphere or existence or "lifeworld"), with Judge William in the Ethical Sphere, withdrew from his active life of seeking the maximum amount of pleasure, into a world of only reflecting and dreaming about pleasures in order to avoid the real risks of pursuing real-life pleasure that might be disappointing or elusive. "Judge William" lived in a lifeworld with self-defining commitments to being the sole definer and arbiter of all meaning in his world. This detachment brought him a sense of control over the risks involved in being connected, related, and human, but it also caused a sense of meaninglessness when nothing outside himself could lay claim on his attention and be meaningful in its own terms.

I confronted similar meaning, stress, and coping issues in caring for persons who dwelt in different lifeworlds, in ways that shaped their suffering, anxiety, and fears related to their illnesses and recovery. Note, this came through understanding rather than explanation, but understanding is essential for understanding human beings dwelling in lifeworlds. I took Professor Dreyfus' Kierkegaard course five times, learning and understanding more each time. His classes were so layered, nuanced, and complex, and I was learning more than I had ever learned in a psychology class on stress and coping. I now had a richer language in which to describe my nursing caring practices. I also took the courses offered by Dreyfus on Philosophy of Science, on Merleau-Ponty's philosophy of embodiment and critique of natural, objectifying sciences to study human beings, and courses on early Heidegger's notions of "being in the world" and engagement and involvement as the most common stance of human beings, rather than Descartes' vision of persons as private, idiosyncratic, subjective atomistic persons, detached and standing over against an objective world. I realized that such a philosophical stance of disengagement and detachment was not a good starting point for understanding caring practices in nursing. It misrepresents human intelligence and perception. I have written in nursing and ethics literature critiquing a Cartesian representational view of the mind, which is currently not accepted as how human beings learn nor a good account of human intelligence in philosophy or the neuro-cognitive learning sciences.

Charles Taylor, a world-renowned philosopher and close friend of Bert Dreyfus, came to engage in thinking, writing, and teaching with Bert often during the next seven years. Charles Taylor was equally influential on my thinking and scholarly work in nursing and ethics. Charles Taylor's teachings on the nature of social practices, and practical reasoning as a perfect analogue for science-using clinical reasoning, had a profound influence on my thinking and writing. Particularly in my work on clinical reasoning as a science-using form of practical reasoning, i.e., reasoning across time about the particular patient through changes in his or her clinical condition, and/or changes in the agents' responsibility to attend to the well-being of the patient.

Charles Taylor's writings and teachings on the interpretative nature of human sciences, in large measure, shaped my development of interpretive phenomenology as a research method for nursing, health care, and human sciences. His book *Explanation and Understanding* effectively ended the dominance of behaviorism in psychology, and influenced my thinking and dialogue with Professor Richard Lazarus, who had a controversial and influential research on the notion of "subception" (which I would later interpret as perceptual grasp and embodied fuzzy recognition). Lazarus' experiment confirmed that subjects' galvanic skin responses correlated with electrical shocks that subjects could not verbally identify.

Collectively and interactively, these philosophical teachings and readings helped articulate my understanding of the relationships between embodied skilled know-how, "fuzzy recognition," family resemblances, and tacit understanding, as well as relationships between practice and theory, the importance of overcoming Descartes' representational theory of the mind with its radical mind, body, world separation and atomistic individualism. I came to realize that while theory can enrich practice, without practice, theorizing cannot sustain itself. Practice is a wellspring of knowledge and knowledge development, gained experientially in practice. The Cartesian legacy required theoretical thinking and theory for the enactment of practice. How often do nurse educators and students cite the sacrosanct phrase "putting theory into practice" without giving thought to learning directly from practice and developing theory based upon practice? This Cartesian view imagined that theory is stamped out on an inert, passive practice. My goal in teaching became to help students articulate their own experiential learning and new insights gained directly from experiential learning in practice. Theorizing in nursing is relatively underdeveloped; however, the practice of nursing is rich, practiced in many contexts, and is highly varied. Nursing knowledge is radically diminished and misunderstood without active strategies for articulating the knowledge embedded in practice, and if it is imagined that practice cannot be a self-improving, knowledge developing practice without being seen as a mere application of theory, efforts won't be made to articulate the nature of actual nursing practice. Expert practice requires the situated *use* of knowledge, and this is more than mere *techne* (rational calculation) applying theory to practice. For example, learning to take blood pressure is a good example of mere application of knowledge. While interpreting blood pressures as trends and trajectories with particular clinical meaning for a patient exemplifies the situated higher-order thinking of *situated use* of knowledge.

Most often nursing knowledge is described in detached, objectified "knowing about and that." But such accounts cannot account for the situated thinking-in-action, situational awareness, and actual clinical reasoning across time through changes in the patient's clinical condition and/or the clinician's understanding of the patient's clinical condition. Notably, "knowing that and about" accounts leave out "knowing how and when." I found that first-person-experience narratives of nurses' actual clinical reasoning and patient care experiences were essential to describing nurses' dynamic clinical reasoning, situational awareness, caring practices, and frontline knowledge embedded in actual practice. First-person-experience near narratives enabled me, other teachers, students, and other nurses to articulate (give a clearer descriptive language) about the knowledge embedded in practice. For example, one year in my theory class for master's level students with about 80 students, we discovered 11 qualitatively distinct narratives on patient advocacy, e.g., "giving the silent patient her voice"; "Following the body's lead for the premature infant or the patient in a vegetative state"; "Running defense for the patient to prevent conflicting tests, therapies, or physician orders," and more. Articulating the knowledge embedded in practice focuses students on practice as both a source of knowledge and as a moral source. In each class, reading and articulating knowledge embedded in first-person-experience narratives made it possible to uncover and articulate knowledge not yet well-described in theoretical or scientific literature. In this case, the narratives shed light on the rich moral tradition and practical knowledge and skilled know-how embedded in practice communities concerned with "patient advocacy."

In studies of nursing expertise in practice, we found that the positive skills of involvement, while avoiding pathologies of helping such as over-involvement, or over-identification, moralism, sentimentalism, and so on, were essential to becoming an expert nurse. By moralism, I mean focusing on one's character virtues or flaws, and instead of once correcting character and skill problems, redirecting one's attentions, project, issue, concern, or relationship, rather than continuing to focus one's own moral intent and character, a continued focus on oneself (a form of incurvature of turning emotions back on the self) instead of focusing on intents and goals embed in the situation. Sentimentalism is similar, since it is an elaboration of the feelings involved in a situation, and turning these emotions back on the self (incurvature) by feeling and acting as if what is happening in another person's world is the same (or even equally impactful), as if it were happening in one's own lifeworld. Excessive detachment and objectification of the patient, such as relating only to the disease and not to the human experience of illness, blocks out needed information for good clinical reasoning, and thus impedes the developing of clinical expertise.

In our research on skill acquisition, we also discovered that beginning in the proficient stage, in the Dreyfus and Dreyfus Model of Skill Acquisition, nurses switch to perceptually grasping similar and dissimilar whole concrete clinical cases for recognizing the nature of familiar clinical situations, rather than using textbook lists of signs and symptoms. This experience-based perceptual grasp of whole clinical situations enabled nurses to provide early warnings for clinical situations, e.g., early compensatory phases of shock, premature infants' intolerance of patent ductus arteriosus, pulmonary embolus, and more. This kind of family resemblance or fuzzy recognition is not infallible, but it is superior to machine-based intelligence that is not very effective at "seeing the big picture" nor at fuzzy recognition, context or frame for particular situations. My goal has been to build in legitimacy and teaching for experience-based perceptual grasp, always staying open to disconfirmation while continually seeking and being open to new evidence. This "real world" understanding is more nuanced, and often involves tacit memory. As the maxim of artificial intelligence (AI) states, "The real world is the best model for the real world."

In skill acquisition research writings and teaching, I have emphasized teaching for a sense of salience, where the situation just stands out with aspects that are more or less important, higher or lower in urgency and priority. From the Novice through the Competent stages nurse educators, much like a good ethnographic guide, must fill in and point out what is most urgent and highest priority, providing the student with an understanding of the role of "salience" in clinical reasoning because they have not yet experienced sufficient clinical cases, nor sufficient "futures" of patients' clinical situations. A second emphasis, based on the Carnegie Study, is a focus on integrating the three professional apprenticeships: 1) the cognitive, the science, technology, and theory of a practice discipline; 2) the practice apprenticeship, the skilled-knowing how and when in the practice; 3) ethical comportment and formation. The practice-based apprenticeship focuses on practice-based ethics, and the built-in agent responsibility to the patient, family, and community in clinical reasoning.

Most of my writings and thinking are concerned with a more current vision of the embodied person engaged in the world, because I find it so relevant to nursing practice, and particularly relevant to caring practices in nursing. To that end I seek to articulate engaged, socially embedded, embodied intelligent agency and inter-subjective understandings between persons and situations. We as human beings, dwelling in lifeworlds, share common meanings, embodied understandings, and experiences. A Cartesian view of empathy imagines that we have to theoretically and mentally imagine what the other person is thinking and feeling as a separate atomistic individual, rather than considering them as a member-participant in a lifeworld that has shared, taken-for-granted meanings, and therefore, intersubjective understandings. Empathy is possible through a shared fellow-human-embodied feeling. Empathy is not primarily or only based on intellectually figuring out the other person's feelings and concerns. The *Primacy of Caring* presents caring, having something matter… have meaning and significance, for the possibility of understanding one another, and the possibility of giving and receiving help. Emotions provide one's access to the world, and human rationality depends on emotional responses to situations, to human interactions, facial expressions, tone of voice and more.

Finally, these philosophical writings and explorations have profoundly influenced and given language to ethics in nursing care. I have sought to articulate a concern for the notions of good and qualitative distinctions in excellent nursing care in my writings in both ethics and nursing literature. In keeping with the Dreyfus and Dreyfus Model of Skill Acquisition, I have never studied expertise as a trait or talent, or the possession of knowledge and skills for particular persons for all situations. Expertise, as I have studied and described in actual situations of well-managed, clinical situations, with situation awareness, early warnings, and excellent clinical grasp and sense of salience about unfolding cases can be demonstrated by direct observation or first-person-experience near narratives with real interventions, observations and outcomes in real time and can be assessed as expert or less than expert practice in the situation.

This nursing perspective on expert practice as a moral source, and a demonstration of the notions of good and qualitative distinctions embedded in actual clinical practice contrasts to an overarching concern in biomedical ethics for rights-based ethics, and breakdown and dilemma-based ethics rather than a realization of the notions of good that guide excellence practice and ethical comportment, and clinical reasoning in nursing, and represent the good behind statement of human rights. It is a problem to study only "practice breakdown ethics"; ethics based only on ethical decision-making rather than excellent, above-standard clinical practice, ethical comportment, responsible care for others, relational ethics, or social ethics, and ethics that attends to the notions of good behind rights-based ethics. The Aristotelian distinction between *techne* and *phronesis* is a key ethical discourse in nursing and health care. Distinctions between *techne* (rational calculation) and *phronesis* (wisdom and skilled know-how) are central to ethical comportment, and formation and the everyday practice of the professional nurse. *Techne* is suited for a) producing or making things; b) can be standardized; c) outcomes can be predicted; d) separating means and ends, not a problem. In *phronesis* (wisdom that is situated), separating means and ends can do violence (e.g., disregarding concerns for how birthing or dying processes are achieved). Situations that require *phronesis*: a) underdetermined, unfolding situations; b) ongoing experiential is involved; c) praxis, character, and skill, habits of attentiveness, thought and action involved; d) mutual influence between patient and clinician may be involved; e) outcomes cannot be reliably predicted. Clinical reasoning, a science-using form of practical reasoning, is always concerned with, in addition to accuracy and effectiveness, solving clinical problems with responsible actions toward the patient. I sat on ethics committees at two major medical centers, presented at scholarly societies on ethics and wrote many articles on this more practice-based, ethical comportment and formation. In the Carnegie Study we critiqued "socialization" as too focused on role messages from others, to fully explicate the process of ethical formation and everyday ethical comportment. Formation requires the agent (nursing student) to take up self-understandings, skills, habits, and practices that need to change in order to be a good nurse. For example, many students in their narratives, and Minnie Woods, in particular, wrote about the transformation of moving beyond their own anxiety, repulsion, concerns for skill-mastery and so on, to come to deeply understand that it is "about the patient," and not "me" as the nurse and thus, switch their focus to the best interests of the patient. This is a common and profound transformation of self-involvement that occurs in most students' self-understanding in relation to nursing practice. It is a formative change involving constituting and expressive theories of meaning, moving beyond the scientific meanings… designative and denotive theories of meanings used by physical and natural sciences.

Janet L. Storch: Canada, Code, Consent, and a Carpenter

Never in a million years would I have thought I would be working at the Canadian Nurses Association as lead nurse for revising the *Code of Ethics for Registered Nurses* 2017. But there I was and thankful for the opportunity to be so involved. The first page of this *Code* also contains a lovely acknowledgment of my work over the years. (Be assured that I did not write this tribute!)

> A special thank you goes to Janet Storch, RN, PhD, for her expertise, ongoing work and support in the development of the CNA code of ethics over many years. Through more than two decades of development and refinement to the CNA code of ethics, she has generously lent her exemplary scholarship, careful judgment and sage advice to strengthen this vital resource for nurses across Canada.[29]

My academic focus was health-care ethics throughout my long period of learning. I studied at the University of Alberta where, at the time, there was limited access to a formal study of health-care ethics, but there were a couple of health ethics faculty members who tutored me along the way.

Dr. Shirley Stinson was key to my launch into ethics. "Shirl" was President of the Canadian Nurses Association when I first formally encountered her and I was a beginning graduate student when I chose her as one of my mentors. At our first meeting she encouraged my pursuit of nursing ethics. On my way out of her office she handed me a package of nursing ethics papers to review, which turned out to be a draft of CNA's first accepted code of ethics, urging me to report back to her my response to the draft.

Another precious mentor of mine was Dr. John Dossetor, a renal transplant surgeon. I met him when I was doing some interviews in Alberta for the Faculty of Law in Edmonton, with the goal of preparing health-care ethics resources for students at the University of Alberta and throughout the Province of Alberta.

I first found John in a lower-level room (i.e., the basement of the hospital) where he was working on his transplant research. My assigned task was to learn what resources he had as well as his level of interest in clinical ethics. As I sat there, John had stories to tell. One of his favorite stories was about doing research in India while serving in the army during the war, and how easy it was as a physician to simply tell recruits and others waiting in line to see him to engage in medical testing, because they were captive. From my own early learning, my first question was, "Did you get consent from them?" He looked at me in amazement and said, "Why would I get consent?" That interview began a long period of John and I co-learning more about health-care ethics, medical ethics, and nursing ethics. We jointly, and with others, helped grow a Bioethics Center at the University of Alberta as well as the national Canadian Bioethics Society, both of which continue today.

One of my early ventures was to write a book about health-care ethics which I called *Patients' Rights: Ethical and Legal Issues in Health Care and Nursing* (1982).[30] That book was undertaken in my master's in health services administration program and was based upon my thinking of specific patient rights to include, i.e., the right to be informed, to be respected, to participate, and to equal access to care. With few other Canadian resources available to students, this book was published by McGraw-Hill Ryerson and it was released at a helpful time.

As my own sense of ownership of health ethics developed, I tried to attend ethics seminars in the US and in Canada, offered by Tom Beauchamp and James Childress, and by Edmund Pellegrino. I utilized their books extensively. I also visited their Ethics Centre in New York and later I spent a semester in Washington, DC as a guest of their Ethics Centre, with Dr. Pellegrino serving as my mentor. These wonderful opportunities often had me working overtime to keep abreast of the rapidly growing faculty responsibilities and the rapidly growing program of nursing ethics. This meant I was often working overtime.

One evening as I was working late, a young man with a large drill arrived to fix the door of my office. He viewed my desk loaded with papers and asked me what I was reading. I told him I was studying various codes of ethics for health professionals to see if the nurses' code was missing something important. He responded immediately to say that his "profession" should have a code of ethics, and they did not have one. He then asked if he could borrow some of the papers. I told him I could not let any of the papers go, but they could be copied. His response was that he would very much like to copy them, and he was set to go to the copier which was one floor above. I told him again that, unfortunately, I could not give any of the papers to him because many were irreplaceable and I did not know what I would do if he failed to bring them back. For that excuse, he had a solution. He said he would leave his drill on my desk until he returned. He did so, and "we had a deal."

Learning about health-care ethics from the above sources, and as my confidence grew, I began a more focused program of reading and meeting nurses involved in clinical ethics and nursing ethics. I had the good fortune to meet Verena Tschudin in Vancouver as I arrived at the International Nursing Conference in Vancouver, BC. She was setting up a display for the new journal called *Nursing Ethics*.[31] Later, Verena invited me to serve on the Editorial Review Board, which was a delight.

I have been so blessed to have happenstances that have connected me to "ethics involved people" seemingly by chance. Through Anne Davis, I became involved in ten days at the Rockefeller Center in Bellagio, Italy, to work on a book titled *Ethics, Women and Incarceration*.

My move to British Columbia in 1990 brought me into close working relationships with Dr. Paddy Rodney and Dr. Rosalie Starzomski, who had recently joined the faculty at the University of Victoria. Having known them through involvement in ethics seminars and other engagements across Canada, we quickly formed a three-some to develop health and nursing ethics resources, and to date we have published two editions of texts, with invited guests, called *Toward a Moral Horizon: Nursing Ethics for Leadership and Practice*[32] (2004, 2018). We have recently finalized the third edition of our Open Access text so that our students and others will not have to pay "an arm and a leg" for this book.

Laurie Badzek: At the Intersections of Law, Ethics, and Nursing

I often reflect on how our past has shaped us and how different the world looks through eyes that have seen and studied multiple iterations of the *Code of Ethics for Nursing*. Most of the time, I have been in search of an ethical environment where nurses learn, grow professionally, and practice in a resilient and joyful manner. Even in trying to create such an environment in my own space, I have faced constraints, but I still ask us to be nurses, remain nurses, and recruit nurses—we need nurses now more than ever in our history. We, collectively, are truly the pathway to health. Why nursing? For me it was a strong desire to be helpful in a meaningful way. An opportunity to care for those most vulnerable as part of a profession that is viewed as the most trusted year after year, a profession that requires both individual and collective relationships to "do good."

Recently, I had cause to talk with students—the next generation of nurse leaders—about nursing ethics and the importance of our ANA *Code of Ethics for Nurses*. I shared with them my experience in developing not one, but two versions of the *Code*. Now, enough time has passed, and enough changes have occurred—a pandemic, greater social networking, a more global and nurse-traveled world—that the time has come, once again, to reexamine our *Code* and what changes are necessary for our ethical code to match and guide our ever-changing practice.

The state of our lives is evolving. Life is not static, problems are not static, and health, information, and technology are changing by the minute as we age. As I reflect back to my start in nursing, as a much younger me, the changes were less apparent than they are today. It is hard to imagine a bed you crank or drips you count without the help of a monitor or an IV pump. Often, I wonder how my patients survived in a world where health care and nursing care was so different, lacking in cell phones, MRIs, and assistive technologies.

But then I ask, was it really that different? Even almost a half century ago the focus was on the patient and the family and was inclusive of the community for those of us who served the needs of patients beyond the walls of the hospital or clinic. We valued the needs of those in our care beyond the physical care to encompass something more. As nurses, we considered safety, human rights, dignity, individual uniqueness, and vulnerability as key components of our primary commitments as nurses.

I recall the stress of caring for those for whom we had no answers, a dying group, whose disease we feared was contagious. We dressed as if our lives depended on it, with gowns and gloves and masks. We later called the illness HIV/AIDS. I watched in wonder the parallels of the COVID-19 pandemic with my own experiences years prior. The similarities were uncanny, but the remarkable care of others prevailed even when the fears were great. I think how proud those nurses from earlier pandemics and illnesses must be, recognizing the persistence and resilience that brought us through yet another challenge.

I never remember even thinking that I would resign my position because the fear was too great or the risk to carry out needed nursing care was beyond my capacity. I do remember reflecting on my own mortality and the possibility that it could be transmitted to me and to my family. I do remember working together with other nurses within my workspace and at clinical specific meetings throughout nursing in general to create an environment where we would feel most protected. Whether it was use of PPE for TB, HIV, or to avoid the consequences of toxic chemotherapeutic agents, we made new policies to push our profession forward in a manner that kept us as safe as possible while minimizing risk to ourselves and our patients. All of us, together, pushed to create new paths that focused on better outcomes, and together felt the sadness when despite our efforts the outcome was an inevitable part of the life cycle. Many of these experiences came full circle as we again faced something bigger, something unknown in my lifetime, an unparalleled pandemic, and an all-embracing social crisis.

We learned and acknowledged the importance of self-care for ourselves and our profession, thus increasing our life spans as individuals and as a profession. We also learned that there were distinct differences among us, and that I am privileged to live a life with a skin color and postal zip code that places me inside a world where my personal outcomes in life and health would be favored. I also came to know that my profession and I needed to acknowledge and apologize to others for the disparities and injustices that exist in our history, but more so I needed to work toward equity, inclusion, and belonging to change the path of our profession moving forward.

Additionally, my early research in advance directives and shared decision making strengthened my focus on why clinical ethics are so central to our work as nurses engaged with patient's lives that extend beyond the clinical setting. Recent work using gaming for selection of decision makers with cell phones shows how little we have moved the mark in the world of advance directives and how far we have come in thinking about health-care surrogates.

Thankfully, I, with other nurses, focused on our practice as a profession. We focused on the impact and interconnectedness of our work with the work of others in providing responsible and accountable care within the boundaries of our profession. Often, we were pushing up against the wave of technology that was both a gift and a curse as we aspired to be better. And now innovative technology, a global social network, and the genomic revolution are creating a future for self-care and care of others that is the new reality. However, we continue to see vast disparities and recognize our need for a deepened commitment to fostering dialogue and making real change in order to achieve justice.

My innate abilities and perhaps more than a bit of stubbornness have allowed me to focus on nursing in unique ways. My interest in ethics and the boundaries of nursing practice were amplified by my pursuit of a law degree, followed quickly by graduate study in health policy and ethics as I completed a nursing master's with a focus on education. My love of mentoring and sharing knowledge moved me to a path in nursing education and ultimately to academic administrative leadership. While working at ANA on the *Code of Ethics for Nurses*, multiple ethics position statements and even improvements in how the Center for Ethics and Human Rights operates are experiences I had the privilege to lead. We worked to make applicable and practical the ever-evolving guides and guardrails for our professional practice. Years of involvement in groundbreaking work in genomics health education and, more recently, work to encourage assessment of our ability to use and translate genomics in nursing practice across the world is creating change and forging new paths.

On this winding nursing path, my desire to help others placed me at the bedside, studying the narratives in order to find ethical solutions to the difficult challenges and conflicts in health care. For me, leadership was about people and helping each individual or group find the niche where who they are and what they say and do is in harmony with their passion. This is defined as "happiness" by Gandhi and by me as "joy." When your work and your passion collide—that is joy. Law, ethics, and nursing for me created this collision and this intersection was always a place where I could do my best work.

And now back to our beginning. The words of Nightingale, *Notes on Nursing*, resound, especially the part about using data to create changes! Mary Seacole, Harriet Tubman, Clara Barton, Mary Eliza Mahoney, Lillian Wald, Annie Goodrich, Virginia Henderson, and so many more pathfinders and innovators on whose shoulders we stand have created for us a professional moral compass. Their works provide many practical lessons on pathways for change. More recent colleagues, living legends, and living inductees to the ANA Hall of Fame, many of whom I had the distinct pleasure of knowing, have similarly shaped my practice, teaching, and leadership as they have shared their stories of improvement and change. Both groups challenged me, challenge us to move nursing in a direction that both honors our profession and those we serve. We seek to optimize health and well-being as we provide care for all others. Opportunities abound for nurses to be innovators and change agents. As I reflect on my own contributions to the profession, they pale in comparison to the giants who have enabled me to forge a new side path or two that have expanded nursing.

As an education leader and dean, I am honored each day to mentor the nursing workforce of the future and share visions about the future. I appreciate my colleagues and hold dear those moments of their recognition that humble and delight, yet also confront the fear of the imposter syndrome. Those occasions are always a bold reminder that our work is rarely individual, but is the result of our powerful, collaborative connections.

So again, I reflect on ethics in nursing. Nursing has no boundaries in the good that we can do, through our practice, research, education, or administration. Often, we experience these in combination influenced by our art and science, working to create ethical environments and exerting ourselves together, as one, to advance health for all. All of society and the next generation of nurses is trusting us to provide care as only we can. Be well.

Andrew Jameton: Eulogy for a Friend

This concluding chapter is a series of personal narratives by friends whom I have known from the early days of bioethics. Andy's narrative was to be the last pages in my book. He was working on his narrative but was having some health challenges (as he called them). I suggested that he set it aside and focus on his health, but he emailed back immediately and said, emphatically, "no," that working on it was helpful and he would have it to me within the week. Typical Andy. Shortly thereafter, I received word that he had died. I was undone.

Andy was a dear friend of over 40 years, more a friend than colleague, but that as well. We seemed to start projects together but somehow mostly did not manage to finish them, providing an ongoing excuse to work together to not finish them again. And again. It was always more fun to cavort together, hither and thither, through the recesses of the mind, recalling that there was a poem or editorial cartoon about that, whatever "that" was. Andy was an unparalleled and acute intellectual provocateur.

We spent no small amount of time in elasticizing and reimagining ethics, like toying with pre-Lockean political theory as it might interact with notions of informed consent, or not. In the mid-1980s we had collected 2,500 nurses' first-hand cases of clinical ethics, got started on typologizing them, and then decided that going to a museum would be more fun, or going for Chinese food, than writing a tiny program to transpose two letters in a word-processing document, and then speculating whether a dog, his black dog, would circle its bed in the opposite direction in the Southern Hemisphere—you know, the truly momentous and profound philosophical questions that had to be addressed. Somehow, we never finished the typology of the cases, but we finished the Chinese takeout, though we never came to philosophical truth about the dog circles. Notwithstanding, we accomplished some engaging mental work and collaboration. He was generous that way. He was also good fun and a good person.

Andy was an ardent supporter of nursing, which put him outside the mainstream of philosophers in bioethics, and at cross-purposes or odds with some. But he was his own person. While Andy is credited with distinguishing between moral uncertainty, moral dilemma, and moral distress, there are some ways in which that was the least of his contributions to nursing, and to focus there terribly understates his contributions and who he was as a person. Andy was a kind, supportive, and exceedingly generous colleague to all, and patient and affable with both those who did not know enough, or should have known better. He could be gently stern. He was a person of good humor and great warmth. I deeply miss Andy and in some ways his death is a marker of the passing of the generation of those of us early-into-the-field, to the next generation of scholars and practitioners of ethics in nursing whom we hope will greatly exceed our own accomplishments. Even though his vignette for my book was unfinished, I close these remarks and this book with his own heartfelt words:

> Nursing is the morally central health profession. Philosophies of nursing, not medicine, should determine the image of health care and its future directions. In its anxiety to control the institutions and technology of health care, medicine has allowed the central values of health care—health and compassion—to fall to the hands of nurses. Nurses thus supply the real inspiration and hope for progress in health care, and among health professionals, represent the least equivocal commitment to their clientele.[33]

Notes

1 https://bioethicsarchive.georgetown.edu/pcsbi/studies.html
2 Eiji Maruyama, "Clinical Ethics Committee: Past, Present, and Near Future." Symposium Presentation, the 33rd Annual Conference of Japan Bioethics Association, 2021.
3 Mitsuhiro Nakamura, Mariko Suzuki, Michiko Yahiro, et al, "Promoting Happiness in Nursing Students' Clinical Practice: Suggestions from Three Cases," *Journal of Japanese Nursing Ethics* 7, no. 1 (2015): 89–91.
4 Anne J. Davis, "Dancing on the Margins to a Different Tune: Reflections on Opportunities and Relationships," at Nagano College of Nursing, Japan, 1995–2001. Prof. Anne J. Davis Swan Song Lecture and Publications, Nagano College of Nursing.
5 Emiko Konishi (ed.), *Nursing Ethics: A Guide to Good Nurse and Good Nursing*, 1st ed. (Tokyo: Nankodo Publishing, 2007).
6 Ibid.
7 Megan-Jane Johnstone, *Bioethics: A Nursing Perspective*, 6th ed. (Sydney: Elsevier, 2015), 16.
8 Miki Ono, "Reconsidering 'Nursing Ethics' in the Time of Multidisciplinary Collaboration," *Journal of Japanese Nursing Ethics* 11, no. 1 (2019): 1–2.
9 M.D. Fowler, "Why the History of Nursing Ethics Matters," *Nursing Ethics* 24, no. 3 (2017): 292–304.
10 S. Fry, "Guest Editorial: Defining Nurses' Ethical Practices in the 21st Century," *International Nursing Review* 49 (2002): 1–3.
11 Pamela J. Grace, "An Argument for the Distinct Nature of Nursing Ethics," in M. Deem and J. Lingler (eds.), *Nursing Ethics: Normative Foundations, Advanced Concepts and Professional Responsibility in Advanced Practice* (Burlington, MA: Jones and Bartlett Learning, 2022).
12 Pamela J. Grace, *Nursing Ethics and Professional Responsibility in Advanced Practice*, 3rd edition (Sudbury, MA: Jones & Bartlett, 2018).
13 Ibid.
14 Of course, now I realize that there were good reasons why black people would indeed prefer their own churches. But these are not the reasons my mother had in mind, I am sure! My memory of this exchange is so strong that I am transported to the back seat of the car when I asked the question, "No seat belts?" and sat on the edge of the seat to lean closer to my mother in the passenger seat, eager for an answer to my question.
15 For a wonderful account of this history of Hawaii, see Sarah Vowel's "Unfamiliar Fishes": https://www.amazon.com/Unfamiliar-Fishes-Sarah-Vowell/dp/159448564X/ref=tmm_pap_swatch_0?_encoding=UTF8&qid=1648303841&sr=8-1

16 https://www.allclassical.org/the-songs-of-liliuokalani-queen-of-hawaii/

17 Many years later the Hawaii education system corrected this travesty and now all public schools teach the Hawaiian language and translations of music lyrics.

18 https://www.britannica.com/biography/Liliuokalani

19 https://www.britannica.com/biography/James-Cook

20 My son's Hawaiian heritage originates from a great-great Hawaiian grandmother whose husband, and father of her children, was a Welsh whaler.

21 See https://imagesofoldhawaii.com/punahou/

22 Barack Obama's white grandparents, in order to assure their grandson the best education possible, paid the extremely high costs for middle- and high-schooler Barack to attend mostly white Punahou. He was the only black kid, and one of very few other children of color in his class, but he writes positively about his experience despite being in a clear minority.

23 See https://www.ksbe.edu/education/kapalama/high_school/history_culture/.

24 See https://nursemanifest.com/ongoing-overdue-reckoning-on-racism-in-nursing/ for details on this project led by African-American nurse Lucinda Canty, along with two of us who are white: Christina Nyirati and myself. More details about each of us is provided on the website.

25 Robin DiAngelo provides an excellent model of an accountability statement, and explains "affinity groups" on her website: https://www.robindiangelo.com/accountability-statement/.

26 See"Resources"here:https://nursemanifest.com/ongoing-overdue-reckoning-on-racism-in-nursing/launch-overdue-reckoning-on-racism-in-nursing/resources-for-overdue-reckoning-on-racism-in-nursing/

27 See the "Building Authentic Relationships" section here: https://www.robindiangelo.com/accountability-statement/

28 Carol Gilligan, *In a Different Voice* (Cambridge, MA: Harvard University Press, 1982).

29 Canadian Nurses Association, *Code of Ethics for Registered Nurses* (Ottawa, 2017), 1. https://cna.informz.ca/cna/pages/download_the_code

30 Janet Storch, *Patients' Rights: Ethical and Legal Issues in Health Care and Nursing*, (Toronto: McGraw-Hill Reyerson, 1982).

31 https://journals.sagepub.com/home/nej

32 Janet Storch, Paddy Rodney, and Rosalie Starzomski, *Toward a Moral Horizon: Nursing Ethics for Leadership and Practice* (Ontario: Pearson Education Canada, 2004).

33 Andrew Jameton, *Nursing Practice: The Ethical Issues.* (Englewood Cliffs, NJ: Prentice Hall, 1984), xvi.

AFTERWORD

The Nurses Are Up to Something

They were four aces in a deck stacked against them. Elizabeth, Philippa, Iris, Mary. Going up to Oxford University as women, they came down as philosophers. Not just philosophers, but philosophers of distinction, who had the temerity to upturn the regnant philosophy. Uppity women, uppity scholars. Elizabeth Anscombe, Philippa Foot, Iris Murdoch, Mary Midgley (and a bit later Mary Warnock), remarkably different from one another, together became "metaphysical animals," fast friends, enduring colleagues, and trenchant critics of the philosophy that they had come to study.[1] They found themselves at Oxford at a time when a majority of the men were away for the war, and the colleges were populated by women, men too old to serve in the war, ordinands, and some male conscientious objectors. Male absence worked strongly to their benefit, affording them full attention they might not otherwise have received from the dons.

In the face of the Nazi horrors, the graphically documented depravities, and the obscenity of war in general, Elizabeth, Philippa, Iris, and Mary found the prevailing philosophical theories and discourses inadequate to the task of addressing the realities of war and its atrocities. But it was also sterile when it came to the daily lives of women. Together, and in their own separate domains, they broke the Oxford orthodoxy, and moved philosophy forward. "The women are up to something," was the catchphrase when it was found out that the women would stand against Oxford University administration in awarding an honorary doctorate to Harry Truman. He had ordered that the atomic bomb be dropped on Hiroshima and Nagasaki, intentionally killing civilians, an action that they denounced as evil.

They could hardly have been more different. Elizabeth was a devout convert Roman Catholic; Philippa, a woman born to privilege, and atheist; Iris, progressive, artistic, nonconformist; and Mary a stay-at-home mom-philosopher with a love of animals. Elizabeth focused her scholarly energies on analytic philosophy, ethics, and metaphysics, and is credited with coining the term "consequentialism." Her work *Modern Moral Philosophy*² is of particular importance to nursing ethics. Among others, her work influenced Alasdair MacIntyre, Charles Taylor, and John McDowell. Philippa, deeply moved by photos of Nazi atrocities, searched for an ethical response in Aristotle. She worked to renew Aristotle's ethics against the entrenched deontological and consequentialistic theories. Among others, her work influenced Bernard Williams, Rosalind Hursthouse, and Judith Jarvis Thompson. Her work became pivotal in restoring normative ethics within analytical philosophy. Iris's work in reinterpreting Aristotle, and in moral philosophy, influenced Martha Nussbaum among others. Mary's work was innovative and multidisciplinary, and brought biosciences to bear upon philosophy in dealing with human nature. She fought reductionist approaches to ethics and insisted that human and non-human life were interconnected and complex. Her work influenced Peter Singer, Martha Nussbaum, and others—including the public. Believing that the work of philosophy belonged to all persons, she became the UK's best-known public philosopher. Mary's work earned her the 2011 *Philosophy Now* "Award for Contributions in the Fight Against Stupidity."³ Commenting in an interview on the nature of philosophy, Mary remarked:

> I think it is much more like plumbing—the sort of thinking that people do even in the most prudent, practical areas always has a whole system of thought under the surface which we are not aware of. Then suddenly we become aware of some bad smells, and we have to take up the floorboards and look at the concepts of even the most ordinary piece of thinking. The great philosophers of the past didn't spend their time looking at entities in the sky. They noticed how badly things were going wrong, and made suggestions about how they could be dealt with.⁴

That is exactly what our magical metaphysical four did—noticed a malodor and took up the floorboards of ethics to fix its plumbing. The smell was coming from logical empiricism or logical positivism that would purge human subjectivity from ethics, leaving it, well, empty. Anscombe, Foot, Murdoch, and Midgley's work reattached ethics to human life and experience by installing Aristotle's plumbing. They are credited with restoring and renewing Aristotelianism and more specifically Aristotle's virtue ethics to philosophy—the very stream that nursing ethics had been founded upon.

Anscombe, Foot, Murdoch, and Midgley, at tea, on bicycles, in pubs, in living rooms, at parties, at lectures, punting on the Thames, in the common room, in their apartments and homes, walking in the meadow, were personal friends and intellectual friends, who challenged, provoked, questioned one another, sharpening both their skills and their philosophical work. They were very different women, with very different lives and perspectives, who came together in a particular season to look at what was under the floorboards and to invigorate ethics. And they did. The women were, indeed, up to something.

Philosopher Benjamin Lipscomb asks:

How did Anscombe, Foot, Midgley, and Murdoch all follow a path that was virtually unmarked? How did they stick together, different as they were? And how did they work their way toward a set of ideas sharply at odds with what nearly everyone around them thought? For these four were doubly outsiders. Besides being women in an almost exclusively male discipline, they were advocates of an approach to ethics that was deeply out of fashion.[5]

We nurses, too, should we so choose, could be "up to something." We too could have our own Elizabeth–Philippa–Iris–Mary brain trust. We too could be advocates for an approach to ethics that is deeply out of fashion. We too could lift the floorboards of bioethics and look at the concepts underneath and make suggestions for how to put them right. I call upon us to do so.

In the weeks and months to come...

Let's meet and together let's devise a plan. We could challenge bioethics to a bake-off. To do so, we would need to update our 1919 recipe to suit more contemporary tastes, for recipes do become dated.

Old Recipe for Making a Good Nurse: Mix together equal parts of pluck and good health with well-balanced sympathy, stiffen with energy and soften with the milk of human kindness. Use a first-class training school as a mixer. Add the sweetness of a smile, a little ginger, and generous amounts of tact, humor and unselfishness, with plenty of patience; pour into the mouth of womanhood, time with enthusiasm, finish with a cap and garnish with ambition. The sauce of experience is always an improvement to this recipe, which, if followed closely, should be very successful and exceedingly popular.[6]

I have a cookbook with a new recipe we could try:

Improved Recipe for How to Make a Good Nurse, Flourishing People, and a Good Society: Take one cup each of NeoAristotelian Virtue Theory, Social Ethics, and Nursing Tradition; mix in assorted MacIntyre fruit to taste. Add ½ cup of Progressivism, 3tsp. of whole-grain modern Pragmatism, cut in a knob of stiff curriculum, a glug of thick narrative molasses, and slowly stir in the fluid of Care Ethics. Add a pinch of salt, and a dash of Taylor to taste; leaven with Benner. Allow to proof in the practice oven. Then knead in seeds of liberation, a dash of activist spunk, one tsp. pluck, and two tsp. of grit and resolve. Bake in a very hot oven until the interior is soft and resilient, and an artisan crust forms. Slice and serve to the community, spread generously with a rich dollop of nursing identity.

The nurses could be up to something. The nurses should be up to something. Yes, and well they should be!

Notes

1 Clare Mac Cumhaill and Rachael Wiseman, *Metaphysical Animals: How Four Women Brought Philosophy Back to Life* (New York: Doubleday, 2022).
2 G.E.M. Anscombe. "Modern Moral Philosophy," *Philosophy* 33, no. 124 (Jan. 1958): 1–19.
3 The Philosophy Now Award for Contributions in the Fight Against Stupidity. https://philosophynow.org/award
4 Liz Else, "Mary, Mary Quite Contrary," *New Scientist* 172, no. 2315 (Nov. 3, 2001): 48–51. https://www.newscientist.com/article/mg17223154-800-mary-mary-quite-contrary/
5 Benjamin Lipscomb, *The Women Are Up to Something: How Elizabeth Anscombe, Philippa Foot, Mary Midgley, and Iris Murdoch Revolutionized Ethics* (Oxford: Oxford University Press, 2022).
6 Anon., "Recipe for Making a Good Nurse," *Pacific Coast Journal of Nursing* XV, no. 5 (May 1919): 268.

INDEX

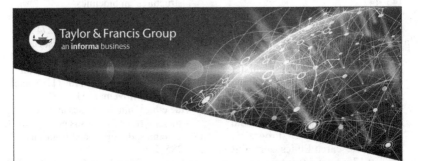

Printed in the United States
by Baker & Taylor Publisher Services